Developing Clinical Competence

··

A Workbook for the OTA

SECOND EDITION

Developing Clinical Competence

A Workbook for the OTA

Marie J. Morreale, OTR

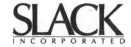

SLACK
INCORPORATED

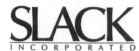

SLACK Incorporated
6900 Grove Road
Thorofare, NJ 08086 USA
856-848-1000   Fax: 856-848-6091
www.slackbooks.com
978-1-63091-896-5
© 2022 by SLACK Incorporated

Senior Vice President: Stephanie Arasim Portnoy
Vice President, Editorial: Jennifer Kilpatrick
Vice President, Marketing: Mary Sasso
Acquisitions Editor: Brien Cummings
Director of Editorial Operations: Jennifer Cahill
Vice President/Creative Director: Thomas Cavallaro
Cover Artist: Katherine Christie
Project Editor: Joseph Lowery

Instructors: *Developing Clinical Competence: A Workbook for the OTA, Second Edition* includes ancillary materials specifically available for faculty use. Included are PowerPoint Slides. Please visit www.efacultylounge.com to obtain access.

Marie J. Morreale *has no financial or proprietary interest in the materials presented herein.*

Printed in the United States of America.

Last digit is print number: 10   9   8   7   6   5   4   3   2   1

Dedication

This book is dedicated to OTA students everywhere, with the hope that you will find much joy and success throughout your occupational therapy journey.

Contents

Developing Clinical Competence: A Workbook for the OTA, Second Edition includes ancillary materials specifically available for faculty and clinician use. Please visit http://www.efacultylounge.com or email educomps@slackinc.com to obtain access.

Acknowledgments

I would like to thank Debbie Amini, EdD, OTR/L, FAOTA, for her knowledge, friendship, and support over many years. I am grateful for her collaboration, expertise, and valuable contributions to *The Occupational Therapist's Workbook for Ensuring Clinical Competence* from which some material is integrated into this new OTA text. Appreciation goes to Brien Cummings at SLACK Incorporated for his positivity and support for all my book projects throughout more than a decade. Finally, my husband, Richard, deserves special thanks for all his love, patience, and help, without which this book would not have been possible.

About the Author

Marie J. Morreale, OTR graduated Summa Cum Laude from Quinnipiac College (now Quinnipiac University) with a B.S. in occupational therapy. Throughout her professional career, Marie worked in a variety of practice settings, including inpatient and outpatient rehabilitation, skilled nursing facilities, adult day care, home health, cognitive rehabilitation, and hand therapy. Marie held the designation of Certified Hand Therapist for 25 years. She also served several years on a home health professional advisory committee, consulting on quality assurance issues. Marie was adjunct faculty for 17 years at the Occupational Therapy Assistant Program at Rockland Community College, State University of New York in Suffern. There she taught a variety of courses, including Professional Issues and Documentation, Geriatric Principles, Occupational Therapy Skills, Advanced Occupational Therapy Skills, Therapeutic Activities, and Advanced Therapeutic Activities. Marie was also involved with OTA curriculum development and served briefly as interim coordinator of the OTA Program.

Marie created the first edition of *Developing Clinical Competence: A Workbook for the OTA*. She also co-authored *The Occupational Therapist's Workbook for Ensuring Clinical Competence* and the second, third, and fourth editions of *The OTA's Guide to Documentation: Writing SOAP Notes*. In addition, she wrote a chapter on documentation for *The Occupational Therapy Manager, Fifth Edition* and published several occupational therapy articles. For the past several years Marie has been a test item writer for American Occupational Therapy Association (AOTA) continuing education products. She is active in her condo community and enjoys anything travel related.

Introduction

How to Use This Book

This workbook is designed to help occupational therapy assistant (OTA) students and new practitioners demonstrate the "practical" problem-solving and "real-life" skills essential for fieldwork and clinical practice. The workbook is intended as a user-friendly resource to help the reader apply occupational therapy concepts, improve professional (clinical) reasoning, and measure attainment of knowledge and skills needed for successful transition to fieldwork and entry-level practice. The worksheets, learning activities, and suggested worksheet answers are written in an easy-to-read format and include a variety of methods such as multiple choice, matching, and true/false questions; case studies; vignettes; fill in the blanks; and experiential activities. Competencies are broken down into smaller units and explained step-by-step to allow for easy, independent study. Thoroughly explained worksheet answers are provided so that readers can check their responses with suggested best practices.

This manual will help the reader work through a wide range of situations commonly encountered in occupational therapy for various practice areas. Many helpful tips are presented to guide the reader in occupational therapy clinical decision making, professional conduct, and meeting standards of care. Although the exercises in each chapter are presented in a logical progression, each chapter is fully independent of the others. Thus, the reader can skip around and complete individual chapters or specific exercises in the order most conducive to one's individual learning needs. This book can be used as a companion text for multiple classes throughout an OTA educational curriculum. Many of the exercises can be used to help measure attainment of knowledge and skills for specific educational standards delineated by the Accreditation Council for Occupational Therapy Education (ACOTE, 2018). The worksheets and learning activities are also conducive for role-playing exercises, studying in small groups, and as a study aid when preparing for fieldwork or the national certification exam.

The instructional methods, learning activities, and worksheets presented in this book stem from the author's 17 years of experience teaching OTA students. This text addresses fundamental areas of occupational therapy practice for a wide variety of conditions, situations, and practice settings. Topics presented include professionalism, ethical behavior, effective communication, roles and responsibilities, cultural sensitivity, supervision, occupation-based interventions, therapeutic methods and tasks, assessment of client function, safety, documentation, group process, department management, evidence-informed practice, and much more. Many of the questions and learning activities were developed to specifically address common mistakes or difficulties exhibited by OTA students during their academic coursework and fieldwork so that the reader can avoid making the same errors.

Worksheets and learning activities are designed so that readers can practice problem-solving and organizational skills, improve clinical and professional reasoning, demonstrate understanding of professional behaviors, and learn effective communication strategies. The reader will also be able to test attainment of knowledge and skills for various conditions, interventions, and practice areas. Answers to the worksheet exercises are explained clearly and simply at the end of each chapter. However, as it is impossible to present or predict every possible scenario or intervention, it is important to realize that these answers are often examples of best practice. It is possible that you may come up with other best practice examples that could also be correct. This workbook is not meant to be a book on theory, nor an instruction manual for technical hands-on skills. Thus, it is expected that the reader will have some fundamental understanding of occupational therapy theory and basic technical skills. Readers should utilize pertinent resources as needed to fill in any personal gaps in knowledge or practical skills that may become apparent when completing exercises in this workbook.

New in the Second Edition

This second edition includes updated references and revised exercises that reflect more current terminology and clinical practice standards. Also incorporated into this text are concepts and principles from the new *Occupational Therapy Practice Framework: Domain and Process, Fourth Edition* (OTPF—4; AOTA, 2020c). Effort has been made to also include more questions that represent different practice areas such as behavioral health and pediatrics. Many new topics have been added to this second edition, such as infection control, amputations and prosthetics, wheeled mobility, development of hand function, medical procedures/devices, wound care basics, chronic conditions, spinal cord injury, human trafficking, neglect/abuse, quality improvement, and others. Additional worksheets and learning activities have also been created to expand upon the areas of professional behaviors, effective communication, supervision, cultural sensitivity, occupation-based practice, physical agent modalities, feeding and eating, evidence-informed practice, and more.

Guiding Principles

The specific roles and responsibilities of the occupational therapist (OT) and OTA in the areas of evaluation, intervention, and outcomes are delineated in the AOTA's *Guidelines for Supervision, Roles, and Responsibilities During the Delivery of Occupational Therapy Services* (2020b) and *Standards of Practice for Occupational Therapy* (2015). The OTA works under the supervision of an OT and partners with the OT to perform selected, delegated tasks for which the OTA demonstrates service competency and is in accordance with state and federal regulations (AOTA, 2015, 2020b). Considering that each client is unique with individual circumstances, OTs and OTAs use a holistic, client-centered approach. A variety of methods and interventions are implemented to work toward the goal of contributing to a client's or population's occupational performance as described in the *OTPF—4* (AOTA, 2020c) and *Scope of Practice* (AOTA, 2014). The services that occupational therapy practitioners provide are also guided by the *AOTA 2020 Occupational Therapy Code of Ethics* (AOTA, 2020a), relevant laws, facility policies, third-party payer requirements, and evidence-informed practice.

While this book presents sound examples of best practice, an occupational therapy practitioner must always use professional reasoning to determine the methods, interventions, or recommendations that are most appropriate for a client's personal situation. OTs and OTAs must carefully consider the client's health status and circumstances; specific client factors, skills and contexts that hinder or support performance; relevant precautions/contraindications; safety concerns; available methods; and current evidence supporting clinical practice. It is important to realize that a "standard" intervention for a particular condition, such as a specific physical agent modality, orthosis, exercise protocol, communication strategy, assistive technology or adaptive device, may not be appropriate for all clients with the same diagnosis. Also, an intervention plan might delineate more than one device or method as a specific kind of intervention. For example, a condition that necessitates use of an orthotic device, such as a flexor tendon repair, might entail using both a nighttime static positioning orthosis and a daytime dynamic mobilization orthosis.

The scenarios presented are representative of situations commonly encountered in clinical practice. The names and specific details have been fabricated to create optimal learning exercises, so any specific resemblance to an actual person is purely coincidental. It is the author's intent that this workbook serves as a useful resource to help OTA students succeed academically and become competent, ethical practitioners.

References

Accreditation Council for Occupational Therapy Education. (2018). 2018 Accreditation Council for Occupational Therapy Education (ACOTE) standards and interpretive guide (effective July 31, 2020). *American Journal of Occupational Therapy*, *72*(Suppl. 2), 7212410005. https://doi.org/10.5014/ajot.2018.72S217

American Occupational Therapy Association. (2014). Scope of practice. *American Journal of Occupational Therapy*, *68*(Suppl. 3). https://doi.org/10.5014/ajot.2014.686S04

American Occupational Therapy Association. (2015). Standards of practice for occupational therapy. *American Journal of Occupational Therapy*, *69*(Suppl. 3), 6913410057. http://dx.doi.org/10.5014/ajot.2015.696S06

American Occupational Therapy Association. (2020a). AOTA 2020 occupational therapy code of ethics. *American Journal of Occupational Therapy*, *74*(Suppl. 3), 7413410005. https://doi.org/10.5014/ajot.2020.74S3006

American Occupational Therapy Association. (2020b). Guidelines for supervision, roles, and responsibilities during the delivery of occupational therapy services. *American Journal of Occupational Therapy*, *74*(Suppl. 3), 7413410020. https://doi.org/10.5014/ajot.2020.74S3004

American Occupational Therapy Association. (2020c). Occupational therapy practice framework: Domain and process (4th ed.). *American Journal of Occupational Therapy*, *74*(Suppl. 2), 7412410010. https://doi.org/10.5014/ajot.2020.74S2001

Communicating Effectively

Good verbal and nonverbal communication skills are essential traits for occupational therapy practitioners. Occupational therapists (OTs) and occupational therapy assistants (OTAs) must incorporate therapeutic use of self throughout the occupational therapy process in addition to displaying empathy (American Occupational Therapy Association [AOTA], 2020c). This chapter presents worksheets and learning activities to help you learn to problem solve and respond professionally to common situations with clients, families, significant others, caregivers, and other professionals. Practical communication tips are provided to help you make a good first impression, explain your role effectively to different audiences, ask open-ended questions, actively listen, and show empathy. Suggested answers to worksheet exercises are provided at the end of the chapter.

Contents

Morreale, M. J. *Developing Clinical Competence:*
A Workbook for the OTA, Second Edition (pp. 1-44).
© 2022 SLACK Incorporated.

Worksheet 1-1

Initial Client Encounter

Sandra Seenyer is 80 years old and sustained a right cerebrovascular accident 1 week ago, resulting in left hemiparesis. She was recently admitted to a skilled nursing facility for rehabilitation and was referred to occupational therapy. The OT determined that Sandra requires moderate assistance for activities of daily living (ADLs) such as self-care and transfers. Melissa, an OTA, will be providing intervention today and is meeting Sandra for the first time. Consider Melissa and Sandra's initial conversation. What suggestions would you make regarding the OTA's interaction with the client?

OTA: Hey Sandra, I'm Melissa, your therapist for today. It is nice to meet you. Any problems now?

Client: Well, the television isn't working and my breakfast was terrible! The eggs and coffee were completely cold. Who are you again?

OTA: I'm your OTA for today and I am here to help you get dressed.

Client: What's an OTA?

OTA: Well, I'm from the occupational therapy department. We are similar to physical therapy except they work on walking and the lower extremities and we work on the upper extremities and ADLs. Are you ready to begin therapy now, Sweetie?

Provide suggestions to improve this interaction:

1.

2.

3.

4.

Worksheet 1-1 (continued)
Initial Client Encounter

5.

6.

7.

8.

9.

10.

Learning Activity 1-1: Communication Basics

Over the course of your professional career as an OTA, you will have the opportunity to meet and work with many clients in occupational therapy. It is useful to practice some standard opening lines ahead of time to help you display confidence and make a positive first impression.

In the following space, write several sentences you might use initially when introducing yourself to a new client, such as Susan Smythe, a 70-year-old female who had total hip replacement surgery 3 days ago.

OTA introduction:

Now check your introductory statement against the following suggestions to determine if all the necessary elements are present.

For an initial encounter with an adult client, it is more respectful for an OTA to use an appropriate title such as "Mr." or "Mrs." and the client's last name. Use proper titles and pronouns for the gender the client identifies as and ensure you are pronouncing the client's name correctly. For the above client, Susan Smythe, her last name could be pronounced either with a short or long "i" sound in the middle. It is courteous to ascertain which pronunciation is correct. Next, tell the client your name and discipline. It is important to realize that an OTA should be referred to as an "occupational therapy practitioner" or "occupational therapy assistant" and not as a "therapist" (AOTA, 2015, 2020b; Centers for Medicare & Medicaid Services [CMS], 2014, 2019). Also acknowledge your working relationship with the client's OT and/or physician who referred the client to occupational therapy and the other team members involved, such as physical therapy personnel or your fieldwork educator (Morreale & Amini, 2016). The OTA might also determine whether the client understands occupational therapy and/or ask how the client is feeling. Of course, each client encounter will be a little different depending on the circumstances. Here are some examples of introductory statements that an OTA might use with a client recovering from hip surgery:

- *Hello, Mrs. Smythe, I am Vera Veracity, an OTA student. Am I saying your last name correctly? It is very nice to meet you. I have been working with your OT, Karen, and she asked me to see you today to review your hip precautions and teach you how to manage putting on your socks and shoes. How are you feeling today?*

- *Good morning, Mrs. Smythe. My name is Vera Veracity, and I am from the occupational therapy department. Dr. Smith ordered occupational therapy to help you recover from your hip surgery and learn the skills you need to be safe at home. I am an occupational therapy assistant student working with Karen Karing, the therapist who evaluated you yesterday. Would you like me to explain further what occupational therapy is or do you have any questions before I teach you how to get out of bed into this wheelchair safely?*

- *Hello Mrs. Smythe. I am Sally Smiley, an occupational therapy assistant. Am I pronouncing your last name correctly? Your occupational therapist, Karen, asked me to work with you today to review your hip precautions and teach you how to get dressed without bending your hip too much. This equipment I brought will allow you to put on your socks and shoes safely. Before we start, tell me how you are feeling today.*

Morreale, M. J. (2022). *Developing clinical competence: A workbook for the OTA* (2nd ed.). SLACK Incorporated.

- *Hello, Mrs. Smythe. I am Sally Smiley, an occupational therapy assistant. Am I saying your last name correctly? Your surgeon referred you to occupational therapy so we can teach you how to manage safely at home with your hip precautions. I work closely with Karen Karing, your occupational therapist. Karen asked me work with you today on transferring on and off the toilet using the walker. Do you have any questions before we begin?*

- *Good morning, Mrs. Smythe, it is nice to meet you. I am Sally Smiley, your occupational therapy practitioner for today. Karen, the occupational therapist whom you have been working with this week, asked me to teach you how to get dressed safely with your hip precautions. Do you remember what equipment Karen gave you yesterday to help you dress?*

Now write an introduction you might use for John Valorie, a 72-year-old male whom you are meeting for the first time to provide occupational therapy. He had a left below-knee amputation 5 days ago due to a non-healing wound and was evaluated by the OT yesterday.

Learning Activity 1-2: What Is Occupational Therapy?

Clients, caregivers, members of the public, or other professionals are not always aware of occupational therapy or may not fully understand what the profession entails. The OT will typically explain what occupational therapy is during the initial client contact or evaluation. However, while coping with an illness, injury, or other challenging circumstances, clients and families/significant others usually encounter multiple health team members and may also feel overwhelmed, confused, anxious, or exhausted dealing with their personal situation. As a result, the distinct value of occupational therapy may remain unclear to them at this time. Thus, the OTA must be ready to provide a clear and simple definition of occupational therapy appropriate to the client's situation and explain briefly how this service can be beneficial. The AOTA website (www.aota.org) and official documents, such as *Philosophical Base of Occupational Therapy* (AOTA, 2017) and *Occupational Therapy Practice Framework: Domain and Process, Fourth Edition (OTPF—4;* AOTA, 2020c), are useful resources to help you define occupational therapy for different audiences. Also, Table 1-1 presents practical suggestions for communicating with clients and others effectively.

Create a brief definition of occupational therapy that you might use with clients or family/caregivers.

Occupational therapy is...

Now develop a brief definition that you might use to explain occupational therapy to other professionals or service providers (i.e., medical interns, teachers, school administrators, optometrists).

Occupational therapy is...

Table 1-1
Suggestions for Initial Client Encounters and Occupational Therapy Definition

Do

- Make a sincere effort to have eye contact with the person you are addressing, particularly if you must review paperwork, jot down notations, or enter information on the computer during the encounter.
- Pay close attention to what the person is saying or doing.
- Use simple, easy-to-understand language.
- Make your definition brief and uncomplicated.
- Explain what "occupation" means.
- Relate to the individual client's condition, situation, or problem.
- Discuss how occupational therapy can help.
- Differentiate occupational therapy from other disciplines.
- Consider what is appropriate for that practice setting, time frames, and reasonable for the client's circumstances.
- Clarify the focus of your intervention for that particular client relating to occupation, such as enabling independence, remediating particular client factors to improve function, facilitating skills or occupational adaptations, assessing safety, providing caregiver education, modifying the environment, and improving comfort or quality of life.
- Provide examples or describe briefly the use of therapeutic methods and tasks, activities and occupations, adaptive equipment, or other specialized interventions indicated for this client.

Don't

- Don't appear preoccupied with other matters, such as personal problems, casual conversations with staff, or paperwork.
- Don't use technical jargon or abbreviations (unless you explain them). Clients may not know what ADL, COTA, OTR, CVA, and so forth stand for, or the meaning of words such as "activities of daily living," "dysphagia," "sensory integration," and "myocardial infarction."
- Don't talk down to the client or act as if the client is unintelligent.
- Don't refer to an adult client with nicknames such as "honey" or "sweetie."
- Don't refer to an OTA as a "therapist."
- Don't use an identical explanation for each client. Not all clients will achieve complete independence or improved functional abilities, as some conditions are irreversible or terminal. However, occupational therapy can help clients maintain function and manage chronic conditions for improved quality of life. The focus of occupational therapy interventions may be different according to various circumstances, but will contribute to occupational performance in some way.
- Don't guarantee results, but instead explain areas that will be addressed or may realistically improve based on sound clinical knowledge.
- Don't overwhelm the client with too much information.
- Don't ask the client a question you really do not want an answer to. For example, if you say, "Do you want to come to therapy today?" that sets up the client to refuse treatment. It might be better to say, "It is time for your occupational therapy session now." If you ask the client, "How was your day today?", be prepared to hear about bland hospital food, a noisy roommate, or how the television or phone did not work properly. You might decide it is better to target a question toward the client's condition, such as, "How does your hip feel today?"
- Don't lie or create false hope or unrealistic expectations. However, how you temper the truth can have a significant effect in helping to prevent client hopelessness and despair.

Worksheet 1-2

It Looks Like You Play All Day

A group of physicians are taking a tour of the rehabilitation department. When they arrive at the busy occupational therapy clinic, the physicians observe the following client interventions happening:

- A 45-year-old female client baking cookies
- A 65-year-old male client using a reacher to pick up socks from the floor
- A 77-year-old female client navigating a power mobility scooter around an obstacle course made of cones
- A 53-year-old female client making a mosaic tile trivet
- A 38-year-old female client standing and placing cans of food into an upper cabinet
- A 22-year-old male client playing checkers with an OTA

One of the physicians comments, "*It looks like you must play with toys all day in here.*" How might an OTA respond to this?

Learning Activity 1-3: Explaining Occupational Therapy's Distinct Value

For each of the following situations, role play with a partner or write a brief paragraph below. Introduce yourself as an OTA or student and explain the distinct value of occupational therapy for that client and the general desired, realistic outcomes that may be attainable. For this exercise, assume each client has been evaluated by the OT and is just beginning the first intervention session.

1. **Early intervention**: Lauren Laney is a single parent of 20-month-old Charlotte. Charlotte was recently diagnosed with a developmental delay; is nonverbal; exhibits poor eye contact, oral-motor sensitivity, tactile defensiveness; and does not walk yet.

2. **Outpatient clinic**: Aviva Katz is a 40-year-old married bookkeeper with children ages 2 and 5 years. Aviva sustained a Colles fracture in her dominant upper extremity 6 weeks ago. The cast was removed 5 days ago and she has not returned to work yet. Her hand is swollen, painful, and stiff, causing difficulty with ADLs and instrumental activities of daily living (IADL).

3. **School setting**: Jake Springer is the parent of Henry, a second-grade student with a learning disability. Henry demonstrates poor handwriting abilities, difficulty using scissors, and has challenges with time management and organizational skills. Henry's delayed skills acquisition creates difficulty with various school occupations such as completing class assignments and managing clothing for gym and recess.

4. **Skilled nursing facility**: Karen Kairgiver is the adult child and health care agent of Ruth Rezzydent, a client with moderate stage dementia. Ruth has lived in a long-term care facility for the past year but fell out of bed last week, breaking her hip. She is 1-week status post total hip replacement surgery.

5. **Acute care hospital**: Mike O'Malley, a 75-year-old retired plumber, had a heart attack 5 days ago. He lives with his wife in a single-family home and was independent prior to his hospitalization.

6. **Rehabilitation hospital**: Matthew Billings is an 18-year-old male who sustained a C6 spinal cord injury due to a recent diving accident in his backyard pool. Prior to his injury he was planning to attend college on a sports scholarship.

7. **Inpatient behavioral health setting**: Judy Jones is a 21-year-old female diagnosed with stimulant use disorder (cocaine addiction). She lives at home with her parents, recently dropped out of college, and was arrested for drug possession a few days ago. She was admitted to an inpatient drug rehabilitation program in lieu of going to jail.

8. **Primary care**: Rosa Rosario is a 45-year-old female who works full-time in an elementary school as a teacher's aide. She weighs 280 lb, has Type 2 diabetes, hypertension, and stage 2 kidney disease. Rosa is a single parent with 3 teenage children. She reports having "*no time*" for herself and expresses concern about her "*high stress level*" due to her health problems, work, and family obligations.

9. **Home care**: Lester Flint is an 82-year-old male diagnosed with congestive heart failure. He has poor activity tolerance for standing and requires assistance for meal preparation and lower body dressing and bathing due to low endurance. He lives with his wife Sheila on the 12th floor of a high-rise apartment building.

Worksheet 1-3

Do You Know What You Are Doing?

1. Your client, realizing you are a student or new practitioner, may express concern about your knowledge base or ability to handle their situation. The client may state, *"Have you ever worked with someone like me before?"* or *"Do you know what you are doing?"* How can you respond appropriately while being truthful about your limited experience?

2. You are an OTA student completing Level II fieldwork at an outpatient facility. Earlier this week you sat with and observed your fieldwork educator performing an occupational therapy evaluation with a client diagnosed with tennis elbow (lateral epicondylitis). Today the OT asks you to teach this client some therapy putty exercises and to make a pattern for a volar wrist orthosis. When the client arrives at the clinic, you reintroduce yourself as an OTA student and explain the delegated intervention you will be providing. The client states, *"Honey, you seem very nice. Nothing personal, but I think a real therapist is better for my therapy. You know, someone that is specially trained in this medical stuff—not an aide."* How would you respond?

3. You are an OTA student completing Level II fieldwork at an inpatient rehabilitation unit. This morning your fieldwork educator is planning to teach a client with left hemiparesis safe bathing techniques. The OT introduces you as a student and asks the client for permission to let you participate in the intervention session. The client states, *"Why would you want to watch an old lady like me take a shower? That can't be very interesting."* How would you respond?

Worksheet 1-4

Are You Really Sure You Can Do This?

Clients often experience anxiety and uncertainty regarding their health condition or circumstances. They may express various concerns regarding occupational therapy, other health team members, care received, or upcoming events. It is important that you respond appropriately to help put the client's mind at ease. Consider how you might respond to the following client scenarios. For this exercise, assume that you are competent in the interventions depicted.

1. Your client is concerned about your ability to transfer him safely and states, "*I am a big guy and you are so tiny. I really don't think you can get me into that wheelchair.*"

2. While performing a cooking task in occupational therapy, your client expresses fear regarding functional ambulation and states, "*I am afraid my weak leg will buckle and I will fall.*"

3. As you are about to transfer your client from wheelchair to bed, the client states, "*I don't want you to get hurt moving me.*"

Worksheet 1-5

This Feels Like Kindergarten

Your client, Keith, is a 62-year-old defense attorney whose hobbies include gardening and woodworking. Keith has undergone surgery to repair a lacerated median nerve and is now at the strengthening phase in therapy. He has not returned to work yet due to hypersensitivity in his hand and difficulty grasping and manipulating objects. To implement the occupational therapy intervention plan, you place the client's affected hand in a plastic shoebox filled with uncooked rice and ask him to locate and remove small objects (e.g., blocks, beads) with the affected hand. The client seems offended and states, *"I feel like I am in kindergarten with my grandkids! My children would really laugh if they saw me, a pit-bull defense lawyer, doing this."*

How would you respond to those statements?

To address this client's specific deficits and likely goals, what activities and occupations could you choose that might be more meaningful for this client?

Learning Activity 1-4: Occupational Therapy Versus Physical Therapy

Indicate how an OTA might respond to each of the following situations.

1. You are an OTA working in a skilled nursing facility, and your occupational therapy supervisor has asked you to attend a team meeting today for one of the units. During the meeting the head nurse states, *"Ellen Elderlee in room #468 hasn't had any rehab in a long time. She is developing contractures in her right shoulder and elbow which is making it hard for the aides to dress and bathe her. I wonder if we should get physical therapy (PT) involved."*

2. You are an OTA working in an acute care setting. Helen, a client on your caseload, was admitted 3 days ago due to an exacerbation of multiple sclerosis. The OT evaluated Helen and delegated her intervention to you, which you began implementing yesterday. You go to Helen's room today to provide intervention again and see that she has several visitors. Helen announces to the visitors, *"Oh here's my physical therapist. I guess it is time for my arm exercises now. I hope the physical therapist won't make you all leave now."*

3. You are an OTA working in an inpatient rehabilitation facility. Today you are in the occupational therapy room working with Mr. Getbetta. Your session entails having Mr. Getbetta work on interventions to improve sitting balance, range of motion, and fine-motor skills needed for managing utensils and feeding. As the client is working on tasks such as tossing beanbags and reaching for cones while sitting on a mat, a physical therapist assistant comes to get the client and asks, *"Are you finished playing with Mr. Getbetta? It is time for me to work on ambulation with him so I will have to pull him away from fun and games."*

4. You are an OTA working in a school setting. As you are walking down the hallway, a teacher asks to speak with you and says, *"See that student Emma over there?* [Teacher points to a student in classroom.] *She always fidgets like that, and she can't seem to sit up straight or focus on copying notes from the blackboard. Her desk is always very messy too. Do you think we should try and have her evaluated by the OT or would PT be better? Can therapy even help her?"*

Adapted from Morreale, M. J., & Amini, D. (2016). *The occupational therapist's workbook for ensuring clinical competence.* SLACK Incorporated.

Therapeutic Relationships

The *OTPF—4* (AOTA, 2020c) describes *therapeutic use of self* as an integral aspect, or cornerstone, of the occupational therapy process and an essential component for all interactions with clients. An historical perspective regarding the therapeutic use of self in occupational therapy is presented in Taylor's (2020) *The Intentional Relationship: Occupational Therapy and Use of Self, Second Edition.* Taylor (2008, 2020) created the Intentional Relationship Model, which outlines the interpersonal dynamic between the occupational therapy practitioner and client. According to Taylor (2020), effective therapeutic use of self is defined by empathy and intentionality. Six interpersonal communication modes that occupational therapy practitioners use frequently in therapeutic relationships are delineated, at length, by Taylor (2008, 2020). These six ways of relating to clients include advocating, collaborating, empathizing, encouraging, instructing, and problem-solving (Taylor, 2008, 2020). In clinical practice, OTs and OTAs utilize a professional "toolbox" of therapeutic qualities and methods to foster appropriate and helpful client relationships. Various therapeutic qualities are summarized on the following pages along with practical tips. Chapter 8 contains additional information about interventions used in occupational therapy mental health practice.

Adapted from Morreale, M. J., & Amini, D. (2016). *The occupational therapist's workbook for ensuring clinical competence.* SLACK Incorporated.

Therapeutic Qualities and Tips (Morreale & Amini, 2016)

Attending: Actively centering on the client allows occupational therapy practitioners to make astute observations and glean important clues as to how the client is feeling (Cole, 2018). The occupational therapy practitioner develops initial impressions and expectations of client abilities and needs from these cues using professional reasoning skills. Cole (2018, p. 72) describes this as "the attentive physical presence the therapist focuses on the client…Taking note of appearance, body language, posture, seating position, eye contact and facial expression are all part of attending."

Active listening: During client interactions, the occupational therapy practitioner should strive to show genuine interest in the client and demonstrate a caring approach. Active listening can be conveyed by eye contact, facial expression, not interrupting, and nonverbal communication, such as an appropriately relaxed posture, not fidgeting, and nodding to various client statements (Froehlich, 2017a). It is also useful for OTs and OTAs to occasionally pause and allow for silences which enable the person talking to "fill the space with what weighs heavily on him or her.…If the speaker is struggling with what else to say the simple phrase, 'Tell me more' or 'What else?' may be all the speaker needs to hear in order to continue talking about what is on his or her mind" (Froehlich, 2017a, p. 111).

Genuine caring approach: When speaking to a client or family/significant others, an OTA's nonverbal communication, tone of voice, and choice of words can either convey genuineness or give the impression that the OTA is disinterested or just going through the motions (Morreale & Amini, 2016). Thus, it is important to spend adequate quality time with the client, actively listen, follow through with promises, demonstrate compassion, and provide competent, effective care. Showing kindness and paying attention to detail might include the OTA taking the time to obtain a blanket or drink for the client as needed, neatly folding the client's clothing during a bathing or dressing intervention, carefully adjusting the bedcovers, being respectful of the client's belongings, and positioning the call bell and phone for easy access at the end of the session (Morreale & Amini, 2016). Also, an OTA who makes a genuine effort to point out the "little things" can help clients to feel special, well-cared for, and valued. For example, for a client in a nursing home or home care setting, the OTA might compliment the client's new manicure, comment positively on the family photo on a nightstand, acknowledge the pretty bouquet of flowers the client received, and praise incremental progress or client effort during a particular task or procedure (Morreale & Amini, 2016).

Respect and cultural sensitivity: Occupational therapy practitioners should demonstrate cultural sensitivity and avoid personal bias or judgment regarding a client's gender, age, race, sexual orientation, socioeconomic status, level of education, appearance, diagnosis, and so forth. (AOTA, 2020a, 2020c; Froehlich, 2017a, 2017b). It is essential to understand and be respectful of the client's cultural background and possible implications for emotional expression and personal space requirements. For example, a client's relevant cultural factors could include a more stoic nature, limited eye contact, avoidance of touch, special rituals, and so forth. (Morreale & Amini, 2016). Occupational therapy practitioners should strive to believe in the dignity and worth of each person despite the client's problems or challenging situations (Froehlich, 2017b).

Empowerment: Occupational therapy practitioners believe in the client's potential for change. It is important to foster a client-centered atmosphere that gives the client hope and empowers the client to overcome obstacles and be an active part of their own solution (Froehlich, 2017b). This might include teaching the client specific coping strategies and communication skills such as assertiveness and self-advocacy.

Empathy: Empathy is a vital quality OTs and OTAs use to connect emotionally with clients, enabling a more open dialogue to assist them with current life circumstances (AOTA, 2020c). Primary accurate empathy is recognizing the feelings of the client. A helpful way for OTs and OTAs to convey empathy is by using the statement, "You feel _____because_____" (Cole, 2018, p. 74). Realize that the different kinds of emotions (i.e., bad, glad, sad, mad) all have varying levels of intensity (mild, moderate, high) so it is important that occupational therapy practitioners identify the accurate emotion (Cole, 2018). For example, Cole (2018, p. 74) describes the emotion of anger as a spectrum "from low intensity, like annoyed or perturbed, to very high intensity, like rage" and the emotion of "fearful" as varied levels going from mild (worried) to severe (petrified). Additional techniques such as reflective listening and advanced accurate empathy enable occupational therapy practitioners to form an educated guess or hypothesis about the underlying feelings, topics, or concerns that the client is hinting about (Cole, 2018; Froehlich, 2017a).

Restatement: This technique, which often uses the form of a question, rephrases what the speaker said to reflect that the client was heard or understood (Froehlich, 2017a).

Humor: Besides the physiological benefits of true laughter, humor can be used by occupational therapy practitioners as an effective tool in specific situations to "break the ice," motivate clients, manage difficult situations, reduce client anxiety, or make the OTA or OT seem more approachable (Morreale & Amini, 2016).

Redirection: The OTA must recognize when the session is veering off in an unintended direction due to client inattention, lack of focus, verbosity, or difficulty in answering questions clearly and directly (Morreale & Amini, 2016). Redirection is needed if the client goes off on a tangent or asks the OTA inappropriate or excessive personal questions. The OTA must tactfully and respectfully manage the undesired behavior by directing the client's attention back to the desired intervention activity/topic or close the session as appropriate (Morreale & Amini, 2016).

Therapeutic self-disclosure: Indirect self-disclosure conveys to the client or significant others a sense of the occupational therapy practitioner's approval or disapproval regarding their statements or behavior through nonverbal communication such as nodding yes or no, smiling or frowning, exhibiting tension or laughter, and so forth (Cole, 2018). An OT or OTA might also use direct self-disclosure, as appropriate, to help the client with a specific challenging situation. This technique involves the occupational therapy practitioner relating a personal vignette with a similar theme to provide a different perspective, describe how it was resolved, or present the coping mechanisms/strategies used (Cole, 2018). This technique must be used judiciously, not just as an opportunity for the OT or OTA to vent (Cole, 2018).

Maintain professional boundaries: Unlike personal relationships, which involve reciprocal give-and-take, the OTA's professional client relationships should never make clients feel the need to provide any type of support to the OTA (Drench et al., 2012). Besides limiting disclosure of personal information, occupational therapy practitioners must also limit the extent of emotional involvement to maintain professional judgment and objectivity (Drench et al., 2012). Any use of comforting or therapeutic touch must be in accordance with facility policy, culturally sensitive, and critical that it cannot be misinterpreted as inappropriate personal touch (Drench et al., 2012; Froehlich, 2017b). It is also respectful to ask the client's permission before any essential procedures involving physical touch are performed, such as range of motion, positioning of limbs, retrograde massage, or assessment of areas covered by bedding or clothing (Morreale & Amini, 2016). Maintain client modesty with proper draping during intervention or procedures. Also, gifts from clients should not be hinted at or expected. Many facilities have policies in place which clearly prohibit acceptance of client gifts. Some facilities may allow staff to accept nominal gifts such as candy, cookies, or flowers, but it is inappropriate to accept money or "tips" from clients (Morreale & Amini, 2016). For clients insistent on showing their appreciation for care received, facility policy might allow for donations to the facility's charitable foundation or to benefit the rehabilitation department or other unit.

Adapted from Morreale, M. J., & Amini, D. (2016). *The occupational therapist's workbook for ensuring clinical competence.* SLACK Incorporated.

Worksheet 1-6

I Want to Walk

Consider the therapeutic communication techniques you might use when responding to the following client situations.

1. You are working with Hector, a 22-year-old carpenter who recently sustained a C6 spinal cord injury due to a fall from a roof. As you are discussing his occupational therapy goals for the next few weeks, Hector tells you the doctors are wrong, and his main goal is to walk again. You know this is unrealistic based on the medical reports. What would you say to him?

2. You are working with Omar, a 68-year-old male with a total hip replacement. He has partial–weight-bearing status for his affected lower extremity and is presently using a walker with moderate assistance. Today you are trying to teach Omar how to don his socks and shoes using adaptive equipment. He tells you that the equipment is "silly," his wife can help him dress, and that his only goal is to walk again. What would you say to him?

Learning Activity 1-5: I Don't Want Therapy

Consider the therapeutic communication techniques you might use as an OTA when responding to the following situations.

1. A 65-year-old client was admitted to an acute care hospital recently with an exacerbation of chronic obstructive pulmonary disease. Your occupational therapy supervisor evaluated this client yesterday and delegated today's intervention to you. You enter the client's hospital room and state it is time for occupational therapy. The client replies, *"Please go away. I just did a lot of leg exercises and walking in physical therapy. I am too tired for any more therapy."* What would you say to this client?

2. Your client is an 80-year-old male diagnosed with rheumatoid arthritis. He has pain and stiffness in both upper extremities, causing difficulties with ADLs and IADLs. Today he arrives at the outpatient clinic accompanied by his wife who states, *"My husband doesn't need all this. He had therapy before and it did not help. I don't know why the doctor made us come here."* What would you say to them?

3. Your client in home care is a 67-year-old male who has terminal pancreatic cancer. During the occupational therapy intervention session he states, *"What's the use of all this therapy? The doctor told me I only have 6 months to live. This is a complete waste of time."* What would you say to him?

4. You are an OTA working on an acute behavioral health unit. Your OT supervisor delegated a female client to you who has depression and suicidal ideation. You go to the client's room this morning to take her to a scheduled occupational therapy activity group. The client says, *"Please go away. I just want everyone here to stop bothering me and let me stay in my room by myself. Besides, I am awful with crafts so there is really no point in me going. I don't want to waste your time."* What would you say to her?

5. You are an OTA working in an outpatient clinic. Today a 56-year-old client diagnosed with a rotator cuff tear has been delegated to you by the OT. The client identifies as a devout follower of a religion with strict, conservative beliefs and practices. When the client arrives at the scheduled appointment time, you notice the client does not make eye contact and purposely avoids shaking the hand you extend when introducing yourself. You begin to explain you will be providing today's intervention, which includes passive range of motion, but the client abruptly interrupts and says, *"I am sorry, but I must leave now. It is not appropriate for someone of the opposite gender, besides my spouse, to be touching me. That would be very immoral."* How would you respond?

6. Your client is a 75-year old male with Medicare who lives alone in senior housing. He recently had left total knee replacement surgery and was admitted to a skilled nursing facility for short-term rehabilitation. To implement the OT intervention plan, you go to the client's room to bring him to an upper extremity exercise group. The client states, *"Oh, I don't need all that. I already did that group with the stretchy bands yesterday. I promise I'll do some arm exercises by myself later. I just want to watch the* Judge Judy *show coming on now. Besides, I'm on a fixed income and can't afford all this therapy."* What would you say to him?

Learning Activity 1-6: I Don't Need a Job

Clients who are unfamiliar with occupational therapy often take the word occupation literally, erroneously believing the profession entails finding jobs for people. Consider how you might respond to the following situations.

1. A 22-year-old college student was admitted to the hospital 2 days ago with bilateral leg fractures and internal injuries due to a motor vehicle accident. He was evaluated by the OT yesterday and is on your caseload today. You enter the client's hospital room and tell him it is time for occupational therapy. The client states, *"I don't need a job now. What I need is to get out of here to finish up my bachelor's degree and go to law school in the fall."* How would you respond to those statements?

2. Your client is 78 years old and diagnosed with Parkinson's disease. He has decreased bilateral upper extremity range of motion and strength, along with a history of falling. Today he arrives at the outpatient clinic accompanied by his wife who states, *"My husband certainly doesn't need a job at his age. He hasn't worked in years! I don't know why the doctor made us come here."* How would you respond to those statements?

3. A toddler diagnosed with a developmental delay started receiving early intervention services last week. Today the child's father took the day off from work to observe his daughter's therapy program. As you are introducing yourself as an occupational therapy practitioner, the father interrupts you and says, *"Do you always start training disabled kids this early for a job? My daughter is only 2! How do you know what she is going to want to be years from now?"* How would you respond to those statements?

4. Your client is a 55-year-old plumber who recently had cardiac bypass surgery. During the occupational therapy intervention session he states, *"What's the use of this job therapy? Forget about me getting a job. The doctor told me I won't be able to go back to work. This is all a waste of time."* How would you respond to those statements?

5. Your client is a 28-year-old male admitted to a behavioral health unit this week following a heroin overdose. You go to the client's room, introduce yourself as an OTA, and tell him it is time for his occupational therapy activity group. The client responds, *"Hey, I already told the shrink I am not interested in learning any job stuff. I get by okay with the government money I get every month, and my Nana lets me stay at her house because I help with the yard sometimes. Look, I'm real tired right now and going to take a nap, so just leave me alone."* How would you respond to those statements?

6. Your client is a 26-year-old female admitted to an inpatient rehabilitation unit yesterday due to orthopedic injuries sustained in a fall. She is married, has two children under the age of 3 years, and identifies as a devout follower of a traditional, conservative religion. When you go to her room to take her to occupational therapy, the client states, *"Is this occupational stuff really necessary? I don't work and do not need to get a job. My husband has a really good job that supports our family and I just love being a wife and stay-at-home mom. All my kids are going to be home-schooled."* How would you respond to those statements?

Worksheet 1-7

Open-Ended and Closed-Ended Questions

One essential role of the OTA is to assist the OT in gathering relevant client data throughout the occupational therapy process. You may find that some clients will provide vague, limited, or possibly, disingenuous responses when queried about their condition, emotional state, or circumstances. The use of open-ended questions will help the OTA elicit additional pertinent information, encourage more detailed client communication, and better clarify the client's perception regarding their situation (Cole, 2018). Asking clients closed-ended questions will typically elicit a simple "yes" or "no" (or perhaps only a limited one-to-two word) reply. However, they can be appropriate for situations that require only a specific, basic response, for example, determining if the client had a flu shot this year, finding out the client's age, or ascertaining if the person wears hearing aids or glasses.

To avoid a simple "yes" or "no" response when asking a client questions, Cole (2018) suggests using the words "how" or "what" at the start of the question. The OTA might also use phrases such as, "Tell me about, Describe what, I would like to learn more about, Help me to understand" that encourage the client to elaborate. Use caution with the word "why" as that could be perceived as judgmental and avoid starting questions with phrases such as "Do you, Can you, Would you, Are you, Have you" because these can easily elicit just a "yes" or "no" response (Cole, 2018, p. 74).

For each of the following sentences, indicate if it is an open-ended question (O), closed-ended question (C), or neither (N).

1. _____ Do you wear dentures?

2. _____ What caused you to fall?

3. _____ How would you describe your child's personality?

4. _____ Did you take your insulin this morning?

5. _____ I notice that you seem tired today.

6. _____ Tell me about your use of pain killers from the beginning.

7. _____ It looks like you ate all your breakfast this morning.

8. _____ Do you feel you drink too much on weekends?

9. _____ Describe a situation at home that might cause you to become angry and "lose it."

10. _____ What do you notice about your child that is concerning to you?

11. _____ Do you think you get enough exercise?

Worksheet 1-7 (continued)
Open-Ended and Closed-Ended Questions

12. _____ I see that you got a haircut.

13. _____ Describe some things you do for leisure.

14. _____ Are you having difficulty dressing yourself after your stroke?

15. _____ Did you check your blood sugar level this morning?

16. _____ What are the responsibilities you have at work?

17. _____ I would like to learn more about how you are managing at home after hip surgery.

18. _____ Tell me about your exercise routine.

19. _____ It seems like you handled that situation well.

20. _____ Please describe what a typical day of yours is like.

21. _____ Do you use any mobility devices?

22. _____ How many children do you have?

23. _____ What year were you born?

24. _____ I see that you are using a walker.

25. _____ Would you be willing to tell me about your living situation?

Adapted from Morreale, M. J., & Amini, D. (2016). *The occupational therapist's workbook for ensuring clinical competence.* SLACK Incorporated.

Worksheet 1-8

Asking Open-Ended Questions

For each of the following client statements, develop several open-ended questions to obtain pertinent information from the client.

1. My shoulder hurts.

2. I can't do anything right.

3. I fell in my apartment.

4. My life is a charade.

5. I never thought I would turn out like this.

6. My hand is useless.

7. I'm so confused.

8. I lost my job.

9. I hate school.

10. I am no good in gym class.

Adapted from Cole, M. (2018). *Group dynamics in occupational therapy: The theoretical basis and practice application of group intervention* (5th ed.). SLACK Incorporated.

Learning Activity 1-7: Asking Open-Ended Questions—More Practice

For each of the following client statements, develop several open-ended questions to obtain pertinent information from the client, family/significant other or caregiver.

1. My hand feels numb.

2. My daughter is really a handful.

3. I wish my husband would get some help for his drinking.

4. I have a lot of trouble getting dressed.

5. The teacher does not like my child.

6. I can't handle my elderly mother anymore.

7. Something is wrong with my wrist.

8. I feel like such a burden for my kids.

9. I don't want an aide at home.

10. I have trouble walking sometimes.

Adapted from Cole, M. (2018). *Group dynamics in occupational therapy: The theoretical basis and practice application of group intervention* (5th ed.). SLACK Incorporated.

Worksheet 1-9

Eliciting Information Efficiently

Nick, an OTA, is meeting his client, Jean Jones, for the first time. Jean is a 60-year-old female recently hospitalized and diagnosed with Guillain-Barré syndrome. Yesterday Jean was transferred from acute care to a rehabilitation hospital and subsequently evaluated by the OT, Karen. Today the OT asked Nick to obtain further information about the client's living situation. Consider Nick and Jean's initial conversation below. What suggestions would you make regarding the OTA's interaction with the client?

OTA: Hello Jean, I am Nick, an occupational therapy assistant. It is very nice to meet you. Your occupational therapist, Karen, asked me to work with you today. Are you feeling better today?
Client: No.
OTA: Why do you say that?
Client: I'm terrible. Don't you know how weak I am? I can't do anything!
OTA: That's not true. When I came in here, I saw that you were doing a pretty good job feeding yourself with that device Karen gave you.
Client: Well, I spilled half of my food.
OTA: The nurses will be in soon to get you cleaned up. Anyway, can I ask you some questions?
Client: I would rather be left alone.
OTA: This won't take too long. Where do you reside?
Client: 1374 East Main Street—just a few blocks from here.
OTA: I mean, do you live in a house?
Client: No.
OTA: An apartment?
Client: No, a condo.
OTA: Do you have any stairs?
Client: Yes.
OTA: How many stairs?
Client: Do you mean inside or outside?
OTA: Both.
Client: Three steps outside and about 10 steps to the second floor.
OTA: Okay, now tell me about your bathroom situation.
Client: Well, I occasionally get constipated so I have to drink a lot of prune juice.

Suggestions to improve this OTA's interaction with the client:

1.

2.

Morreale, M. J. (2022). *Developing clinical competence: A workbook for the OTA* (2nd ed.). SLACK Incorporated.

Worksheet 1-9 (continued)
Eliciting Information Efficiently

3.

4.

5.

Revise the interaction to incorporate more useful questions from the OTA:

Learning Activity 1-8: Developing an Emotions Vocabulary

Many feelings can be divided into the categories of "glad," "bad (fearful)," "sad," and "mad" and within each of those categories are varying levels of emotional intensity (Cole, 2018). For example, glad feelings might be described as satisfied or pleased on the mild end of emotion and euphoric on the high end. Low intensity mad feelings might be identified as annoyed or frustrated, whereas high intensity mad feelings might be described as rage or fury (Cole, 2018).

This exercise will help you to identify a range of emotions and develop a vocabulary of "feelings" terms to express them. Having a repertoire of words to choose from is beneficial when using empathy with your clients. For each of the following scenarios, choose a word that would most clearly describe your feelings if you were in that situation. You can use a thesaurus but do not use any "emotion" term more than once.

Examples:

Anxious You are stuck in traffic while driving to your first day of fieldwork.

Concerned You woke up with a 101° temperature this morning.

1. _____ A friend visits and brings a small gift or flowers while you are in the hospital.

2. _____ Your parent/guardian or spouse/significant other makes you your favorite dinner or dessert that you have not had in months.

3. _____ You failed a test you studied very hard for.

4. _____ You just won the million-dollar lottery.

5. _____ You come home and discover that your house was burglarized.

6. _____ You find out your spouse or significant other has been cheating on you.

7. _____ You received 10 spam phone calls today.

8. _____ You just reached your goal of losing 10 lb.

9. _____ You get a flat tire while driving to the grocery store today.

10. _____ You are trying to swat away a small swarm of mosquitoes that keep flying around you while you are taking a walk outdoors today.

11. _____ The doctor's office just called to notify you that the results of your mammogram or prostate test were atypical and you need to repeat the test.

12. _____ You were just served legal papers notifying you that you are being sued for a person's injuries sustained in the fender bender you had last month.

13. _____ You were just notified a close family member has died suddenly.

14. _____ You earned all A's in your OTA classes this semester.

15. _____ You are awaiting the results of your certification exam.

16. _____ You must give a presentation in front of the class this week.

17. _____ You must cancel your vacation tomorrow because you have the flu.

18. _____ You lost your wallet.

19. _____ A telemarketing call woke you up early on your day off today.

20. _____ You (or your spouse/significant other) had a miscarriage after trying for 3 years to finally become pregnant.

21. _____ Your spouse/significant other had an accident today and sustained third-degree burns over half their face and body.

22. _____ You are flying cross country and experiencing severe turbulence causing the plane to dip rapidly multiple times.

23. _____ You just found out you inherited $500,000 from a long-lost relative.

24. _____ The waitress accidentally spilled a drink on your brand-new shirt.

25. _____ You are playing ball in the backyard and accidentally break a neighbor's window.

Adapted from Cole, M. (2018). *Group dynamics in occupational therapy: The theoretical basis and practice application of group intervention* (5th ed.). SLACK Incorporated.

Worksheet 1-10

Interaction OTA—Elementary School Student

Marisol is an entry-level OTA who works at an elementary school. Her client, Chrystal, is a second-grade student with a learning disability. Marisol and Chrystal had the following conversation during an intervention session. Clearly, the OTA's interaction with the student is inappropriate, insensitive, and unethical (AOTA, 2020a). The OTA's improper conduct could result in disciplinary action and possible job termination. What suggestions would you make to improve the OTA's communication with the student so that it is a more professional and productive exchange?

OTA: Okay Chrystal, we are going to work some more on your handwriting today. Let's start with this worksheet.
Student: Do we have to?
OTA: Yes. You know your parents and teacher would like your work to be much neater. It will only get better if you practice.
Student: Writing is boring. Can't we do something else?
OTA: Not today. Would you like to choose a colored pencil from the box?
Student: No.
OTA: Chrystal, pick up a pencil. Any color you would like.
Student: Nope.
OTA: Don't be difficult. Please grab one of the pencils.
Student: What if I don't?
OTA: Well, you'll be sorry.
Student: What does that mean?
OTA: Do you want to see your parents again?
Student: Yes.
OTA: Well, you can't go home until you pick up a pencil and finish this worksheet.
Student: You can't make me stay here.
OTA: Oh yeah, Missy? I will tie you to the chair if I need to. Now pick up a pencil. Why are you crying now?
Student: You are yelling at me. I don't like that.
OTA: I am not yelling. I am just talking in a loud voice because you are being a bad girl. Come on now, start this worksheet. I will give you a sticker when you are finished.

Suggestions to improve this OTA's interaction with the client:

1.

2.

Worksheet 1-10 (continued)
Interaction OTA—Elementary School Student

3.

4.

5.

6.

7.

8.

Learning Activity 1-9: Nonverbal Communication

With a partner, choose a contemporary television talk show (e.g., *The View, The Talk, The Five*) that has a panel of diverse hosts who discuss current events or controversial subjects. Watch the opening segment of the show with the sound off and observe how the talk show hosts interact with each other. Jot down the nonverbal behaviors you observed during the exchange and determine if you can ascertain the overall tone of the conversation. Can you tell which panelists seem to agree or disagree with the others? Did you and your partner interpret what you saw in the same way? What are the specific behaviors you and your partner each observed to reach your conclusions? After you complete this worksheet, watch the segment again—but with the sound on, so you can determine if your interpretation of nonverbal behaviors was correct.

Positive Nonverbal Behaviors Observed	*Negative Nonverbal Behaviors Observed*

- If you felt the panel's tone was congenial, did you observe any panelists smiling, nodding, hugging, lightly touching each other affectionately, or waiting to speak one's turn?

- If you felt the tone was aggressive or argumentative, did you observe panelists standing up, pointing, or exhibiting "in your face" behavior? Were people speaking over each other at the same time? What facial expressions did you observe? What behaviors indicated that people may have been shouting?

- Did any of the panelists "tune out" by looking away or moving elsewhere, crossing arms, sighing, or not actively participating?

Learning Activity 1-10: Communication Styles

Watch a one-on-one television interview performed by a celebrity interviewer who is perceived to have a more gentle or empathetic approach (e.g., Barbara Walters or Oprah Winfrey). Also watch an episode of a show where real people are interrogated by someone with a more direct style or tougher reputation (e.g., Dr. Phil, Judge Judy, Robert Irvine *[Restaurant Impossible]*). Compare and contrast the two styles of questioning and the nonverbal behavior of the interviewers. Consider the following as you are watching the two interviews:

- What did the interviewers do or say to elicit the information they were trying to obtain?

- What specific open- or closed-ended questions did they ask?

- What tone of voice did the interviewers use?

- Were the styles of both interviewers equally effective?

- How did the persons being questioned respond verbally and nonverbally? Did they appear comfortable or uncomfortable?

- Was information freely shared or were responses vague and resistant?

- Do you feel any of the interviewers' questions or behaviors were inappropriate? Why or why not?

- Which interviewer appeared more sympathetic to an individual's situation, and why?

- Did an interviewer specifically acknowledge or guess at what the person was feeling? If so, was the interviewer's interpretation correct?

- What judgmental or empathetic words were used by the interviewers?

- How was active listening evident?

- Was either of the interviewer's approaches too soft or too tough?

- Which approach do you like better and why?

Worksheet 1-11

Better Communication

For each of the following scenarios, choose which of the two statements would likely be the better response from an occupational therapy practitioner. Write one to two sentences to explain your rationale for choosing each answer.

1. You go to a client's hospital room with the intent to transport the client to the occupational therapy room for therapy.

   _____ Would you like to come to therapy now?

   _____ It is time for occupational therapy now.

2. You are beginning an intervention session with a client who had hip replacement surgery.

   _____ Do you have hip pain today?

   _____ How are you today?

3. During an occupational therapy session, a client diagnosed with a cerebrovascular accident is having difficulty transferring to a commode and begins to cry.

   _____ What is making you cry?

   _____ Why are you so upset?

4. A child who is overweight is holding back tears and mentions the other students call him "fatty."

   _____ Just try to ignore them.

   _____ You feel sad because the other children are calling you names.

5. A 22-year-old female client with conservative religious beliefs mentions she is engaged and is looking forward to kissing her fiancé for the first time on her wedding day.

   _____ It is nice you have something special to look forward to.

   _____ How do you know you and your fiancé will be compatible?

Worksheet 1-11 (continued)
Better Communication

6. An older client was admitted due to injuries sustained in a fall at home.

    _____ Tell me what happened to cause you to fall.

    _____ Did you fall because you were not using your walker?

7. An outpatient client with three young children mentions that her family does not celebrate Halloween because of their religious beliefs.

    _____ Do your kids feel like they are missing out?

    _____ I understand that many people prefer not to celebrate certain holidays.

8. An outpatient client states that she experienced pain while performing the new exercise program at home that the OTA told her to do.

    _____ Don't worry—no pain, no gain.

    _____ Show me how you are doing your exercises.

9. An OT working with a 3-year-old child in a preschool program would like the child to work on fine-motor activities to improve play skills.

    _____ If you are a good girl today you can pick a prize from the prize box.

    _____ If you complete these activities, I will give you a prize.

10. A client who sustained third-degree burns and has severe facial scars was admitted to a behavioral health program due to depression over his appearance. He is being evaluated by the OT.

    _____ I am sorry your scars make you feel depressed.

    _____ How have your injuries impacted you?

Reproduced with permission from Morreale, M. J., & Amini, D. (2016). *The occupational therapist's workbook for ensuring clinical competence.* SLACK Incorporated.

Answers to Worksheets

Worksheet 1-1: Initial Client Encounter

1.   It is more respectful to call the older client "Mrs. Seenyer" rather than her first name.

2.   *"Hey"* in the opening statement is not very professional. "Hello" or "Good morning" is more appropriate in this situation. Use appropriate language for the particular context and geographical area.

3.   It is incorrect and unethical for that OTA to refer to herself as a "therapist." The OTA should use the terms *occupational therapy practitioner* or *occupational therapy assistant* instead (AOTA, 2015, 2020b; CMS, 2014, 2019).

4.   The question *"Any problems now?"* is not specific enough so the client responds about issues unrelated to her diagnosis.

5.   The OTA uses unfamiliar abbreviations, such as ADLs and OTA, which the client is not familiar with.

6.   The OTA does not acknowledge her working relationship with the OT, physician, or mention that Sandra was evaluated by the OT.

7.   The purpose of the session, *"help you get dressed,"* does not reflect skilled therapy, as an aide or family member could help the client dress.

8.   The OTA does not adequately explain what occupational therapy is, such as the meaning of "occupation" or goals of improving the client's function. There also needs to be a better distinction between the disciplines of occupational therapy and physical therapy.

9.   Calling an adult client "Sweetie" is disrespectful.

10. The OTA did not acknowledge the client's complaints.

Worksheet 1-2: It Looks Like You Play All Day

You might explain how occupational therapy practitioners use everyday objects and adaptive equipment to work on remediating various client factors and skills to improve a client's performance in daily living tasks (occupations). Without breaching client confidentiality, you might relate the use of craft activities to improve specific motor functions, such as shoulder and elbow range of motion, cylindrical grasp, tip pinch, or other essential skills, such as crossing midline and coordination. Cooking activities, checkers and obstacle courses might be used to teach or restore specific occupational skills (e.g., home management, functional mobility, leisure) by addressing specific cognitive/perceptual deficits, such as unilateral neglect or problems in sequencing, problem solving, spatial relations, and safety awareness. Standing and putting weighted cans on a shelf may help to restore balance, range of motion, strength, and endurance, all of which are necessary for performing functional, daily activities. **However, the occupational therapy department might internally use this experience to reflect upon whether enough occupation-based interventions are being implemented on a regular basis.**

Worksheet 1-3: Do You Know What You Are Doing?

In clinical practice, if you are expected to do a task you are very unsure of, you should discuss this with your supervisor (AOTA, 2020b). It is unethical to perform interventions for which you are not competent (AOTA, 2015, 2020a). Assuming you are competent with the specific intervention, your communicative style should convey confidence in your abilities and professionalism. However, an OTA student or practitioner should never exaggerate or fabricate information about one's credentials or experience (AOTA, 2020a). As an OTA student, you might explain to the client that you have professional education in this area, are closely supervised, and would not do anything that would knowingly put the client in danger. As a new OTA, you might add that you have fieldwork experience, have passed a national certification exam, and are licensed by that state. If the client still appears concerned, you might ask another colleague or your supervisor to intervene and oversee or assist with the task.

For clients that are asking why you are there observing or participating as a student, you might explain that this is a standard part of your college education/professional training and you are grateful for these learning opportunities with clients. You might add that these lengthy clinical rotations (i.e., fieldwork) are required for you to graduate, become certified and licensed in this field, and that you consider every client interaction to be a valuable educational experience.

Worksheet 1-4: Are You Really Sure You Can Do This?

For these kinds of situations, it is imperative that the client feels safe and that you demonstrate understanding of the client's concerns, such as fear of falling or getting hurt. Your demeanor and communication should convey confidence and professionalism, but you have an ethical obligation to only attempt tasks that you are competent to perform (AOTA, 2015, 2020a). You might convey your professional education, practice, and experience. Reassure the client that you would not knowingly do anything that would be unsafe. Explain the procedure and address the client's specific concerns such as, "*I will support your knee with my leg so it can't buckle*" or "*I have experience transferring a lot of people much bigger than you and will not let you fall. This transfer belt will help ensure your safety.*" If the client still appears concerned, you might ask another colleague or your supervisor to stand by or assist with the task. Sometimes a humorous approach can be an effective method with select clients such as, "*I am a lot stronger than I look—this lab coat is hiding my huge muscles!*"

Worksheet 1-5: This Feels Like Kindergarten

If a client seems offended performing an intervention task that is otherwise not normally age appropriate, you might say something like, "*It sounds like you might be feeling a bit insulted doing this. I'm sorry—that is not my intent.*" Acknowledge that, although the activity might appear "juvenile" on the surface, there is indeed a specific therapeutic purpose. When implementing interventions to support occupations, you should make it a point to relate the task to the specific client factors and performance skills you are remediating and also explain how this relates to occupational performance. In this scenario, the task was chosen to help reduce hypersensitivity and improve manipulation skills of the affected hand to enable occupations such as writing, using a computer keyboard, and performing desired hobbies. **Better yet, incorporate activities and occupations into the client's intervention program whenever possible.** Rather than presenting this client with the aforementioned task that offended him, this client may have benefited more from a "real-life" task such as handling soil for a gardening activity, using a sanding block to sand wood, or utilizing a built-up pen for writing.

Worksheet 1-6: I Want to Walk

1. Sometimes clients have great difficulty accepting the reality of a situation. They may be scared, confused, angry, or in denial. You might acknowledge and validate the client's feelings, but without giving false hope. Cole (2018) provides useful tips for therapeutic communication such as attending, effective listening, asking open questions, using primary and advanced accurate empathy, immediacy, showing encouragement, and respect. The following useful formula is suggested for occupational therapy practitioners to show empathy and understand feelings:

   "You feel _____ because _____ " (Cole, 2018, p. 74).

   You might say, "*You feel angry and overwhelmed because this is a huge life-changing event and you don't know how you will be able to cope. Is that correct?*" However, it is a balancing act to gently acknowledge the truth while not causing hopelessness and despair. During the exchange you might add, "*You had a very serious injury. We need to first focus on some of your other goals during the next few weeks like being able to feed yourself and operate a wheelchair. Of course, we will continue to look at your progress along the way and work towards making you as independent as possible*" or "*I realize this situation is very challenging for you and you feel discouraged. I am so sorry that your injury is not likely to make walking a feasible goal. However, we are all here to help you become as independent as possible and will teach you other ways to get around by yourself. I can tell that you are quite determined and will be able to manage many things on your own.*" Of course, you can encourage the client to continue to express feelings and promote the benefits of support groups and counseling as appropriate.

2. It is important to reinforce how the client can benefit from occupational therapy. The intervention plan should include client-centered goals that the OTA can review with the client. The client's frustration can also be acknowledged, *"You feel frustrated because you have to go through all this effort when you just want to be up and about."* You might then go on to say, *"Tomorrow we will be working on arm exercises so you can have enough strength and endurance to manage using your walker at home"* or *"The doctor said you are not allowed to bend for several months because of your surgery. This equipment will allow you to be independent again at home, like you were before your surgery. I am sure your wife would appreciate that."*

Worksheet 1-7: Open-Ended and Closed-Ended Questions

For each of the following sentences, indicate if it is an open-ended question (O), closed-ended question (C), or neither (N).

1. C. Do you wear dentures?

2. O. What caused you to fall?

3. O. How would you describe your child's personality?

4. C. Did you take your insulin this morning?

5. N. I notice that you seem tired today.

6. O. Tell me about your use of pain killers from the beginning.

7. N. It looks like you ate all your breakfast this morning.

8. C. Do you feel you drink too much on weekends?

9. O. Describe a situation at home that might cause you to become angry and "lose it".

10. O. What do you notice about your child that is concerning to you?

11. C. Do you think you get enough exercise?

12. N. I see that you got a haircut.

13. O. Describe some things you do for leisure.

14. C. Are you having difficulty dressing yourself after your stroke?

15. C. Did you check your blood sugar level this morning?

16. O. What are the responsibilities you have at work?

17. O. I would like to learn more about how you are managing at home after hip surgery.

18. O. Tell me about your exercise routine.

19. N. It seems like you handled that situation well.

20. O. Please describe what a typical day of yours is like.

21. C. Do you use any mobility devices?

22. C. How many children do you have?

23. C. What year were you born?

24. N. I see that you are using a walker.

25. C. Would you be willing to tell me about your living situation?

Worksheet 1-8: Asking Open-Ended Questions

Here are some suggestions, although you may come up with other questions.

1. My shoulder hurts.
   - *Describe your shoulder pain—or—What does your shoulder pain feel like?*
   - *What makes your shoulder pain better or worse?*
   - *How does the pain affect your daily activities?*
   - *When does the pain occur?*
2. I can't do anything right.
   - *What do you mean by that?*
   - *Tell me from the beginning when you started feeling this way.*
   - *Describe a situation that causes you to feel that way.*
   - *What would you like to change?*
3. I fell in my apartment.
   - *What caused you to fall in your apartment?*
   - *What happened after you fell?*
   - *Tell me about your history of falling.*
   - *What might you have done differently to prevent falling?*
4. My life is a charade.
   - *What do you mean by that statement?*
   - *How is your life a charade?*
   - *Tell me about your plans for the future.*
   - *What are some things you wish you had done differently?*
5. I never thought I would turn out like this.
   - *How do you see yourself?*
   - *Tell me your thoughts about how other people see you.*
   - *How do you feel about… (i.e., your arrest, use of cocaine, homelessness)?*
   - *How do you think you could turn things around?*
   - *What are your goals?*
   - *What would you like to change?*
6. My hand is useless.
   - *What specific problems are you having with your hand?*
   - *When did you start having difficulty with your hand?*
   - *How does your hand condition affect your daily activities?*
   - *What types of things are hard to do with your hand?*

7. I'm so confused.
    - *What things are confusing you?*
    - *What else are you feeling?*
    - *What would help you to understand?*
    - *How can you get more information?*
8. I lost my job.
    - *What are your plans?*
    - *How does that affect you and your family?*
    - *What happened that caused you to lose your job?*
    - *What might have happened differently to avoid getting fired?*
9. I hate school.
    - *What do you hate about school?*
    - *What would you like to change about school?*
    - *Describe what makes you feel that way about school.*
    - *How long have you felt this way?*
10. I am no good in gym class.
    - *What specific things in gym class are hard for you?*
    - *Tell me how that makes you feel.*
    - *What would you like to be better at?*
    - *What are some things you feel you are good at in school?*

Worksheet 1-9: Eliciting Information Efficiently

Clearly, in this scenario, the OTA is not using appropriate open-ended questions to elicit the desired information in a timely manner. Cole (2018, p. 74) suggests that to prevent a simple "yes" or "no" response, the OT should avoid the following as question starters: "*Do you, Can you, Would you, Are you, and Have you.*" Here are some additional suggestions for improving this client interaction:

1. It is more respectful to call the client Mrs. Jones rather than Jean.
2. The OTA should explain the purpose of the session.
3. The OTA should demonstrate empathy and address the client's concerns when she reports feeling "terrible" or expresses frustration regarding spilling her food.
4. The OTA should acknowledge the client is experiencing specific emotions but, instead, he insinuates that Mrs. Jones should not feel that way.
5. The OTA should use open- rather than closed-ended questions.
6. The OTA needs to phrase questions more clearly to target the desired information in a more clear and concise manner.

Here is the same exchange in a more useful format:

OTA: Hello Mrs. Jones, I am Nick, an occupational therapy assistant. It is very nice to meet you. Your occupational therapist, Karen, asked me to work with you today to discuss your living situation so we can start planning how you will manage at home. How are you today?
Client: Terrible.
OTA: What is making you feel terrible?

Client: Don't you know how weak I am? I can't do anything!

OTA: You are feeling very frustrated because your illness is making everything more difficult for you. Is that correct? [Client nods her head yes.] However, I can tell by the way you were just feeding yourself that you are a very determined person. I am sure you will make a lot of progress here.

Client: Do you really think so?

OTA: Absolutely. Now please tell me about your living situation—what type of place do you live in and who might be around to help?

Client: I live with my husband in a condo. My daughter lives a few miles away and I have a good friend who lives next door to me.

OTA: That's great. I would like to know more about the physical layout of your condo, such as the number of steps and how the bathroom is situated.

Client: I have three steps outside and about 10 steps to the second floor. There is a powder room on the first level and a full bathroom on the second level, next to my bedroom.

The OTA would continue interviewing the client in this manner until all the desired information is obtained.

Worksheet 1-10: Interaction OTA—Elementary School Student

1. Schools strive to create a welcoming and safe environment for all students. Policies are created to prevent harassment, intimidation, and bullying (HIB) of students and schools will typically provide various resources to students, parents, and staff, some of which are readily available on school district public websites (New Jersey Department of Education, 2019; Ohio Department of Education, 2019). The OTA in this scenario is intimidating the student with language that is completely unacceptable. Scaring the student by threatening, "*I will tie you to the chair*" and "*I will not let you see you parents*" can cause emotional harm to the student. The OTA's behavior is clearly unprofessional, unethical, and may result in disciplinary action or possibly getting fired.

2. The OTA is not maintaining professional composure as she is yelling at the student.

3. Do not ask a client if they "want" to do a task if the answer "no" would not be a desired response.

4. It may be better to offer a specific choice to the student such as "*What color pencil do you want to use today—the red or green one?*" or "*Choose one of these two worksheets to work on today.*"

5. It might be better for the OTA to present the activity more positively, such as "*Let's show your parents how much better you are doing with your handwriting*" or "*We are going to do this worksheet in pretty rainbow colors. You can use a different colored pencil for each line.*"

6. By using appropriate verbal and nonverbal communication, the OTA must "set the tone" that they are an authority figure that deserves respect. However, it is not productive or professional to lose one's temper, yell, or get into an argument with a student.

7. Do not call a student "bad." It is the child's specific behavior and language that are unacceptable. The OTA might say, "*You are talking back to me and not following directions. That is not acceptable.*"

8. Use therapeutic communication techniques such as therapeutic use of self, behavior modification, or even making the activity into a "game." Here are some examples:

   "*If you form all the letters correctly today, I will give you a special prize today.*"

   or

   "*If you can finish this worksheet before the timer goes off, I will give you an extra sticker.*"

   or

   "*After you finish this worksheet, I will put it on my bulletin board because I am proud of how hard you have been working on your handwriting this month.*"

   or

   "*You feel writing is boring because it is not easy for you and you don't like to practice—is that right? I understand. Let's just work on this for only 10 minutes and then we will do something fun.*"

Worksheet 1-11: Better Communication

For each of the following scenarios, choose which of the two statements would likely be the better response from an occupational therapy practitioner.

1. You go to a client's hospital room with the intent to transport the client to the occupational therapy room for therapy.

   _____ Would you like to come to therapy now?

   ___*___ It is time for occupational therapy now.

   Do not ask a question for which the answer "no" would be unacceptable. However, clients do have the right to refuse therapy.

2. You are beginning an intervention session with a client who had hip replacement surgery.

   _____ Do you have hip pain today?

   ___*___ How are you today?

   An open-ended question would elicit more information rather than just a simple "yes" or "no" response.

3. During an occupational therapy session, a client diagnosed with a cerebrovascular accident is having difficulty transferring to a commode and begins to cry.

   ___*___ What is making you cry?

   _____ Why are you so upset?

   The word "why" may sound judgmental and give the impression the therapist is insinuating the client should not be feeling the way they are feeling (Cole, 2018).

4. A child who is overweight is holding back tears and mentions the other students call him "fatty."

   _____ Just try to ignore them.

   ___*___ You feel sad because the other children are calling you names.

   An empathic response acknowledges the child's feelings. The OT must also adhere to facility policies and procedures regarding reporting of the bullying.

5. A 22-year-old female client with conservative religious beliefs mentions she is engaged and is looking forward to kissing her fiancé for the first time on her wedding day.

_____*_____ It is nice you have something special to look forward to.

_____ How do you know you and your fiancé will be compatible?

It is important to respect this client's moral and religious beliefs and not inject personal bias.

6. An older client was admitted due to injuries sustained in a fall at home.

_____*_____ Tell me what happened to cause you to fall.

_____ Did you fall because you were not using your walker?

In this scenario, an open-ended question would sound less judgmental and elicit more information rather than just a yes or no response.

7. An outpatient client with three young children mentions that her family does not celebrate Halloween because of their religious beliefs.

_____ Do your kids feel like they are missing out?

_____*_____ I understand that many people prefer not to celebrate certain holidays.

It is important to respect this client's moral and/or religious beliefs and not express personal bias.

8. An outpatient client states that she experienced pain while performing the new exercise program at home that the OTA told her to do.

_____ Don't worry—no pain, no gain.

_____*_____ Show me how you are doing your exercises.

It is important to ascertain if the client is performing the exercises accurately and safely. The OT also needs to determine whether the pain is typical and expected or is a concern that needs to be addressed.

9. An OT working with a 3-year-old child in a preschool program would like the child to work on fine-motor activities to improve play skills.

_____ If you are a good girl today you can pick a prize from the prize box.

_____*_____ If you complete these activities, I will give you a prize.

Do not label a child as good or bad. Focus on the behavior instead.

10. A client who sustained third-degree burns and has severe facial scars was admitted to a behavioral health program due to depression over his appearance. He is being evaluated by the OT.

_____ I am sorry your scars make you feel depressed.

___*___ How have your injuries impacted you?

An open-ended question will help elicit the client's feelings rather than reinforcing the negativity of the scars.

Reproduced with permission from Morreale, M. J., & Amini, D. (2016). *The occupational therapist's workbook for ensuring clinical competence.* SLACK Incorporated.

References

American Occupational Therapy Association. (2015). Standards of practice for occupational therapy. *American Journal of Occupational Therapy, 69*(Suppl. 3), 6913410057. http://dx.doi.org/10.5014/ajot.2015.696S06

American Occupational Therapy Association. (2017). Philosophical base of occupational therapy. *American Journal of Occupational Therapy, 71*(Suppl. 2), 7112410045. https: //doi.org./10.5014/ajot.2017.716S06

American Occupational Therapy Association. (2020a). AOTA 2020 occupational therapy code of ethics. *American Journal of Occupational Therapy, 74*(Suppl. 3), 7413410005. https://doi.org/10.5014/ajot.2020.74S3006

American Occupational Therapy Association. (2020b). Guidelines for supervision, roles, and responsibilities during the delivery of occupational therapy services. *American Journal of Occupational Therapy, 74*(Suppl. 3), 7413410020. https://doi.org/10.5014/ajot.2020.74S3004

American Occupational Therapy Association. (2020c). Occupational therapy practice framework: Domain and process (4th ed.). *American Journal of Occupational Therapy, 74*(Suppl. 2), 7412410010. https://doi.org/10.5014/ajot.2020.74S2001

Centers for Medicare & Medicaid Services. (2014). *Medicare benefit policy manual.* (Pub. 100-02: Ch. 15, Section 230.2). https://www.cms.gov/Regulations-and-Guidance/Guidance/Manuals/Downloads/bp102c15.pdf

Centers for Medicare & Medicaid Services. (2019). *Medicare benefit policy manual.* (Pub. 100-02: Ch. 15, Section 220). https://www.cms.gov/Regulations-and-Guidance/Guidance/Manuals/Downloads/bp102c15.pdf

Cole, M. (2018). *Group dynamics in occupational therapy: The theoretical basis and practice application of group intervention* (5th ed.). SLACK Incorporated.

Drench, M., Noonan, A. C., Sharby, N., & Ventura, S. H. (2012). *Psychosocial aspects of health care.* (3rd ed.). Pearson Education.

Froehlich, J. (2017a). Effective communication. In K. Jacobs & N. MacRae (Eds.), *Occupational therapy essentials for clinical competence.* (3rd ed., pp. 99-132). SLACK Incorporated.

Froehlich, J. (2017b). Therapeutic use of self. In K. Jacobs & N. MacRae (Eds.), *Occupational therapy essentials for clinical competence.* (3rd ed., pp. 133-147). SLACK Incorporated.

Morreale, M. J., & Amini, D. (2016). *The occupational therapist's workbook for ensuring clinical competence.* SLACK Incorporated.

Ohio Department of Education. (2019). *Anti-harassment, intimidation and bullying resources.* Retrieved June 22, 2021, from http://education.ohio.gov/Topics/Student-Supports/Anti-Harassment-Intimidation-and-Bullying-Resource

State of New Jersey Department of Education. (2019). *Harassment, intimidation, & bullying (HIB).* NJ Department of Education. Retrieved June 22, 2021, from https://www.state.nj.us/education/students/safety/behavior/hib/

Taylor, R. R. (2008). *The intentional relationship: Occupational therapy and use of self.* F. A. Davis Company.

Taylor, R. R. (2020). *The intentional relationship: Occupational therapy and use of self* (2nd ed.). F. A. Davis Company.

Demonstrating Professionalism

Professional behaviors for occupational therapy practitioners include traits such as dependability, punctuality, conscientiousness, a well-groomed appearance, and appropriate demeanor. Occupational therapists (OTs) and occupational therapy assistants (OTAs) must meet professional standards for attire, workplace conduct, oral and written communication, and safety. In addition, it is essential that OTs and OTAs demonstrate ethical conduct, professional boundaries, respect, integrity, good time management, and organizational skills. This chapter presents worksheets and learning activities to help you understand and practice professional behaviors and skills essential for fieldwork and clinical practice. Suggested answers to worksheets are provided at the end of the chapter.

Contents

Morreale, M. J. Developing Clinical Competence:
A Workbook for the OTA, Second Edition (pp. 45-107).
© 2022 SLACK Incorporated.

Worksheet 2-1

Scheduling Fieldwork

Always follow your academic fieldwork coordinator's specific instructions regarding the scheduling of fieldwork, such as if you should contact your fieldwork educator by phone or email.

For this exercise, consider the following information when answering questions 1 and 2.

Imagine you have just been assigned Level I fieldwork for the spring semester. Your academic fieldwork coordinator provided the facility name and address, fieldwork educator name, and contact information (i.e., phone number and email address). You must contact the site directly to schedule your fieldwork. The fieldwork consists of 3 full days, which do not have to be consecutive but must be completed by May 15th. It is now February 1st.

1. You would really like to complete your fieldwork during Spring Break (the third week of April this year) when you do not have classes. When should you first attempt to contact the fieldwork site to set up your fieldwork dates?
   A. One week before you plan on completing the fieldwork
   B. One month before you plan on completing the fieldwork
   C. Beginning of February
   D. Beginning of March
   E. Beginning of April

2. You called your fieldwork site as directed, but your fieldwork educator was not available at that time. You left a message with the department secretary asking the fieldwork educator to call you back. It is now 2 days later and you have still not heard back. Which of the following is your best course of action?
   A. Contact your academic fieldwork coordinator
   B. Wait another day or two for the fieldwork educator to call back
   C. Wait another week for the fieldwork educator to call back
   D. Call again and leave another message if your fieldwork educator is again unavailable
   E. Call again and ask to speak with the rehabilitation director if your fieldwork educator is still unavailable

3. Your fieldwork educator told you that Hannah Happie, OTR will be your Level II fieldwork educator at a local facility. You are very pleased because you heard from other students that Hannah always provides an excellent learning experience and never fails anyone. However, when you contact Hannah to schedule fieldwork, she tells you there must be a mistake because you are assigned to someone else at that site. Which of the following is your best course of action?
   A. Tell Hannah that you are very disappointed and would like to cancel fieldwork there because you only wanted her as your fieldwork educator
   B. Thank Hannah and inform your academic fieldwork coordinator that you would like a new fieldwork site because Hannah does not want to supervise you
   C. Thank Hannah and notify your academic fieldwork coordinator of the change
   D. Express politely that the change is not acceptable because you need to complete the fieldwork exactly as it was assigned to you
   E. Ask to speak with the rehabilitation director there

Worksheet 2-1 (continued)

Scheduling Fieldwork

4. You contacted your fieldwork educator several weeks ago to schedule your Level I fieldwork. The fieldwork is supposed to begin tomorrow, but you just became ill with a bad stomach virus that is causing severe nausea and diarrhea. Which of the following is your best course of action?
   A. Contact the site immediately to inform your fieldwork educator that you are ill and must reschedule
   B. Take some medicine, get a good night's sleep, and attend fieldwork even if you still are having symptoms
   C. Contact your academic fieldwork coordinator and ask that person to notify the site about your pending absence tomorrow
   D. Ask a family member or friend to call the site and notify your fieldwork educator about your pending absence tomorrow
   E. Bring a doctor's note to fieldwork tomorrow to prove your illness and ask your fieldwork educator if you have to stay or not

5. A week before you are to begin Level II fieldwork, your fieldwork educator calls to inform you that, due to several staff members on sick leave, your fieldwork must be rescheduled to 1 month later than you were originally scheduled to begin. This will conflict with your next Level II fieldwork. Which of the following is your best course of action?
   A. Thank the person for calling but state that you must now cancel fieldwork at that site
   B. Thank the person for calling but state you will need to discuss this with your academic fieldwork coordinator
   C. Let the fieldwork educator know this will inconvenience you greatly and indicate it is unfair this happened so close to your scheduled starting date
   D. Insist strongly that you must complete the fieldwork during the exact dates that were assigned to you
   E. Ask to speak with the rehabilitation director

6. You contact your Level I fieldwork educator, Carrie Capable, by email. Carrie sends the following reply, *"Dear Student, I am sorry, but the rehabilitation director has already assigned another fieldwork student to me at this time. However, I have forwarded your message to Ellen Ethical, OTR, as she will be your supervisor instead. She will contact you by email today or tomorrow."* Which of the following is your best course of action?
   A. Send an email to the rehabilitation director asking if your fieldwork start date can be delayed so that Carrie Capable can remain your fieldwork educator
   B. Reply by email to thank Carrie Capable for the information but state that you would prefer to cancel the fieldwork if she cannot be your fieldwork educator
   C. Reply by email to thank Carrie Capable and then wait several days for the new fieldwork educator to contact you
   D. Call the fieldwork site and ask to speak with Ellen Ethical today as you do not have her email address
   E. Reply by email and ask Carrie Capable if it is possible for her to switch students

7. As directed, you send an email to your fieldwork educator to set up your Level I fieldwork. It is now 1 week later and you have not gotten any reply. Which of the following is your best course of action?
   A. Resend the original email to your fieldwork educator now
   B. Wait several more days for the fieldwork educator to reply
   C. Send another email to the fieldwork educator asking why that person has not replied and if there is a problem with the fieldwork
   D. Send an email to the rehabilitation director and copy the fieldwork educator and your academic fieldwork coordinator on the email
   E. Send an email to your academic fieldwork coordinator asking for assistance

© 2022 SLACK Incorporated.
Morreale, M. J. (2022). *Developing clinical competence: A workbook for the OTA* (2nd ed.). SLACK Incorporated.

Worksheet 2-1 (continued)
Scheduling Fieldwork

8. You contacted your fieldwork educator several weeks ago to schedule your Level I fieldwork. The fieldwork is supposed to begin tomorrow but the weather forecast calls for severe weather conditions (i.e., a tornado, hurricane or snow). You are very nervous about driving in these weather conditions. Which of the following is your best course of action?

    A. Contact the site immediately to inform your fieldwork educator that you are unable to attend fieldwork tomorrow

    B. Get a good night's sleep, and check the weather forecast in the morning to decide if you will attend fieldwork or not

    C. Request that your academic fieldwork coordinator notify the site about your pending absence tomorrow

    D. Follow your college's policy regarding fieldwork absences

    E. Have your parent, guardian, or spouse call to inform the fieldwork educator that you are not allowed to drive in bad weather

9. You are supposed to begin your Level I fieldwork today at 8:30 a.m. However, you are stuck in traffic and will probably not be arriving until about 9:15 a.m. Which of the following is your best course of action?

    A. Once you arrive late, apologize profusely and promise it will not happen again

    B. Only when it is safe to do so, attempt to call, text, or email your fieldwork educator to notify the person of your impending lateness

    C. Turn around to return home and reschedule fieldwork for another day

    D. When you arrive at fieldwork, act as if nothing happened and hope that no one notices that you were late

    E. Once you arrive late, tell the fieldwork educator it really was not your fault that you were late and complain about all the traffic you encountered

10. Your Level I fieldwork is scheduled to begin tomorrow. However, your fieldwork educator contacts you today to inform you she needs to take the day off and must reschedule fieldwork to the following week. This change will cause you to be late handing in your fieldwork paper and timesheet to the academic fieldwork coordinator. Which of the following is your best course of action?

    A. Tell the fieldwork educator that this is not fair as you scheduled the fieldwork way ahead of time and you will now get a bad grade in class

    B. Firmly insist that you be assigned to another person tomorrow so you can complete the fieldwork on time

    C. Once the conversation is completed, hang up and then call your fieldwork educator's supervisor

    D. Reschedule fieldwork and contact your academic fieldwork coordinator to explain the situation

    E. Start crying and hope the fieldwork educator will do something to help you

Worksheet 2-2

Fieldwork Phone Interview

You must call your fieldwork educator as directed to set up your Level I fieldwork schedule. You have never been to this facility before and are not very familiar with the area. For each of the items below, indicate with a Y (yes) or N (no) if it is an appropriate topic for you to ask during the initial phone contact.

1. _____ Directions to the fieldwork site

2. _____ Start and end times for the day

3. _____ Where to meet in the facility

4. _____ If the facility is in a "bad" area

5. _____ Date(s) to complete fieldwork

6. _____ Amount of time for lunch

7. _____ Permission to come in late because you have to drive your kids to school

8. _____ If a lab coat is required

9. _____ Wearing of sneakers

10. _____ Availability of coffee or tea in the morning

11. _____ Permission to use your cell phone so you can monitor your children

12. _____ Permission to come in late or leave early to accommodate your bus or train schedule

13. _____ Permission to leave early to pick up your children from school

14. _____ Permission to leave early due to a dental appointment to get your teeth cleaned

15. _____ Permission to wear a head covering if required by your religion

16. _____ What paperwork to bring

Worksheet 2-2 (continued)

Fieldwork Phone Interview

17. _____ If it will be a very hard fieldwork, because a classmate failed fieldwork there last semester

18. _____ Reimbursement for gas and tolls

19. _____ If the fieldwork will require a lot of homework

20. _____ Types of diagnoses you will observe

Worksheet 2-3

Directions to Fieldwork Site

List at least five ways to obtain directions to your fieldwork site without asking your fieldwork educator.

1.

2.

3.

4.

5.

Worksheet 2-4

Fieldwork Attire

Imagine you have been assigned fieldwork at an inpatient medical setting. You contacted your fieldwork educator, and this person indicated that your client interventions will primarily consist of self-care occupations, transfers, and therapeutic exercises. Your fieldwork educator also informed you that the dress code is "business casual with a lab coat." For each of the following items listed, indicate with a Y (yes) or N (no) whether it is an appropriate choice for a fieldwork student to wear at this site. Explain why you chose each of your answers in the blank space following the item.

1. _____ Scrubs

2. _____ Sneakers

3. _____ Flat, closed-toe shoes with a rubber sole

4. _____ Dressy flip-flops

5. _____ Low-heeled leather sandals

6. _____ Heavy perfume/cologne/after shave

7. _____ Stud earrings

8. _____ Eyebrow piercing

9. _____ Head covering

10. _____ Visible underwear above pants' waistband

11. _____ Neatly pressed dark jeans

12. _____ Khaki pants and a polo shirt

13. _____ Plain black sweatpants/yoga pants

14. _____ Sport t-shirt/jersey

15. _____ Button-down oxford shirt

Worksheet 2-4 (continued)
Fieldwork Attire

16. _____ Dress slacks

17. _____ Cargo pants

18. _____ Polo shirt with collar and small designer logo emblem

19. _____ 32-in. plain gold necklace

20. _____ Charm bracelet

21. _____ Well-groomed, long artificial nails without polish

22. _____ Dark gray suit

23. _____ Name tag

24. _____ Solid color leggings

25. _____ Solid color hoodie

Morreale, M. J. (2022). *Developing clinical competence: A workbook for the OTA* (2nd ed.). SLACK Incorporated.

Worksheet 2-5

Planning for Fieldwork

Your fieldwork is scheduled to begin next week. List at least 10 things you can do to help ensure that you will get to fieldwork on time on your first day.

1.

2.

3.

4.

5.

6.

7.

8.

9.

10.

Worksheet 2-5 (continued)

Planning for Fieldwork

Think of five complete outfits (including footwear) from your existing wardrobe that you feel are appropriate for you to wear to fieldwork. List the specific items below, describing the style and color or pattern of each item you chose (i.e., solid black turtleneck, light blue striped button-down shirt, knee-length navy skirt). You can mix and match items for the 5-day workweek.

1.

2.

3.

4.

5.

Determine if there are any clothing items you will need to purchase (or borrow from friends/family) prior to fieldwork, such as a lab coat, extra slacks, or suitable footwear. List those items here, if applicable, and develop an action plan for obtaining them.

Learning Activity 2-1: Professional Presentation and Traits

Complete the form on the following page. For each item presented in the left-hand column, identify which of the health professionals listed typically wear those items to work and/or have the character traits listed. Multiple health professionals may be selected for each item if applicable. After completing the worksheet, compare answers in small groups. Circle the answers for which group members had differing of opinions before coming to a consensus for that item. Discuss the following:

- What similarities were evident among the professions listed?

- What differences were evident among the professions listed?

- Discuss items for which group members had differing of opinions and identify the possible reasons why (e.g., age, culture, past experiences, stereotypes)?

- Would responses generally be the same or different depending on the practice setting (e.g., inpatient behavioral health, hand therapy clinic, acute care) or type of teacher (e.g., special education, physical education, math teacher)?

- Why is a professional image important?

- Is a personal image different than a professional image? Why or why not?

Professional Presentation and Traits	Doctor	Nurse	Nurse's Aide	OT	OTA	PT	PTA	Speech Therapist	Teacher	Dentist	Social Worker	Psychologist
Clothing Items												
Lab coat												
Scrubs												
Suit or dress												
Khaki pants and polo shirt												
White footwear												
Dress shoes or high-heeled shoes												
Sandals												
Jeans												
Name tag												
Sneakers												
Button-down shirt and tie												
Sweatpants/yoga pants												
Character Traits												
Intelligent												
Easy-going												
Likes children												
Serious												
Detail-oriented												
Fun												
Empathetic												
Advocate												
Sophisticated												
Good listener												
Likes playing sports												
Enjoys research												
Good conversationalist												
Team player												
Organized												
Likes to exercise and eat healthy												

Worksheet 2-6

Professional Conduct

For each of the following professional behaviors, list the professional characteristics or traits it represents (i.e., reliability, veracity, professional boundaries, beneficence).

Professional Behavior	Professional Characteristic
1. Administering a standardized assessment accurately	*Example: Service competency* *Attention to detail*
2. Offering to put your fieldwork educator's clinical notes back into the clients' charts without being asked	
3. Admitting you did not complete your notes on time, apologizing, and offering to stay late or come in early to complete them	
4. Arranging self-feeding interventions pre-dawn or after dusk for an occupational therapy client who is fasting during Ramadan	
5. Switching a client's treatment time so as not to conflict with physical therapy	
6. Addressing an adult client by using "Mr." or "Mrs." and client's surname	
7. Not refusing to work with a client who is positive for HIV or tuberculosis	
8. Writing a thank-you note to your fieldwork educator after your Interview	
9. Arriving to your fieldwork interview 5 minutes early	
10. Asking a senator to vote for a proposed law that improves access to mental health services	
11. Cleaning up water that you notice on floor near the hydrocollator	
12. Preparing and assembling all the information packets in time for a workshop that the occupational therapy department is sponsoring	
13. Noticing that the paraffin unit temperature is too high	
14. Closing the computer screen after entering client information	
15. Not billing Medicare for time the OTA spent documenting or transporting the client	
16. Nodding and maintaining eye contact when a client is answering questions	
17. Participating in an event to raise awareness of a specific disease	
18. Being the "go to" person for solving problems regarding manual wheelchairs	
19. Not dating a cute client your age who asks you out on a date	

Worksheet 2-6 (continued)

Professional Conduct

Professional Behavior	Professional Characteristic
20. Ensuring that all the OTA's notes are co-signed when required by law or facility policy	
21. Knocking on a closed door before entering the client's room or an examination room	
22. Discussing a client's discharge plan with the physical therapist (PT) and social worker	
23. Acknowledging that the client feels disappointed when the client's son did not come for a visit	
24. Not complaining when you must stay late today to order a client's durable medical equipment before the client is discharged home	
25. Writing several drafts of a SOAP note to ensure an accurate, professional presentation before showing it to your fieldwork educator	
26. Reporting suspected child or elder abuse to appropriate personnel/agencies to prevent further harm to the individual	
27. Arranging for an interpreter when the client speaks a different language than you	
28. Checking the chart and asking the client about possible food allergies before planning a cooking intervention	
29. Shredding extra copies of client information rather than throwing them in the trash	
30. Neatly folding or hanging up a client's clothing during a self-care intervention	

Worksheet 2-7

Ethics Sanctions

Occupational therapy practitioners who demonstrate unethical behavior may face disciplinary action at work (including possible termination) and could incur legal consequences depending on the nature and severity of the behavior. In addition, unethical behavior may result in sanctions issued by state licensure boards, National Board for Certification in Occupational Therapy (NBCOT, 2020a, 2020b), and/or American Occupational Therapy Association (AOTA, 2019, 2020). Define the following disciplinary action terms and put them in order from less severe to more severe.

1. Probation

2. Reprimand

3. Revocation

4. Suspension

5. Censure

1. _____

2. _____

3. _____

4. _____

5. _____

Ethical Decision-Making

Kornblau and Burkhardt (2012) developed a multi-step process of ethical decision-making entitled, "The Clinical Ethics and Legal Issues Bait All Therapists Equally (CELIBATE) Method for Analyzing Ethical Dilemmas," which is summarized in Figure 2-1. This method assists OTs and OTAs in identifying ethical problems and related facts, considering the legal and ethical aspects of the situation (plus other pertinent factors), and developing an appropriate action plan (Kornblau & Burkhardt, 2012). Situations can be influenced by personal values and beliefs, but occupational therapy practitioners must always adhere to professional standards and abide by state and federal regulations applicable to occupational therapy, such as licensure laws and practice acts. Practitioners should be cognizant of any mandatory reporting requirements that may be in place concerning child/elder/spousal abuse and human trafficking, in addition to understanding legal and ethical ramifications regarding malpractice, discrimination, privacy, insurance fraud, sexual harassment, theft, copyright violation, and so forth (Kornblau & Burkhardt, 2012).

---

1. What is the problem?
2. What are the facts of the situation?
3. Who are the interested parties?
   - Facility
   - Patient
   - Other therapists
   - Observers
   - Payers
   - Others
4. What is the nature of their interest? Why is this a problem?
   - Professional
   - Personal
   - Business
   - Economic
   - Intellectual
   - Societal
5. Is there an ethical issue?
   - Does it violate a professional code of ethics? Which section(s)?
   - Does it violate moral, social, or religious values?
6. Is there a legal issue?
   - Practice act/licensure law and regulations? Which section(s)?
   - Check the CELIBATE checklist for other possible legal issues.
7. Do I need more information?
   - What information do I need?
   - Is there a treatment, policy, procedure, law, regulation, or document that I do not know about?
   - Can I obtain a copy of the treatment, policy, procedure, law, regulation, or document in writing?
   - Do I need to research the issue further? What does the literature say?
   - Do I need to consult with a mentor, an expert in this area, and/or a lawyer?
8. Brainstorm possible action steps.

Figure 2-1. CELIBATE Method for Analyzing Ethical Dilemmas. (*continued*)

9. Analyze action steps.
    - Eliminate the obviously wrong or impossible choices.
    - How will each alternative affect my patients, other interested parties, and me?
    - Do my choices abide by the applicable code of ethics?
    - Do my choices abide by the applicable practice act and regulations?
    - Are my choices consistent with my moral, religious, and social beliefs?

10. Choose a course of action (considering ethical principles and philosophies).
    - The Rotary Four-Way Test:
      1. Is it the truth?
      2. Is is fair to all concerned?
      3. Will it build goodwill and better friendships?
      4. Will it be beneficial to all concerned?
    - Is it win-win?
    - How do I feel about my course of action?

Figure 2-1 (continued). CELIBATE Method for Analyzing Ethical Dilemmas. (Reproduced with permission from Kornblau, B. L., & Burkhardt, A. (2012) *Ethics in rehabilitation: A clinical perspective* [2nd ed.]. SLACK Incorporated.)

Worksheet 2-8

Ethical Behavior

Determine if the following statements are true (T) or false (F).

1. T ____ F ____ If an OTA is found guilty of committing a severe unethical act, AOTA can take away the OTA's license to practice.

2. T ____ F ____ An occupational therapy volunteer can report an OTA's unethical behavior to NBCOT.

3. T ____ F ____ An OTA student should begin following the Code of Ethics when Level II fieldwork commences.

4. T ____ F ____ An OTA who commits an unethical act could have their name listed publicly as an ethics violator by AOTA or NBCOT.

5. T ____ F ____ AOTA guidelines take precedence over state laws.

6. T ____ F ____ Committing a felony may limit a person's ability to practice occupational therapy.

7. T ____ F ____ If an occupational therapy practitioner did not know about a particular law, the OT or OTA cannot be sanctioned for an unethical act that violates that law.

8. T ____ F ____ An OTA state license is only affected by occupational therapy ethical infractions and not other legal violations of which an OTA might be guilty.

9. T ____ F ____ An occupational therapy practitioner has an obligation to report a colleague's unethical behavior only if it is occupational therapy related.

10. T ____ F ____ NBCOT implements sanctions within 1 week when a very serious complaint is lodged against an OT or OTA.

11. T ____ F ____ A state can suspend an occupational therapy aide's license for unethical behavior in an occupational therapy clinic.

12. T ____ F ____ A person visiting a hospital patient can file a complaint with an occupational therapy state licensure board.

13. T ____ F ____ An OTA accused of practicing under the influence of drugs automatically loses NBCOT certification if reported to NBCOT.

14. T ____ F ____ An OTA receiving 6 months of probation from an occupational therapy state licensing board cannot practice for the entire 6 months.

15. T ____ F ____ An OTA sanctioned by NBCOT cannot appeal the decision.

16. T ____ F ____ Minimizing a client's progress when documenting is not considered unethical if it helps the person receive essential therapy services from the insurance company.

17. T ____ F ____ An occupational therapy practitioner cannot be disciplined by AOTA, NBCOT, and an occupational therapy state licensure board all at the same time.

Worksheet 2-8 (continued)

Ethical Behavior

18. T ____   F ____   It is acceptable for an OTA to refuse to treat a person with HIV if the OTA is concerned about catching the disease.

19. T ____   F ____   An OTA censured by an occupational therapy state licensure board cannot practice during the time of the censure.

20. T ____   F ____   When an occupational therapy licensure board's sanction is revocation, the occupational therapy practitioner can only practice with daily, direct supervision.

Learning Activity 2-2: Unprofessional Conduct

List several possible consequences for each of the following unprofessional behaviors of an OTA. Consider how the OTA's actions might create specific safety concerns or problems, affect relationships with a client or colleagues, or merit disciplinary action by not complying with facility policy/procedures or professional guidelines such as *NBCOT Professional Practice Standards for COTA and Candidates Seeking the COTA Designation* (2020a, 2020b) or the *AOTA 2020 Occupational Therapy Code of Ethics* (2019, 2020). Also specify the type of trait or conduct each behavior in the following chart represents (e.g., poor safety awareness, carelessness, dishonesty, tardiness, disrespect).

Unprofessional Behavior	Potential Safety Concerns or Problems	Possible Effect on Relationship With Clients or Colleagues	Possible Disciplinary Action That May Result
1. Habitually arriving to work late Trait:			
2. Not putting therapy equipment away when finished using Trait:			
3. Playing games on your work computer while waiting for your outpatients to arrive Trait:			
4. Forgetting to bring your professional name tag to work Trait:			
5. During Level I fieldwork at a hospital, giving a client your home phone number so the client can call to ask questions or just to talk Trait:			
6. Realizing that a pair of scissors is missing after an occupational therapy crafts group in a mental health setting Trait:			
7. Accidentally sending an email containing confidential client information to the wrong email address or leaving a printed copy on the copy machine Trait:			

Unprofessional Behavior	Potential Safety Concerns or Problems	Possible Effect on Relationship With Clients or Colleagues	Possible Disciplinary Action That May Result
8. Telling a client that they look "hot and sexy" in an outfit Trait:			
9. Talking to a colleague about a client while buying candy in the hospital gift shop Trait:			
10. Calling in sick in order to go to a concert with a friend Trait:			
11. Forgetting to fill out the purchase requisition for reachers, sock aids, and long-handled shoehorns Trait:			
12. Not washing hands after treating a client Trait:			
13. Signing a note written by another OTA because the other OTA forgot to sign it before going home Trait:			
14. Casually conversing with colleagues while a client is performing exercises or activities of daily living Trait:			
15. Not informing nursing staff that the client experienced an episode of incontinence in therapy and now has soiled clothing Trait:			
16. Throwing away draft SOAP notes in the garbage pail without shredding or removing identifying information Trait:			

Unprofessional Behavior	Potential Safety Concerns or Problems	Possible Effect on Relationship With Clients or Colleagues	Possible Disciplinary Action That May Result
17. Asking an occupational therapy aide to perform a skilled occupational therapy intervention with a client because you are too busy to manage all the clients today Trait:			
18. Losing occupational therapy paperwork that was previously entered in the client's chart Trait:			
19. Minimizing a client's progress in a treatment note so the insurance company will approve additional sessions Trait:			
20. Forgetting to set a timer when placing a hot or cold pack on a client Trait:			

Learning Activity 2-3: Unprofessional Conduct—More Examples

List several possible consequences for each of the following unprofessional behaviors of an OTA. Consider how the OTA's actions might create specific safety concerns or problems, affect relationships with a client or colleagues, or merit disciplinary action by not complying with facility policy and procedures or professional guidelines such as *NBCOT Professional Practice Standards for COTA and Candidates Seeking the COTA Designation* (2020a, 2020b) or the *AOTA 2020 Occupational Therapy Code of Ethics* (2019, 2020). Also specify the type of trait or conduct each behavior in the following chart represents (e.g., poor safety awareness, carelessness, dishonesty, tardiness, disrespect).

Unprofessional Behavior	Potential Safety Concerns or Problems	Possible Effect on Relationship With Clients or Colleagues	Possible Disciplinary Action That May Result
1. Badmouthing your facility, boss, or colleagues on a social media site Trait:			
2. Peeking at the medical records of a famous person admitted to your facility but who is not on your caseload Trait:			
3. Always recommending a specific durable medical equipment provider to patients because that company pays you a percentage of sales made from the people you referred to them Trait:			
4. Immediately providing a copy of clinical documentation when a client requests it during an intervention session Trait:			
5. Giving a glass of apple juice to an unfamiliar nursing home resident when that person asks you for a drink Trait:			
6. Bringing client paperwork home to complete it Trait:			
7. Jokingly telling a first-grade student that they need to complete all therapy activities now or you will not let that student go home today Trait:			

Unprofessional Behavior	Potential Safety Concerns or Problems	Possible Effect on Relationship With Clients or Colleagues	Possible Disciplinary Action That May Result
8. Telling a post-surgical client with poor recovery that his surgeon is a "quack" with a reputation for botching surgery Trait:			
9. Accepting cash gifts from your client in home care Trait:			
10. Before trying other alternatives, applying a vest restraint to a client at risk for falling out of their wheelchair Trait:			
11. While on break or having lunch at work with colleagues, making fun of patients or staff members who demonstrate peculiar mannerisms or behaviors Trait:			
12. Not reporting or filling out an incident report when a client cuts himself on the sharp edge of a therapy device because the client reports feeling "okay" and only needs a bandage and some antiseptic, which you provided Trait:			
13. Forgetting to lock wheelchair brakes during a client transfer Trait:			
14. Criticizing a colleague's skills in front of clients or staff Trait:			
15. "Borrowing" adaptive equipment or an exercise device from the rehabilitation department because your older relative would benefit from using it after recent surgery Trait:			

Unprofessional Behavior	Potential Safety Concerns or Problems	Possible Effect on Relationship With Clients or Colleagues	Possible Disciplinary Action That May Result
16. Keeping a client on your schedule and billing Medicare for routine range of motion or self-care activities when skilled intervention is no longer necessary Trait:			
17. Attending a 6-hour continuing education seminar but leaving after 4 hours and submitting the full course completion certificate for OTA license renewal or NBCOT certification Trait:			
18. Not informing your OT supervisor that you are not competent in the use of a delegated physical agent modality intervention because you "think" you can figure it out Trait:			
19. Using your cell phone to check personal email or text your friends/family while you are at a rehabilitation department inservice or team meeting Trait:			
20. While you are completing Level I fieldwork at a school setting, giving a batch of your home-made peanut butter cookies to a group of students receiving occupational therapy without first checking with your supervisor Trait:			

Adapted from Morreale, M. J., & Amini, D. (2016). *The occupational therapist's workbook for ensuring clinical competence.* SLACK Incorporated.

Worksheet 2-9

Student and Client Interaction

Laura is an OTA student completing Level II fieldwork at a skilled nursing facility. Her client, Peggy, is 80 years old and has a diagnosis of rheumatoid arthritis. Laura and Peggy had the following conversation at the end of an intervention session. What suggestions would you make regarding the OTA student's interaction with the client?

OTA student: Peggy, as you know, I have to say goodbye to you today as I am finally finished with my 8-week fieldwork here at the nursing home. However, I am sure you are really looking forward to going back home next week.
Client: To tell you the truth, I am a bit nervous about it.
OTA student: Why?
Client: Well, as you know, I live all by myself. My two children would help if they were here, but unfortunately, they both live clear across the country. My sister isn't too far away but she has been kind of sick lately. Unfortunately, my nice neighbor who used to help me every so often just told me she got a new job and is moving away.
OTA student: Honey, don't worry. Everything will be fine. We would not be discharging you unless you were ready.
Client: Yes, but I do not really know anyone else in my apartment building.
OTA student: Now you have an excuse to make some new friends then.
Client: That is not so easy at my age.
OTA student: Oh, Sweetie, you have a such a nice personality. I certainly enjoyed talking with you, and I will miss you. You remind me of my grandma.
Client: I like talking to you too. Maybe we can talk once in awhile after I go home, or you can come visit me and we can have some tea and cookies together. I know chocolate chip is your favorite! Can I have your cell phone number? I wouldn't be able to reach you here, of course, because you are leaving.
OTA student: Sure, let me write it down for you. [Student writes phone number on a piece of paper and hands it to Peggy.]
Client: Also, I have a something for you to show my appreciation. Let me get it out of my pocket. [Peggy removes a $50 bill and hands it to the student.]
OTA student: Peggy, that really isn't necessary.
Client: I insist. Put it toward your certification exam. You have been so nice to me the whole time I have been here.
OTA student: Wow, thank you so much, Peggy. That is very kind of you. [She gives Peggy a hug] Unfortunately, I do have to go now and finish up all my paperwork. Good luck to you. Bye for now.

Suggestions to improve this interaction:

1.

2.

3.

4.

Worksheet 2-9 (continued)
Student and Client Interaction

5.

6.

7.

8.

Adapted from Morreale, M. J., & Amini, D. (2016). *The occupational therapist's workbook for ensuring clinical competence.* SLACK Incorporated.

Worksheet 2-10

People-First Language and Term Usage

People-first language and the appropriate use of diagnostic terms makes a profound difference on the focus and perception that others have on the individual with a disabling condition. In the list that follows, indicate whether the phrase is an appropriate (A) or inappropriate (I) use of descriptive language.

1. _____ The blind people

2. _____ The athetoid child

3. _____ Crazy person

4. _____ Individual who has served in combat

5. _____ Person who has a disability

6. _____ Victim of depression

7. _____ Person who is crippled

8. _____ The child with leukemia is a heroic boy

9. _____ Wheelchair user

10. _____ The epileptic

11. _____ Downs kid

12. _____ The schiz I am working with today

13. _____ The borderline

14. _____ The person with cancer

15. _____ The older man who is mentally retarded

Worksheet 2-10 (continued)

People-First Language and Term Usage

16. _____ Suffers from Alzheimer's

17. _____ Wheelchair-bound

18. _____ Senior who lives in an active adult community

19. _____ Group of old people

20. _____ Client is max assist

Worksheet 2-11

Written Communication

Critique the following email that an OTA student wrote to her professor. List 10 suggestions to improve this note.

Hey Prof Jones,

I don't think it is fare that u failed me on my research paper. I SPEND A LOT OF TIME AND WORKED REALLY HARD ON IT! ☹ I wanna meat with u ASAP to discuss. Thx.

Mary Smith

Suggestions to improve this note:

1.

2.

3.

4.

5.

6.

7.

8.

9.

10.

Morreale, M. J. (2022). *Developing clinical competence: A workbook for the OTA* (2nd ed.). SLACK Incorporated.

Learning Activity 2-4: Professional Communication

Imagine you just had a 1-hour interview with your fieldwork educator, Nick Knack, regarding your upcoming Level II fieldwork experience. You learned you will be working primarily on the spinal cord and traumatic brain injury units. During the interview it was confirmed that you are scheduled to begin fieldwork on the first Monday of next month. Your fieldwork educator requested that on your first day you meet him in the human resources office at 8:00 a.m. to fill out required paperwork. In the space below (or using a computer), write a sample email to the fieldwork educator as a follow-up to your recent interview. Switch notes with a partner and critique each other's notes.

Consider the note created for this exercise. Does it thank the fieldwork educator for his time, demonstrate enthusiasm for the upcoming experience, and confirm the meeting place and time? Is the note free from slang and errors in spelling and grammar? Does the note convey a professional image and include a respectful greeting and an appropriate closing?

Worksheet 2-12

Medical Terminology and Abbreviations

Translate the following diagnoses, abbreviations, and physician's orders into full English phrases or sentences using a medical terminology book or an approved abbreviations list from your facility or OTA program.

1. Child Dx c̄ TBI demonstrates poor graphomotor and scissors skills 2°↓FM Ⓑ UE

2. Client Fx Ⓛ humerus 6 wks ago 2° fall at home. Reports Ⓛ shoulder pain 7/10 & has ↓ P/AROM flex/abd, ER/IR which limit BADLs/IADLs.

3. Pt. c/o chest pain. Hx of MI 2016. EKG and CXR today are –, VS stable. NKA

4. DOA to behavioral health unit 4/10/2021, Dx of depression. Client also has OCD which manifests in frequent washing of hands and personal-care items, impeding proper use of nightly CPAP and orthosis for CTS. PMH: PVD, HTN.

5. X-ray Ⓡ wrist/hand neg. EMG + Ⓡ CTS

6. Dx: COPD: HOB 30°, BRP, OOB c̄ walker

7. Dx: PTSD, PMH: Ⓛ BKA, Ⓡ AKA 2° IED during Iraq deployment

8. 7 y.o. ♀ Dx c̄ ASD, ADHD has an URI

Worksheet 2-12 (continued)
Medical Terminology and Abbreviations

9. OT eval & tx; NWB Ⓛ LE, transfers, ADLs, BUE ther ex; 5 X wk X 2 wks

10. OT 2/wk X 4 wks: US, e-stim to Ⓡ shoulder, ROM, PREs, BADLs/IADLs

Adapted from Morreale, M. J., & Borcherding, S. (2017). *The OTA's guide to documentation: Writing SOAP notes* (4th ed.). SLACK Incorporated.

Learning Activity 2-5: Medical Terminology and Abbreviations—More Practice

Translate the following diagnoses, abbreviations, and physician's orders into full English phrases or sentences using a medical terminology book or an approved abbreviations list from your facility or OTA program.

1. Resident Ⓘ w/c ⟷ commode using SP cane but exhibits DOE

2. Pt. min Ⓐ EOB → commode c̄ WBQC and Ⓛ AFO

3. The IEP indicates that the student uses AE for feeding and requires min Ⓐ to manage clothing for toileting/recess

4. Pt. has ESRD and exhibits SOB at rest and c/o nausea. HR 82, BP 145/95

5. 75 y.o. ♂ Dx c̄ Ⓡ CVA, Ⓛ hemiparesis, CAD. O X 3 but exhibits STM deficits. Requires SBA when AMB and transferring due to unilateral neglect and ↓ safety awareness.

6. Dx: SLE, UTI; PMH: Breast CA

7. Dx: s/p Fx Ⓡ DRUJ c̄ ORIF, CHF

8. Dx: s/p Ⓡ THR 2° DJD, HTN: Avoid IR/Add, no flex > 90°. WBAT using walker. Daily OT X 1/wk for ADL retraining, Ⓑ UE ther ex

9.   OT 3 X wk X 1 mo. for ADL retraining, P/AROM LUE, PAMs PRN

10.   OT 1/X daily: ADLs, bed mobility and transfers, OOB AMB $\bar{c}$ walker $\bar{c}$ SBA, monitor O_2

Adapted from Morreale, M. J., & Borcherding, S. (2017). *The OTA's guide to documentation: Writing SOAP notes* (4th ed.). SLACK Incorporated.

Worksheet 2-13

Avoiding Documentation Errors

Rewrite the following sentences to make them more professional by correcting errors in spelling, abbreviations, grammar, and fundamentals of documentation.

1. The wheelchair bound client was able to preform wheelchair mobility independently to go from his hospital room to the dinning room.

2. The students musical instruments were stored in the band teacher's office.

3. The COPD client stated she becomes OBS when performing heavy activities for more then a few minutes.

4. The Occupational Therapy Assistant instructed the client on therapy puddy exercises.

5. The senile PT. was seen for 30 minutes bedside to help her eat breakfast.

6. The client's dysphasia contributed to his inspiration pnumonia.

7. The child needed modified assistance to donn his orthosis.

8. The client who lives in an apartment for old people stated "he cannot wait to go home."

Worksheet 2-13 (continued)

Avoiding Documentation Errors

9. The client used his bad hand to grasp the bed rail when rolling to the left.

10. The TBI worked on ↓ safety and ↑ left neglect to improve IADL performance.

Adapted from Morreale, M. J., & Borcherding, S. (2017). *The OTA's guide to documentation: Writing SOAP notes* (4th ed.). SLACK Incorporated.

Worksheet 2-14

Avoiding Documentation Errors—More Practice

Rewrite the following sentences to make them more professional by correcting errors in spelling, abbreviations, grammar, and fundamentals of documentation.

1. The student asked if the OTA could help her write her name?

2. The resident exhibited urinary incontinents and stated "I have a urinary track infection."

3. The client was instructed in arom exercises so that her bad arm does not get stiff.

4. The home health aid was adapt at transfering clients.

5. The client's throat was sore because the speech pathologist made the client speak two long in therapy.

6. The pt.'s torn rotary cup required surgery and afterward his deltoid was painful when palpitated.

7. The two OTA's treated the OT's to lunch when they got a promotion.

Worksheet 2-14 (continued)

Avoiding Documentation Errors—More Practice

8. The child griped the toy steering wheel with her dominate right hand and used her left hand to press the horn.

9. The clients' tremers made it unsafe for her to use the parrafin machine.

10. The Autistic toddler exhibited a positive babinski sign.

Adapted from Morreale, M. J., & Borcherding, S. (2017). *The OTA's guide to documentation: Writing SOAP notes* (4th ed.). SLACK Incorporated.

Worksheet 2-15

Documentation Fundamentals

An OTA wrote the following note after contact with a client. Use AOTA's *Guidelines for Documentation of Occupational Therapy* (2018) or other documentation resources to help determine which fundamental elements are incorrect or missing in the OTA's note below.

Really Good Rehabilitation Center
Restful Springs, Florida

Name: Rhezzident, R.   *Date of Birth: 4/1/1932*

Dx: Right mastectomy 2° Breast Cancer   *Physician: Dr. Seth Oscope*

11:30: Client in bed and refusing therapy this morning due to side eff. from chemotherapy. Client stated she vomited ~~two~~ three times this morning and is tired from not sleeping well last night. Plan: attempt therapy again this aft. and instruct client on right upper extremity AROM exercises.

J.W.

1.

2.

3.

4.

5.

6.

7.

Worksheet 2-15 (continued)
Documentation Fundamentals

8.

9.

10.

Adapted from Morreale, M. J., & Borcherding, S. (2017). *The OTA's guide to documentation: Writing SOAP notes* (4th ed.). SLACK Incorporated.

Worksheet 2-16

Managing a Schedule

Imagine you recently started a new OTA job with work hours from 8:30 a.m. to 4:30 p.m. You are allowed a 30-minute lunch break and may also take two 15-minute breaks (one in the morning and one in the afternoon). Your caseload consists of 10 clients, described on the next page, and you have a mandatory 30-minute staff meeting today at 11:00 a.m. In addition, you must also set aside time to collaborate with your occupational therapy supervisor and complete all your daily paperwork and departmental tasks. Fill in your schedule below, including the best time frames for treating your clients.

Time	Client
8:30 a.m.	
9:00 a.m.	
9:30 a.m.	
10:00 a.m.	
10:30 a.m.	
11:00 a.m.	
11:30 a.m.	
12:00 p.m.	
12:30 p.m.	
1:00 p.m.	
1:30 p.m.	
2:00 p.m.	
2:30 p.m.	
3:00 p.m.	
3:30 p.m.	
4:00 p.m.	
4:30 p.m.	

Worksheet 2-16 (continued)
Managing a Schedule

Client Caseload (approximately 30 minutes each session)

1. Mary sustained a stroke and requires instruction in self-feeding. Her schedule includes physical therapy at 9:00 a.m. and speech therapy at 3:00 p.m.

2. Tim has colon cancer and requires instruction in energy conservation. He receives chemotherapy at 1:00 p.m.

3. Mabel sustained a stroke and requires instruction in grooming. She receives physical therapy daily at 10:30 a.m. and speech therapy at 2:00 p.m.

4. Leroy has undergone rotator cuff surgery and requires instruction in post-surgical care of the involved extremity before his discharge at noon.

5. Jim has Parkinson's disease and requires instruction in safe transfers. He is scheduled for physical therapy at 3:00 p.m.

6. Leila sustained a left femur fracture and now must use a walker. She needs recommendations for durable medical/adaptive equipment prior to her discharge at noon. She is scheduled for physical therapy at 8:30 a.m.

7. Natasha has undergone surgery for a right below-knee amputation and needs exercises to increase her upper body strength and endurance. She receives physical therapy daily at 11:00 a.m.

8. Ellen sustained multiple trauma from a motor vehicle accident recently. She needs a right resting hand orthosis today. Physical therapy is scheduled for 2:00 p.m.

9. Mario sustained a stroke and needs activities to decrease his left neglect and improve cognition. He is scheduled for an MRI at 3:00 p.m.

10. Harvey is recovering from pneumonia and is being discharged tomorrow. He needs a home exercise program to increase activity tolerance. He is scheduled for physical therapy at 12:30 p.m.

Learning Activity 2-6: Gathering and Organizing Therapy Items

As OTAs are often pressed for time in a workday, it is important to perform tasks efficiently. To avoid wasting time, gather and organize therapy materials in advance whenever possible, such as when planning to implement a home health or school-based intervention, work with a client bedside, or assess client factors.

Consider the following clients on your caseload. Make a list of all the items you will need to gather and bring with you to implement each client intervention. Be sure to consider any paperwork or documentation materials you may also need.

1. **Home health**: Stanley is a 75-year-old male diagnosed with Parkinson's disease. He was recently discharged from an acute care hospital to home, but never had any occupational therapy during his hospitalization. Stanley exhibits fair plus muscle strength in both upper extremities and fair activity tolerance. He demonstrates decreased dynamic sitting balance and reports dizziness when bending over. The OT evaluated Stanley 2 days ago and, for today's session, has asked you to initiate upper extremity strengthening and to teach Stanley lower body dressing using adaptive equipment.

2. **School setting**: Tamika is an 8-year-old student diagnosed with a developmental delay. She has decreased muscle tone, resulting in poor posture while sitting at her desk. Tamika also demonstrates difficulty holding a pencil properly, maintaining wrist extension, and staying within the lines when writing. The OT has asked you to work with Tamika in the classroom today and provide some adaptations for Tamika's challenges.

3. **Acute care hospital**: Juan was involved as a passenger in a motor vehicle accident and sustained multiple trauma, including bilateral femur fractures, internal injuries, and a wrist sprain. He is presently on bedrest but is conscious and awake. The doctor has ordered an ulnar gutter orthosis for Juan's wrist. Today the OT has asked you to fabricate Juan's orthotic device bedside as the department does not have a prefabricated orthosis that can be used. A rolling cart is available to transport items.

4. **Outpatient clinic**: Margaret is 50 years old and has carpometacarpal osteoarthritis in her right, non-dominant thumb. Today the OT has asked you to assess Margaret's affected hand for thumb active range of motion (AROM), grip and pinch strength, and to work on fine-motor skills.

5. **Behavioral health unit**: Renata is 45 years old and has a history of substance use disorder. Her husband finally convinced Renata to get help because she has had frequent arguments with her family and neighbors, was involved in two recent motor vehicle accidents, and broke her nose in a fall earlier this month, all caused by her drinking alcohol excessively. In today's occupational therapy session, Renata will be working on a homemaking occupation involving making lunch for herself in the unit's patient kitchen. Renata has chosen to make a grilled cheese sandwich and salad. You, the OTA, will need to order and pick up the necessary food ingredients from the facility's food service department ahead of the session, plus double check that the patient kitchen contains all the cooking implements needed.

Answers to Worksheets

Worksheet 2-1: Scheduling Fieldwork

1. C. Attempts to schedule fieldwork should be made as soon as possible, as it could take several weeks just to connect with your fieldwork educator. Also, although you may want to complete fieldwork during a particular time frame, this may not fit with your supervisor's schedule. Your fieldwork educator might be on vacation or have other students already scheduled at that time. If you wait until only a short time before your desired time frame to schedule, you risk not being accommodated and unable to complete fieldwork by your program deadline. Contacting your fieldwork educator promptly after fieldwork is assigned should provide ample time to schedule a mutually agreeable time frame.

2. D. Occupational therapy practitioners are very busy at clinical sites and may not be able to return your call immediately. Also, that person may not have received the message or may forget to call you back. You should try and call again. If you cannot contact your fieldwork educator after three or four attempts over several weeks, then you should discuss this with your academic fieldwork coordinator. It would not be appropriate to ask for the rehabilitation director at this time.

3. C. Due to staffing changes, scheduled vacations, and other factors, the facility may assign a different fieldwork educator to you. You should schedule your fieldwork with this new supervisor, but also immediately inform your academic fieldwork coordinator regarding the change.

4. A. A student should not attend fieldwork with an illness that could be contagious to clients or staff or significantly impact job performance. Educators and supervisors understand that emergencies and illnesses do occur but do expect that situations be handled appropriately. The professional action to take is for you to immediately notify your fieldwork educator that you will be absent, humbly apologize for the inconvenience your illness causes, and ask politely to reschedule. Realize the site might not agree to reschedule and, if this is the case, do not get upset or argue with the site. You should also notify your academic fieldwork coordinator about your illness and absence, and determine whether the site is able to reschedule your fieldwork. If you are planning to see a health professional for treatment of your illness, it is helpful to offer your fieldwork educator and academic fieldwork coordinator medical documentation to verify that you have a valid reason to be absent.

5. B. First of all, do not panic! Fieldwork schedules can change due to a variety of reasons, so this is not an uncommon situation. It would not be productive to argue with the fieldwork educator. Your primary course of action would be to immediately contact your academic fieldwork coordinator who can discuss your situation with the two sites and help you find a workable solution. Perhaps the second site can be rescheduled, or your fieldwork coordinator may be able to substitute a different site for your first or second fieldwork. However, you may need to be flexible with time frames.

6. C. This is not an uncommon situation. Thank the individual for contacting you, notify your academic fieldwork coordinator of the change, and wait a day or two for the new person to contact you as directed. If you do not hear from that individual within several days, be sure to follow up. It would be inappropriate to speak to the rehabilitation director or ask the person to switch students.

7. A. One week is more than adequate time to wait for a reply, so you should follow up immediately and resend your email. The fieldwork educator may have overlooked the email or deleted it accidentally, so do not be defensive or accusatory. There is no need to contact the rehabilitation director. You should make further attempts to contact the fieldwork educator before asking your academic fieldwork coordinator to intervene.

8. D. Follow your college's policy regarding fieldwork absences for inclement weather, emergencies, or other situations. You should also understand the consequences for unexcused absences. Health facilities count on staff being present to provide essential client care but, of course, realize that it may be unsafe or impossible for some staff to get to work in severe conditions. Certainly, a big difference exists between a "possible" inch of snow versus an active blizzard or, a thunderstorm versus hurricane conditions. Another option is to consider other means of getting to fieldwork, such as public transportation or perhaps spending the night at a hotel (or a friend/relative's house) within walking distance of the facility. The weather forecast could change by tomorrow and not even be an issue anymore. It would be unprofessional to have a parent, guardian, or spouse call.

9. B. As soon as you realize you are going to be late, the professional action to take is to attempt to notify your fieldwork educator. However, if you are doing the driving, be sure to follow the rules of the road and only text, email, or call when it is safe and legal to do so, such as pulling over into a parking space. Then, once you arrive late, accept responsibility, apologize profusely, and promise it will not happen again. Do not lie or make excuses. Lateness, particularly on the first day, gives a negative impression. It is prudent to plan beforehand and allow enough travel time for unexpected situations or traffic.

10. D. Emergencies and other situations happen occasionally, so you might find that your fieldwork schedule changes. You should remain patient, understanding, and flexible. It would be unprofessional to cry, whine, or contact the supervisor. Reschedule the fieldwork and contact your academic fieldwork educator to discuss the situation. It is best to not wait until the last minute to complete fieldwork to allow for any unexpected changes.

Worksheet 2-2: Fieldwork Phone Interview

1. N. Directions to the fieldwork site

    Working occupational therapy practitioners are very busy. It may be perceived as unprofessional to ask for non-clinical information you can easily obtain on your own. It is better to obtain directions by other means such as an internet search or by using a navigation system.

2. Y. Start and end times for the day

3. Y. Where to meet in the facility

4. N. If the facility is in a "bad" area

    This type of question is not professional and might be perceived as discriminatory.

5. Y. Date(s) to complete fieldwork

6. N. Amount of time for lunch

    This type of question may be perceived as unprofessional, as it implies you are more interested in breaks. You might ask, "Can you tell me about a typical day's schedule?" It may be prudent to pack a lunch to bring with you the first day as there may not be enough time to purchase lunch offsite or wait in line in the cafeteria.

7. N. Permission to come in late because you must drive your kids to school

    You are expected to be at the site during typical working hours. You should try to make other arrangements for your children.

8. Y. If a lab coat is required

9. N. Wearing of sneakers

    Sneakers are not considered professional attire, so it is best not to initiate asking about them. Plan to wear comfortable low-heeled shoes, preferably with non-slip soles. If your supervisor happens to indicate that sneakers may be worn, realize the sneakers must be clean (no scuff marks or dirt), low profile, and tasteful (i.e., no blinking lights, sparkles, or bright colors).

10. N. Availability of coffee or tea in the morning

    Your focus should be on the clinical experience. Plan to have your breakfast or beverage before coming to the fieldwork site.

11. N. Permission to use your cell phone so you can monitor your children

    Your entire focus should be on the clinical experience while you are at the site. While a brief call at lunchtime should be acceptable, it is best to make alternate arrangements for your children for the rest of the workday.

12. N. Permission to come in late or leave early to accommodate your bus or train schedule

    You are expected to be at the site during typical working hours, even if it is not the most convenient for you. Plan to take an earlier or later bus/train or make other arrangements, such as taking an Uber, taxi, or asking a friend or family member to drive you.

13. N. Permission to leave early to pick your children up from school

    You are expected to be at the site during typical working hours. You should try to make other arrangements for your children.

14. N. Permission to leave early due to a dental appointment to get your teeth cleaned

    You are expected to be at the site during typical working hours. It is not appropriate to leave early for a routine appointment that can be rescheduled.

15. Y. Permission to wear a head covering if required by your religion

    Head coverings are normally not allowed, except for those required for religious reasons. It is prudent to discuss any religious accommodations you might need.

16. Y. What paperwork to bring

17. N. If it will be a very hard fieldwork, because a classmate failed fieldwork there last semester

    It is not appropriate to discuss another student's experience, and this could also be perceived as a negative attitude.

18. N. Reimbursement for gas and tolls

    Commuting costs are typically the student's responsibility.

19. N. If the fieldwork will require a lot of homework

    A question phrased that way could be perceived as a negative attitude. It would be better to ask if there will be any assignments that you might start preparing for now.

20. Y. The types of diagnoses you will observe

Worksheet 2-3: Directions to Fieldwork Site

The following box lists possible suggestions for obtaining directions to your fieldwork site without asking your fieldwork educator.

Obtaining Directions to Fieldwork Site
• Ask a friend or family member for directions.
• Use a cell phone app that provides step-by-step driving directions (e.g., Google Maps or Waze).
• Do an internet search or use a website that provides customized driving directions (e.g., www.Mapquest.com).
• If available, use your car's navigation device/global positioning system (GPS).
• Call the facility's main number and ask the operator or follow the telephone prompts for directions, if available.
• Look for directions on the facility's website.

Worksheet 2-4: Fieldwork Attire

Always check with your facility regarding the required dress code. Although some settings are more formal or casual than others, attire must meet standards for client care and safety. Realize that in many practice settings, such as physical rehabilitation and schools, an OTA might be standing and walking a lot, going up and down flights of stairs, bending, transferring clients, and so forth. Attire should be comfortable, clean, neat, modest (i.e., no low-cut shirts or short hemlines) and allow for safe client care. "Business casual" means clothing that gives a professional appearance but is not overly dressy or formal. Here are some typical guidelines based on the inpatient scenario presented:

1. N. Scrubs

    In this situation, scrubs would not be appropriate as they do not conform to the designated dress code. However, in some settings, scrubs might be the required dress code for rehabilitation staff.

2. N. Sneakers

    Sneakers are not considered business casual attire. However, some settings may allow rehabilitation staff to wear clean, low-profile sneakers.

3. Y. Flat, closed-toe shoes with a rubber sole.

   These are professional and generally safer for client care.

4. N. Dressy flip-flops

   Unacceptable for inpatient client care as they can be a safety hazard during transfers or exposure to bodily fluids. Hosiery and closed-toe shoes are often mandatory.

5. N. Low-heeled leather sandals

   Hosiery and closed-toe shoes are often mandatory for direct care roles. Exposed feet can be a safety hazard during transfers or exposure to bodily fluids.

6. N. Heavy perfume/cologne/aftershave

   Clients may be allergic or sensitive to smell. Also limit use of heavily scented lotions, shampoos, and so forth.

7. Y. Stud earrings

   One or two small, tasteful earrings are usually acceptable.

8. N. Eyebrow piercing

   This does not give a professional appearance. It is best to remove visible facial piercings.

9. N. Head covering

   Typically, only head coverings for religious requirements are allowed. Baseball hats, fedoras, bonnets, and so forth, are not appropriate.

10. N. Visible underwear above pants' waistband

    This looks sloppy and is unprofessional. Also avoid very sheer or tight clothing that allows undergarments to be clearly visible.

11. N. Neatly pressed dark jeans

    Jeans are not professional attire, although some settings may allow them.

12. Y. Khaki pants and a polo shirt

    These are examples of some standard types of garments that occupational therapy practitioners may wear.

13. N. Plain black sweatpants/yoga pants

    These are not professional attire and are better suited for a gym or leisure activities.

14. N. Sport t-shirt/jersey

    These are not professional attire and are better suited for a gym or leisure activities.

15. Y. Button-down oxford shirt

    Example of a standard type of garment that occupational therapy practitioners may wear.

16. Y. Dress slacks

    Acceptable if they are tasteful and not extremely fancy or garish.

17. N. Cargo pants

    These tend to be more casual-looking and generally do not give a professional appearance.

18. Y. Polo shirt with collar and small designer logo emblem

    This is an example of a standard type of garment that occupational therapy practitioners may wear. Of course, no logo is necessary.

19. N. 32-in. plain gold necklace

    While necklaces may not be prohibited, long chains could be an infection control or safety hazard during transfers or bed mobility (such as hitting client in face or getting caught on something). Also, clients may pull on it, possibly harming the health practitioner.

20. N. Charm bracelet

    While bracelets may not be prohibited, dangling charms could be an infection control or safety hazard when handling clients as they may injure skin or catch on client's clothing. The sound of jingling charms could also be a distraction for clients with attentional issues.

21. N. Well-groomed, long artificial nails without polish

    Long nails, particularly artificial nails (of any length), can harbor bacteria (Centers for Disease Control and Prevention, 2002; 2020; WHO, 2009). Long nails may also rupture gloves or injure clients.

22. N. Dark gray suit

    This would generally be considered overdressed.

23. Y. Name tag

    An identification badge is usually required in health care settings per facility policy and/or state regulation.

24. N. Solid color leggings

    These are unprofessional as the only lower body covering. They might be acceptable if worn under a dress or skirt.

25. N. Solid color hoodie

    This is not professional attire and is better suited for a gym, school, or leisure activities.

Worksheet 2-5: Planning for Fieldwork

The following box provides practical suggestions of what you can do ahead of time to help ensure that you will get to fieldwork on time and reduce your stress level on your first day.

Preparing for Your First Day of Fieldwork

- Obtain clear and correct directions to the fieldwork site ahead of time.
- Perform at least one "dry run" beforehand to determine how long it will take to get to your fieldwork site and, also ensure you will not get lost on your first day. Ideally, your practice run should be during the same time frame that you will need to travel for fieldwork.
- On your fieldwork day, allow more time than you deem necessary to travel to your site. This will give you an extra cushion of time if you have several red lights, experience road construction, or get stuck in extra traffic.
- Set an alarm clock or timer the prior evening.
- A day or two ahead of time, make sure you will have enough gas in the car if you are driving.
- Check the weather report to determine if the weather may impact driving conditions.
- At least a week or more ahead of time, look through your wardrobe to ensure you have enough outfits appropriate to wear to fieldwork. Check that they still fit properly and make a list of items you feel you will need to obtain, for example, a lab coat, extra slacks, or appropriate footwear. Be sure to allow yourself enough time to order items online, go shopping, or borrow items from friends or family.
- A day or two ahead of time, make sure you have enough cash for parking, tolls, lunch, and so forth, so you do not have to go to an ATM right before fieldwork.
- A day or two ahead of time, confirm any essential plans such as a babysitter, car availability, train or bus schedule, and so forth.
- Select and prepare your clothes and accessories the evening before fieldwork, making sure they are clean and neatly pressed.
- Pack your lunch the prior evening.
- Gather necessary items such as your name tag, car keys, and wallet the prior evening so you are not searching for them in the morning.
- If a lab coat is required, make sure it fits and is clean and neatly pressed ahead of time.

Worksheet 2-6: Professional Conduct

Resource: AOTA, 2020
You may identify additional pertinent traits/characteristics besides the suggested answers listed.

Professional Behavior	*Professional Characteristic*
1. Administering a standardized assessment accurately	*Example: Service competency* *Attention to detail*
2. Offering to put your fieldwork educator's clinical notes back into the clients' charts without being asked	Initiative
3. Admitting you did not complete your notes on time, apologizing, and offering to stay late or come in early to complete them	Accepts responsibility
4. Arranging self-feeding interventions pre-dawn or after dusk for an occupational therapy client who is fasting during Ramadan	Cultural sensitivity Flexibility
5. Switching a client's treatment time so as not to conflict with physical therapy	Flexibility Cooperation
6. Addressing an adult client by using "Mr." or "Mrs." and client's surname	Respect Courtesy
7. Not refusing to work with a client who is positive for HIV or tuberculosis	Unbiased
8. Writing a thank-you note to your fieldwork educator after your interview	Courtesy
9. Arriving to your fieldwork interview 5 minutes early	Punctuality Dependability
10. Asking a senator to vote for a proposed law that improves access to mental health services	Social justice Advocacy
11. Cleaning up water that you notice on floor near the hydrocollator	Initiative Safety awareness
12. Preparing and assembling all the information packets in time for a workshop that the occupational therapy department is sponsoring	Time management Organizational skills Reliability
13. Noticing that the paraffin unit temperature is too high	Attention to detail Safety awareness
14. Closing the computer screen after entering client information	Confidentiality
15. Not billing Medicare for time the OTA spent documenting or transporting the client	Honesty Veracity Integrity
16. Nodding and maintaining eye contact when a client is answering questions	Active listening
17. Participating in an event to raise awareness of a specific disease	Social justice Altruism Advocacy
18. Being the "go to" person for solving problems regarding manual wheelchairs	Dependability Service competency
19. Not dating a cute client your age who asks you out on a date	Professional boundaries Good judgment

Morreale, M. J. (2022). *Developing clinical competence: A workbook for the OTA* (2nd ed.). SLACK Incorporated.

Professional Behavior	Professional Characteristic
20. Ensuring that all the OTA's notes are co-signed when required by law or facility policy	Attention to detail Conscientious Reliability
21. Knocking on a closed door before entering the client's room or an examination room	Respect Courtesy
22. Discussing a client's discharge plan with the physical therapist (PT) and social worker	Interprofessional collaboration Teamwork Cooperation
23. Acknowledging that the client feels disappointed when the client's son did not come for a visit	Empathetic
24. Not complaining when you must stay late today to order a client's durable medical equipment before the client is discharged home	Good attitude Flexibility Strong work ethic
25. Writing several drafts of a SOAP note to ensure an accurate, professional presentation before showing it to your fieldwork educator	Conscientious Attention to detail
26. Reporting suspected child or elder abuse to appropriate personnel/agencies to prevent further harm to the individual	Beneficence
27. Arranging for an interpreter when the client speaks a different language than you	Autonomy Cultural sensitivity
28. Checking the chart and asking the client about possible food allergies before planning a cooking intervention	Safety awareness Conscientious Nonmaleficence
29. Shredding extra copies of client information rather than throwing them in the trash	Confidentiality
30. Neatly folding or hanging up a client's clothing during a self-care intervention	Courtesy Respect

Worksheet 2-7: Ethics Sanctions

The order of sanctions from less severe to more severe is as follows (AOTA, 2019; NBCOT, 2020b):

1. Reprimand
2. Censure
3. Probation
4. Suspension
5. Revocation

Worksheet 2-8: Ethical Behavior

Resources: AOTA, 2020, 2019; NBCOT, 2020a, 2020b. Also refer to any federal guidelines affecting occupational therapy practice and the state agency that regulates occupational therapy in the state in which you are working or plan to work.

1. F. If an OTA is found guilty of committing a severe unethical act, AOTA can take away the OTA's license to practice.

    AOTA cannot issue state regulatory sanctions but can report the individual's behavior to the appropriate state regulatory agency and implement sanctions regarding AOTA membership.

2. T. An occupational therapy volunteer can report an OTA's unethical behavior to NBCOT.

    Anyone can formally report unethical behavior. However, the volunteer should use judgment to consider the nature of behavior that would warrant a complaint to NBCOT versus simply reporting unprofessional conduct to a supervisor or administrator at that facility.

3. F. An OTA student should begin following the Code of Ethics when Level II fieldwork commences.

    Professional conduct should be exhibited throughout an OTA educational program, including Level I and Level II fieldwork.

4. T. An OTA who commits an unethical act could have their name listed publicly as an ethics violator by AOTA or NBCOT.

    This describes the disciplinary action of censure.

5. F. AOTA guidelines take precedence over state laws.

    State and federal laws are preeminent.

6. T. Committing a felony may limit a person's ability to practice occupational therapy.

    Refer to the NBCOT website (www.nbcot.org) and the state agency that regulates occupational therapy where the individual is practicing.

7. F. If an occupational therapy practitioner did not know about a particular law, the OT or OTA cannot be sanctioned for an unethical act that violates that law.

    An occupational therapy practitioner is expected to be knowledgeable about applicable laws affecting occupational therapy practice.

8. F. An OTA state license is only affected by occupational therapy ethical infractions and not other legal violations of which an OTA might be guilty.

    Committing a felony may limit a person's ability to practice occupational therapy. Refer to the NBCOT website (www.nbcot.org) and the state agency that regulates occupational therapy.

9. F. An occupational therapy practitioner has an obligation to report a colleague's unethical behavior only if it is occupational therapy related.

    For example, an OTA may report the unethical conduct of a nurse or physical therapist.

10. F. NBCOT implements sanctions within 1 week when a very serious complaint is lodged against an OT or OTA.

    The process of information-gathering and appeals require a longer time frame.

11. F. A state can suspend an occupational therapy aide's license for unethical behavior in an occupational therapy clinic.

    Occupational therapy aides are not typically licensed professionals.

12. T. A person visiting a hospital patient can file a complaint with an occupational therapy state licensure board.

    Any member of the public may file a complaint.

13. F. An OTA accused of practicing under the influence of drugs automatically loses NBCOT certification if reported to NBCOT.

    Any complaint must be substantiated, and there is a formal disciplinary process.

14. F. An OTA receiving 6 months of probation from an occupational therapy state licensing board cannot practice for the entire 6 months.

    That is not the definition of probation. Suspension limits practice for a particular time period.

15. F. An OTA sanctioned by NBCOT cannot appeal the decision.

    NBCOT has a formal appeals process.

16. F. Minimizing a client's progress when documenting is not considered unethical if it helps the person receive essential therapy services from the insurance company.

    It is unethical to falsify or "fudge" client information.

17. F. An occupational therapy practitioner cannot be disciplined by AOTA, NBCOT, and an occupational therapy state licensure board all at the same time.

    Each organization has different functions.

18. F. It is acceptable for an OTA to refuse to treat a person with HIV if the OTA is concerned about catching the disease.

    Communicable diseases always pose a concern for health providers whether it is HIV, hepatitis B, tuberculosis, and so forth. However, it is unethical to discriminate based on a person's diagnosis and clients must always be treated with dignity and respect. As health practitioners may not even know if a person has a communicable disease, the health worker must always incorporate standard precautions for infection control as appropriate.

19. F. An OTA censured by an occupational therapy state licensure board cannot practice during the time of the censure.

    A public disapproval statement (censure) does not prevent an OTA from practicing occupational therapy.

20. F. When an occupational therapy licensure board's sanction is revocation, the occupational therapy practitioner can only practice with daily, direct supervision.

    Revocation means the license has been taken away.

Worksheet 2-9: Student and Client Interaction

1. It is condescending to call an adult client such nicknames as "honey" or "sweetie."

2. The student does not use primary accurate empathy to acknowledge the client's feelings about going home and being alone. It might be better to say, *"You feel worried about being home alone because you do not have a support system nearby. Is that correct?"* or, *"You feel like you will be lonely at home because your sister and neighbor are not able to visit. Is that correct?"*

3. The student does not discuss any available community supports.

4. The student does not indicate any follow-up by the OT before the client's discharge.

5. It is unprofessional to state that the client reminds the student of her grandmother. A client may also perceive this statement as an insult.

6. It is not appropriate for the student to give the client her personal phone number or to imply that she will visit the client at home. The student must maintain professional boundaries.

7. **Students and employees must always adhere to the facility's policies and procedures regarding any gifts from clients**. Usually, there are rules in place against accepting "tips" or gifts worth more than a nominal amount. In this scenario, the student should not be accepting this monetary gift. Facilities often only allow acceptance of small items such as flowers or food that can be shared with the department (such as a box of doughnuts, cookies, or candy). If the client would like to express appreciation with a larger gift, the facility might allow a monetary donation to the rehabilitation department (e.g., to purchase a piece of equipment) or the facility's charitable foundation.

8.   Do not make guarantees, such as, *"Everything will be fine"* or *"You will make a complete recovery."* In this situation, it might be better to say something like, *"The health team will try to make your transition home as smooth as possible. We will do our best to address your concerns before you are discharged."*

Worksheet 2-10: People-First Language and Term Usage

People-first language and the appropriate use of diagnostic terms makes a profound difference on the focus and perception that others have on the individual with a disabling condition. In the list that follows, indicate whether the phrase is an appropriate (A) or inappropriate (I) use of descriptive language.

1.   I. The blind people

     This should read "The persons who have blindness."

2.   I. The athetoid child

     This should read "The child who has athetoid cerebral palsy."

3.   I. Crazy person

     This should read "The person who has serious mental illness."

4.   A. Individual who has served in combat

5.   A. Person who has a disability

6.   I. Victim of depression

     People should not be referred to as victims of a disease. A more empowering statement would be "The person who has depression."

7.   I. Person who is crippled

     The word crippled is no longer appropriate for use in conversation. More appropriate terms are "The person who has a disability" or "The client who is unable to ambulate."

8.   I. The child with leukemia is a heroic boy

     People facing a disease process do not typically describe themselves as heroes; they are simply dealing with a disease.

9.   A. Wheelchair user

10. I. The epileptic

     People should not be referred to as a diagnosis. It would be better to say, "The client who has epilepsy."

11. I. Downs kid

     This is not people-first language. It would be better to say "The child who has Down syndrome."

12. I. The schiz I am working with today

     This is not people-first language and also is a derogatory way to say "schizophrenia."

13. I. The borderline

     This is not people-first language and dehumanizes individuals with the diagnosis of borderline personality disorder.

14. A. The person with cancer

15. I. The older man who is mentally retarded

     While this is people-first language, the term "intellectual disability" is preferred (American Psychiatric Association, 2013; Harris, 2013).

16. I. Suffers from Alzheimer's

     It is more appropriate to say "The person who is diagnosed with Alzheimer disease."

17. I. Wheelchair-bound

     The correct term is wheelchair user.

18. A. Senior who lives in an active adult community

19. I. Group of old people

    Terms such as seniors, mature adults, and older clients are more respectful.

20. I. Client is max assist

    The client is not an assist level. It is better to say "Client requires max assist for..." (Morreale & Borcherding, 2017).

Worksheet 2-11: Written Communication

Resources: Davis & Rosee, 2015; Morreale & Borcherding, 2017

1. Proofread written communication. This note contains misspelled words (i.e., correct words are "fair" and "meet" rather than "fare" and "meat") and poor grammar (i.e., correct verb is "spent" rather than "spend").

2. Do not use slang such as "hey" and "wanna."

3. Do not use unprofessional abbreviations such as "u" or "thx."

4. Use a greeting or salutation such as "Dear."

5. Use the person's full, appropriate title (i.e., Professor Jones, Mrs. Jones). Ensure you have spelled the person's name correctly. This author has frequently experienced students spelling the author's surname incorrectly on homework assignments and emails (i.e., "Morreal" or "Morales" rather than the proper spelling of "Morreale").

6. Do not use all capitals in a sentence, as this denotes shouting.

7. The use of emoticons or emojis does not give a professional appearance.

8. Consider the tone of what is written and how it may be perceived. This note conveys an angry and accusatory tone.

9. It is better to spell out standard abbreviations, such as "as soon as possible."

10. Use a closing such as "Sincerely."

Here is the same note written in a more useful format:

Dear Professor Jones,
I would like to meet with you to discuss my research paper grade. Please let me know a time that would be convenient for you. Thank you.
   Sincerely,
   Mary Smith

Worksheet 2-12: Medical Terminology and Abbreviations

Resources: Gateley & Borcherding, 2017; Morreale & Borcherding, 2017, Sames, 2015

1. Child Dx c̄ TBI demonstrates poor graphomotor and scissors skills 2°↓FM Ⓑ UE

   The child diagnosed with traumatic brain injury demonstrates poor graphomotor and scissors skills secondary to decreased fine-motor abilities in both upper extremities.

2. Client Fx Ⓛ humerus 6 wks ago 2° fall at home. Reports Ⓛ shoulder pain 7/10 & has ↓ P/AROM flex/abd, ER/IR which limit BADLs/IADLs.

   Client fractured left humerous 6 weeks ago due to a fall at home. Client reports left shoulder pain level as a 7 on a scale of 1 to 10. Client has decreased passive and active range of motion for flexion/abduction, and external/internal rotation which limit basic and instrumental activities of daily living.

3. Pt. c/o chest pain. Hx of MI 2016. EKG and CXR today are –, VS stable. NKA

   Patient complains of chest pain. Client has a history of myocardial infarction in 2016. Electrocardiogram and chest x-ray performed today were both negative. Vital signs are stable. There are no known allergies.

4. DOA to behavioral health unit 4/10/2021, Dx of depression. Client also has OCD which manifests in frequent washing of hands and personal-care items, impeding proper use of nightly CPAP and orthosis for CTS. PMH: PVD, HTN.

   4/10/2021 is client's date of admission to behavioral health unit with diagnosis of depression. Client also has obsessive compulsive disorder which manifests in frequent washing of hands and personal-care items, impeding proper use of nightly continuous positive airway pressure device, and orthosis for carpal tunnel syndrome.

5. X-ray Ⓡwrist/hand neg. EMG +ⓇCTS

   X-rays of right wrist and hand were negative. Electromyogram is positive for right carpal tunnel syndrome.

6. Dx: COPD: HOB 30°, BRP, OOB c̄ walker

   Diagnosis is chronic obstructive pulmonary disease. Head of bed needs to be raised at 30 degrees, client is allowed bathroom privileges and can get out of bed but must use a walker.

7. Dx: PTSD, PMH:ⓁBKA,ⓇAKA 2° IED during Iraq deployment

   Diagnosis is post-traumatic stress disorder. Client's past medical history includes a left below-knee amputation and right above-knee amputation due to injury from an improvised explosive device while deployed in Iraq.

8. 7 y.o.♀Dx c̄ ASD, ADHD has an URI

   The 7-year-old girl diagnosed with autism spectrum disorder and attention deficit hyperactivity disorder has an upper respiratory infection.

9. OT eval & tx; NWB ⓁLE, transfers, ADLS, BUE ther ex; 5 X wk X 2 wks

   Physician's orders: Occupational therapy evaluation and treatment. Left lower extremity status is non–weight-bearing. Treatment to include transfers, activities of daily living, bilateral upper extremity therapeutic exercise. Five times per week for 2 weeks.

10. OT 2/wk X 4 wks: US, e-stim toⓇshoulder, ROM, PREs, BADLs/IADLs

    Physician's orders: Occupational therapy 2 times per week for 4 weeks for ultrasound and electrical stimulation to right shoulder, range of motion, progressive resistive exercises, basic and instrumental activities of daily living.

Worksheet 2-13: Avoiding Documentation Errors

Here are some corrections and suggestions for professional documentation: Gateley & Borcherding, 2017; Merriam-Webster, 2001; Morreale & Borcherding, 2017; Sames, 2015

1. The <u>wheelchair bound client</u> was able to <u>preform</u> wheelchair mobility independently to go from his hospital room to the <u>dinning</u> room.

   The client was able to perform wheelchair mobility independently to go from his hospital room to the dining room.

2. The <u>students musical</u> instruments were stored in the band teacher's office.

   This sentence does not indicate whether only one student had multiple instruments stored (e.g., The student's musical instruments were stored in the band teacher's office) or if multiple students had their instruments stored (e.g., The students' musical instruments were stored in the band teacher's office).

3. The <u>COPD client</u> stated she becomes <u>OBS</u> when performing heavy activities for more <u>then</u> a few minutes.

   Use people-first language: The client with COPD stated she becomes SOB when performing heavy activities for more than a few minutes.

   (OBS is abbreviation for organic brain syndrome. SOB is abbreviation for shortness of breath.)

4. The <u>Occupational Therapy Assistant</u> instructed the client on therapy <u>puddy</u> exercises.

    The sentence may vary depending on the intended audience or purpose of the notation:

    The occupational therapy assistant instructed the client on therapy putty exercises.

    The client received skilled instruction on therapy putty exercises.

    The client was instructed in therapy putty exercises by the OTA.

    The occupational therapy assistant instructed the client in exercises using therapy putty.

5. The <u>senile PT. was seen</u> for 30 minutes bedside to <u>help</u> her eat breakfast.

    The pt. with cognitive impairment participated in therapy 30 minutes bedside for skilled feeding instruction during breakfast.

    The pt. diagnosed with Alzheimer's disease participated in 30-minute therapy session bedside for skilled instruction in self-feeding at mealtime.

    The pt. with dementia was able to participate in therapy for 30 minutes bedside, with session focusing on skilled feeding interventions at mealtime.

    (PT stands for physical therapist or physical therapy. "Help" does not denote a skilled intervention.)

6. The client's <u>dysphasia</u> contributed to his <u>inspiration pnumonia</u>.

    The client's dysphagia contributed to his aspiration pneumonia.

7. The child needed <u>modified assistance</u> to <u>donn</u> his orthosis.

    This sentence needs a standard term for assist level, such as, "The child needed moderate assistance to don his orthosis" or "The child donned his orthosis with modified independence."

8. The client who lives in an <u>apartment for old people stated "he</u> cannot wait to go home."

    The client who lives in senior housing stated, "I cannot wait to go home."

    The client expressed that he could not wait to go back home to his retirement community.

    The client temporarily resides at an assisted living facility and states that he "cannot wait" to go home.

9. The client used his <u>bad</u> hand to grasp the bed rail when rolling to the left.

    The client used his affected hand to grasp the bed rail when rolling to the left.

    The client used his weak hand to grasp the bed rail when rolling to the left.

10. The TBI worked on ↓ safety and ↑ left neglect to improve IADL performance.

    Use people-first language: The client with TBI worked on ↑ safety and ↓ left neglect to improve IADL performance.

Worksheet 2-14: Avoiding Documentation Errors—More Practice

Here are some corrections and suggestions for professional documentation (Gateley & Borcherding, 2017; Merriam-Webster, 2001; Morreale & Borcherding, 2017; Sames, 2015).

1. The student asked if the OTA could help her write <u>her</u> name<u>?</u>
    The student asked if the OTA could help her write the student's name.

2. The resident exhibited urinary <u>incontinents</u> and <u>stated "I</u> have a urinary <u>track</u> infection<u>".</u>
    The resident exhibited urinary incontinence and stated, "I have a urinary tract infection."

3. The client was instructed in <u>arom</u> exercises so that her <u>bad</u> arm does not get stiff.
    The client was instructed in AROM exercises to prevent stiffness of her affected arm.
    The client was instructed in AROM exercises to prevent stiffness of her weak upper extremity.

4. The home health <u>aid</u> was <u>adapt</u> at <u>transfering</u> clients.
    The home health aide was adept at transferring clients.

5. The client's throat was sore <u>because the speech pathologist made the client speak two long in therapy.</u>
    It is best to write objectively and avoid criticizing or blaming another professional, student, or colleague in a therapy note (Kettenbach, 2009; Scott, 2013). Also, "two" should be "too."
    The client reported throat soreness following his speech therapy session.
    The client reported that his sore throat started around 3:00 p.m.

6. The pt.'s torn rotary <u>cup</u> required surgery and afterward his deltoid was painful when <u>palpitated</u>.
The pt's torn rotator cuff needed surgical repair, after which the patient reported pain in deltoid upon palpation.

7. The two <u>OTA's</u> treated the <u>OT's</u> to lunch when they got a promotion.
In the above sentence it is not clear who got the promotion:
The two OTAs treated the OTs to lunch when those OTs got a promotion.
The two OTAs treated the OTs to lunch when those OTAs got a promotion.

8. The child <u>griped</u> the toy steering wheel with her <u>dominate</u> right hand and used her left hand to press the horn.
The child gripped the toy steering wheel with her dominant right hand and used her left hand to press the horn.

9. The clients' <u>tremers</u> made it unsafe for her to use the <u>parrafin</u> machine.
The client's tremors made it unsafe for her to use the paraffin machine.

10. The <u>Autistic</u> toddler exhibited a positive <u>babinski</u> sign.
The toddler with autism exhibited a positive Babinski sign.

Worksheet 2-15: Documentation Fundamentals

Resources: AOTA, 2018; Gateley & Borcherding, 2017; Morreale & Borcherding, 2017; Sames, 2015

1. No case number present
2. Client's full name not delineated
3. Date of client contact not indicated
4. Time does not indicate if it is a.m. or p.m.
5. Department of occupational therapy not indicated
6. Type of note not delineated (contact note)
7. Initials are not acceptable for OTA signature
8. OTA credentials not indicated with signature
9. Note is not co-signed by OT (when required by law or facility policy)
10. Error not corrected properly (not initialed or dated)
11. Blank space exists between end of note and signature
12. Nonstandard abbreviations used (i.e., eff. and aft.)
13. Note does not relate AROM to occupational performance

Worksheet 2-16: Managing a Schedule

Daily schedules will vary based on factors such as: actual number of clients, length of intervention sessions, unexpected circumstances, amount of real time spent on chart review, supervision, staff communication, client transport, documentation, and so forth. In the following examples, the two blank time frames (mid-morning and mid-afternoon) allow for breaks and catching-up if needed. While there are several different time frames that would work for the caseload presented, here are two suggested schedules:

Time	Sample Schedule A	Sample Schedule B
8:30 a.m.	Organize workday/collaborate with OT supervisor	Organize workday/collaborate with OT supervisor
9:00 a.m.	Mabel	Mabel
9:30 a.m.	Leroy	Leila
10:00 a.m.	Leila	Leroy
10:30 a.m.		Tim
11:00 a.m.	Meeting	Meeting

Time	Sample Schedule A	Sample Schedule B
11:30 a.m.	Tim	
12:00 p.m.	Lunch	Mary
12:30 p.m.	Mary	Lunch
1:00 p.m.	Ellen	Jim
1:30 p.m.	Jim	Mario
2:00 p.m.	Mario	Natasha
2:30 p.m.	Harvey	
3:00 p.m.		Ellen
3:30 p.m.	Natasha	Harvey
4:00 p.m.	Complete paperwork/collaborate with OT supervisor	Complete paperwork/collaborate with OT supervisor
4:30 p.m.	Workday ends	Workday ends

1. Mary sustained a stroke and requires instruction in self-feeding. Her schedule includes physical therapy at 9:00 a.m. and speech therapy at 3:00 p.m.
    It is preferable to do a feeding session at mealtime. Scheduling Mary at lunch time today should be appropriate.

2. Tim has colon cancer and requires instruction in energy conservation. He receives chemotherapy at 1:00 p.m..
    Tim may feel ill following his chemotherapy, so therapy should be implemented prior to that time.

3. Mabel sustained a stroke and requires instruction in grooming. She receives physical therapy daily at 10:30 a.m. and speech therapy at 2:00 p.m.
    A good time would be during normal morning self-care. The suggested schedule allows for Mabel to have a rest period before physical therapy.

4. Leroy has undergone rotator cuff surgery and requires instruction in post-surgical care of the involved extremity before his discharge at noon.
    Leroy must be seen in the morning.

5. Jim has Parkinson's disease and requires instruction in safe transfers. He is scheduled for physical therapy at 3:00 p.m.
    He should be allowed time for a rest period before or after physical therapy; after physical therapy would probably be too late in the day.

6. Leila sustained a left femur fracture and now must use a walker. She needs recommendations for durable medical/adaptive equipment prior to her discharge at noon. She is scheduled for physical therapy at 8:30 a.m.
    Therapy must begin after 9:00 a.m. (after physical therapy session) and by 11:30 a.m. (before noon discharge).

7. Natasha has undergone surgery for a right below-knee amputation and needs exercises to increase her upper body strength and endurance. She receives physical therapy daily at 11:00 a.m.
    Natasha's time frame is flexible but occupational therapy cannot conflict with physical therapy.

8. Ellen sustained multiple trauma from a motor vehicle accident. She needs a right resting hand orthosis today. Physical therapy is scheduled for 2:00 p.m.
    Ellen's time frame is flexible but cannot conflict with physical therapy.

9. Mario sustained a stroke and needs activities to decrease his left neglect and improve cognition. He is scheduled for an MRI at 3:00 p.m.
    It is prudent to schedule Mario at least 1 hour prior to his MRI to complete his session.

10. Harvey is recovering from pneumonia and is being discharged tomorrow. He needs a home exercise program to increase activity tolerance. He is scheduled for physical therapy at 12:30 p.m.
    Harvey will require a rest period between therapy sessions.

References

American Occupational Therapy Association. (2018). Guidelines for documentation of occupational therapy. *American Journal of Occupational Therapy, 72*(Suppl. 2), 7212410010. https:// doi.org/ 10.5014/ajot.2018.72S203

American Occupational Therapy Association. (2019). Enforcement procedures for the AOTA occupational therapy code of ethics. *American Journal of Occupational Therapy, 73*(Suppl. 2), 7312410003. https://doi.org/10.5014/ajot.2019.73S210

American Psychiatric Association. (2013). *Diagnostic and statistical manual of mental disorders* (5th ed.).

American Occupational Therapy Association. (2020). AOTA 2020 occupational therapy code of ethics. *American Journal of Occupational Therapy, 74*(Suppl. 3), 7413410005. https://doi.org/10.5014/ajot.2020.74S3006

Centers for Disease Control and Prevention. (2002, October 25). *Guideline for hand hygiene in health-care settings: Recommendations of the healthcare infection control practices advisory committee and the HIPAC/SHEA/APIC/IDSA hand hygiene task force.* https://www.cdc.gov/mmwr/PDF/rr/rr5116.pdf

Centers for Disease Control and Prevention. (2020). *Hand hygiene guidance.* Retrieved May 12, 2020, from https://www.cdc.gov/handhygiene/providers/guideline.html

Davis, L. & Rosee, M. (2015). *Occupational therapy student to clinician.* SLACK Incorporated

DeIuliis, E. D. (2017). *Professionalism across occupational therapy practice.* SLACK Incorporated.

Gateley, C. A., & Borcherding, S. (2017). *Documentation manual for occupational therapy: Writing SOAP notes* (4th ed.). SLACK Incorporated.

Harris, J. C. (2013). New terminology for mental retardation in DSM-5 and ICD-11. *Current Opinion in Psychiatry, 26*(3), 260-262. http://www.medscape.com/viewarticle/782769

Kettenbach, G. (2009). *Writing patient/client notes: Ensuring accuracy in documentation* (4th ed.). F. A. Davis Company.

Kornblau, B. L., & Burkhardt, A. (2012). *Ethics in rehabilitation: A clinical perspective* (2nd ed.). SLACK Incorporated.

Merriam-Webster. (2001). *Merriam-Webster's guide to punctuation and style* (2nd ed.).

Morreale, M. J., & Amini, D. (2016). *The occupational therapist's workbook for ensuring clinical competence.* SLACK Incorporated.

Morreale, M. J., & Borcherding, S. (2017). *The OTA's guide to documentation* (4th ed.). SLACK Incorporated.

National Board for Certification in Occupational Therapy. (2020a). *NBCOT professional practice standards for COTA and candidates seeking the COTA designation.* https://www.nbcot.org/-/media/NBCOT/PDFs/Practice-Standards-COTA.ashx?la=en&hash=7D24D031D583DBE15E6585A707F2702A84B2DF21

National Board for Certification in Occupational Therapy. (2020b). *Procedures for the enforcement of the NBCOT candidate/certificant code of conduct.* https://www.nbcot.org/-/media/NBCOT/PDFs/Enforcement_Procedures.ashx?la=en&hash=8EAADDC6A7013BC159A4CCE14EF6965D01FFEBF2

Sames, K. M. (2015). *Documenting occupational therapy practice* (3rd ed.). Pearson Education.

Scott, R. W. (2013). *Legal, ethical, and practical aspects of patient care documentation: A guide for rehabilitation professionals* (4th ed.). Jones & Bartlett Learning.

World Health Organization. (2009). *WHO guidelines on hand hygiene in health care: A summary.* https://www.who.int/publications/i/item/9789241597906-summary

References

Understanding Professional Roles and Responsibilities

Professional roles and responsibilities in occupational therapy include maintaining professional credentials, enabling appropriate, collaborative supervision, demonstrating cultural sensitivity, and performing services competently (American Occupational Therapy Association [AOTA], 2015a, 2015b, 2020a, 2020b). Occupational therapy practitioners also have a professional duty to behave ethically, attain on-going professional development, help victims of abuse, advocate for the profession, collaborate interprofessionally, and use evidence-informed practice (AOTA, 2015b, 2017, 2020a). This chapter presents worksheets and learning activities to help you understand professional roles, responsibilities, and expectations for fieldwork and clinical practice. Worksheet answers are provided at the end of the chapter.

Contents

Morreale, M. J. Developing Clinical Competence:
A Workbook for the OTA, Second Edition (pp. 109-163).
© 2022 SLACK Incorporated.

Worksheet 3-1

Roles and Responsibilities

For each of the following tasks, indicate if it is a skilled role/responsibility of an occupational therapist (OT) and/or occupational therapy assistant (OTA). For this exercise, assume the occupational therapy practitioner is competent in the designated tasks.

	Task	*OT*	*OTA*
1.	Instruct client in a home exercise program		
2.	Develop the occupational therapy intervention plan		
3.	Determine if a client performs a cooking task safely		
4.	Gait training		
5.	Teach positioning techniques to a parent of a child with cerebral palsy		
6.	Upgrade an exercise program		
7.	Determine discharge from occupational therapy		
8.	Respond to a referral to occupational therapy		
9.	Implement occupational therapy interventions		
10.	Teach one-handed shoe-tying		
11.	Complete the occupational therapy initial evaluation report independently		
12.	Administer a standardized assessment		
13.	Interpret initial evaluation results		
14.	Fabricate an orthosis		
15.	Customize a resident's wheelchair with specialized inserts		
16.	Administer superficial thermal modalities as the sole client intervention during a session		
17.	Document occupational therapy treatment		
18.	Provide intervention to a home care client		
19.	Instruct client in workplace ergonomics		
20.	Provide specialized instruction in self-care		
21.	Help a student put on boots for recess		
22.	Develop goals for an Individualized Education Program (IEP)		
23.	Assess transfer skills		
24.	Provide occupational therapy in a neonatal intensive care unit		
25.	Attain certification in hand therapy		
26.	Attain AOTA board certification in pediatrics		
27.	Use evidence-informed practice		
28.	Make recommendations to a teacher regarding compensatory techniques for a student receiving occupational therapy services		
29.	Delegate aspects of an occupational therapy initial evaluation		
30.	Write short-term goals in a treatment note as a sub-step toward implementing an established intervention plan		
31.	Update a client's intervention plan		

Worksheet 3-1 (continued)
Roles and Responsibilities

	Task	OT	OTA
32.	Write a discharge report independently		
33.	Adapt an ADL device to improve a client's self-care performance		
34.	Assess range of motion using a goniometer		
35.	Teach nursing staff how to apply a client's orthotic device		
36.	Provide a handout on cardiac precautions		
37.	Supervise a rehabilitation aide		
38.	Supervise a volunteer in the occupational therapy department		
39.	Supervise a Level I OTA student		
40.	Supervise a Level II OTA student		
41.	Supervise a Level I OT student		
42.	Supervise a Level II OT student		
43.	Lead an occupational therapy group in a behavioral health setting		
44.	Observe a child color a picture		
45.	Recommend durable medical equipment upon client's discharge home		
46.	Assess a client's orientation to person, place, and time		
47.	Inform nursing staff about a client's report of pain		
48.	Provide an inservice to the rehabilitation staff about an evidence-informed practice article		
49.	Assess vital signs		
50.	Attend a team meeting to discuss a client's care and progress		

Worksheet 3-2

Supervision

1. Steve, an OTA, was recently hired to work at a facility that has two OTs and three other OTAs on staff. Steve feels he needs more supervision from his supervising OT than he has been receiving since starting work 2 weeks ago. What primary action should Steve take?

   A. Ask coworkers how much supervision time they each receive

   B. Discuss concerns with the rehabilitation director

   C. Discuss concerns with his supervising OT

   D. Wait and see if supervision improves over the next several weeks

2. Huma, an OTA student, is performing Level II fieldwork in a school setting. During the first week, her fieldwork educator asked her to perform various standardized formal assessments on clients without direct supervision. Because Huma has never administered those specific assessments and did not learn about them in school, she informed her fieldwork educator about her inexperience. The fieldwork educator responded that the caseload is much busier than normal this week, she is confident in Huma's abilities, and those assessments really need to be completed. The fieldwork educator also apologized for not having the time to watch Huma perform those assessments this week but suggested that Huma take the assessments home to review them ahead of time. What should Huma's primary action be?

   A. Contact her academic fieldwork coordinator

   B. Take the assessments home to review them

   C. Quit fieldwork

   D. Speak to the rehabilitation director

3. The OT has delegated a client intervention to an OTA today. The OTA feels the intervention is not in the best interest of this client and is very uneasy about implementing it. When discussing these concerns with the OT, the OTA is told not to worry and to perform the intervention with the client, despite the OTA's continued apprehension. What should be the OTA's primary action?

   A. Perform the delegated intervention

   B. Ask another colleague to perform the intervention

   C. Quit and go home

   D. Speak to the OT's supervisor

4. An entry-level OTA was hired recently to work in an inpatient rehabilitation setting. The OTA is a bit overwhelmed and is running behind with today's schedule. The occupational therapy aide, who has worked there for 15 years and is very good with clients, offers to help. Which of the following tasks is more suitable for the OTA to delegate to the aide?

   A. Teaching a client with a recent total hip replacement how to use a sock assist

   B. Reviewing a client's home exercise program for accurate performance

   C. Asking a client with a recent lower limb amputation to fill out a leisure inventory

   D. Determining if the client requires any durable medical equipment for home

Worksheet 3-2 (continued)
Supervision

5. An OTA is supervising a volunteer in the outpatient OT department. The volunteer is enrolled in college and studying to be an OTA. As a result, the volunteer is familiar with how to use adaptive equipment. The volunteer is at the site because of wanting to learn more about occupational therapy but it is not a fieldwork experience. Which of the following is more appropriate for the OTA to allow the volunteer to do?
    A. Cut out Velcro tabs for orthotic devices
    B. Review charts to learn more about OT documentation
    C. Teach a client how to use a buttonhook
    D. Provide hand-over-hand assistance to help a client with decreased hand strength learn to use a reacher

Morreale, M. J. (2022). *Developing clinical competence: A workbook for the OTA* (2nd ed.). SLACK Incorporated.

Learning Activity 3-1: Supervision Situations

Imagine you are an OTA with 15 years of experience working at various skilled nursing facilities. The occupational therapy department at your current facility consists of you, one OT, plus an occupational therapy aide who is employed by the nursing home. You have worked at this site for 9 years, but your OT supervisor is a recent graduate and 20 years younger than you. The rehabilitation director is a physical therapist. Reflect on the following scenarios described, considering these two different employment situations.

> Employment situation #1: You are a full-time employee of the nursing home, but the OT is contracted through an agency
>
> Employment situation #2: You and the OT are both employed full-time by the nursing home

As you complete the questions, determine if the actions you would take would be the same or different if working at either of the two jobs.

1. Upon meeting the OT for the first time to discuss expectations and a supervision schedule, what might you say to help set the tone for a positive collaborative working relationship?

2. The OT wants to learn more about the facility and keeps asking you questions about facility policies, procedures, and how to use the electronic documentation system and some of the rehabilitation equipment. This is negatively affecting your productivity levels, and some days you almost feel like you are supervising the OT instead of the other way around. What are your thoughts about this and what would you do?

3. You would like to implement some new evidence-based procedures for occupational therapy client interventions that you learned at a recent AOTA conference. You are really looking forward to trying out these techniques, but the OT tells you, *"I never even heard about that in school or on fieldwork so I think we will pass on that."* How might you respond?

4. The OT has arrived 30 minutes late to work 3 days this week, which has limited your supervision time. How would you handle this situation?

5. You are working in a state that allows OTs and OTAs to use electrotherapeutic agents. You are competent in the use of neuromuscular electrical stimulation [NMES] because you attended several courses to learn its use and have experience implementing it under OT supervision at your prior OTA job. You ask your OT supervisor if you can try using NMES on a current client who has shoulder subluxation resulting from a stroke. The OT responds by saying, *"Oh, I think I read something about that when I was in OT school, so maybe it could help. Unfortunately, I never actually learned how to use that modality."* What would you do if the client could potentially benefit from this specialized intervention?

6. Although you feel the OT is a very nice person, you do not have much in common with this individual due to the large age gap and your different political and/or religious views. What could you do to promote a congenial working environment?

7. You observe the OT fabricate and issue several orthotic devices that have significant cosmetic defects. You believe you can do a better job making these orthoses because you have much more experience with this. What would you do?

8. Due to some unplanned meetings at work today, the OT is unable to treat several of the patients. You already have a very full caseload with no time for additional clients, so the OT tells you, *"Just grab some cognitive worksheets for the aide to use with my patients at bedside to address unilateral inattention and poor problem solving. This way you can document that these clients had some OT today and I'll sign off on it later. Administration is already on our case this month because they think our productivity levels are too low."* You know this is not ethical, but you do not want to get in trouble with your boss. What do you do?

Adapted from Morreale, M. J., & Amini, D. (2016). *The occupational therapist's workbook for ensuring clinical competence.* SLACK Incorporated.

Learning Activity 3-2: State Regulation

Each state has its own requirements regarding occupational therapy practice. Information on credentialing and links to individual state regulatory boards can be found on the AOTA website (www.aota.org), National Board for Certification in Occupational Therapy (NBCOT) website (www.nbcot.org), or by doing an internet search. It is important to realize that individual states may differ in the amount or type of mandatory continuing education hours and/or professional development activities needed to maintain licensure in that state. These requirements may also differ from the professional development/continuing education requirements needed to maintain NBCOT certification. Occupational therapy practitioners have a professional obligation to participate in on-going professional development activities, maintain appropriate credentials, and be competent in the relevant skills needed for ethical occupational therapy practice (AOTA, 2015a, 2015b, 2017). The questions that follow will help you learn more about occupational therapy licensure in the state in which you plan to work. You can also complete Learning Activity 3-4 to develop a professional development plan for your own continuing competence.

Instructions: Consider the state in which you plan to work as an OTA. Visit the website of the agency that regulates occupational therapy practice there and answer the questions that follow.

State in which you plan to work as an OTA: _____

Licensure

How does that state regulate occupational therapy practice for OTAs?
☐ Licensure   ☐ Authorization   ☐ State certification   ☐ Not regulated
What department in that state has jurisdiction over occupational therapy? In New York, for example, occupational therapy is regulated by the New York State Education Department, Office of the Professions. Occupational therapy in the state you wish to work in is regulated by: _____

_____

_____

What is the contact information for OTA regulatory information for the state in which you want to work?
Website address: _____
Phone number: _____
Does that state require passing the NBCOT exam in order to practice as an OTA in that state? ☐ Yes   ☐ No
Does that state offer an option of a temporary license or limited permit allowing OTA practice before the NBCOT exam is taken or passed? ☐ Yes   ☐ No
If applicable, what is the cost to apply for a temporary license or limited permit? _____
If applicable, how long is a temporary license or limited permit good for? _____
What is the cost to apply for licensure? _____
In that state, licensure must be renewed every _____ years.
What continuing education or other requirements are needed in order to maintain licensure in that state?_____

_____

_____

_____

Scope of Practice

Does that state require a prescription in order for an occupational therapy evaluation to be performed?
☐ Yes   ☐ No
Does that state require a prescription in order for an occupational therapy treatment program to be implemented?
☐ Yes   ☐ No
What health professionals can legally write a prescription for occupational therapy in that state (i.e., physician, nurse practitioner, optometrist)? _____

_____

Can an OTA perform an evaluation in that state? ☐ Yes   ☐ No
Explain briefly:_____
_____
_____
_____
_____

What supervision requirements for an OTA are specified in that state? _____
_____
_____
_____
_____

What types of interventions are specified under the scope of occupational therapy practice in that state? _____
_____
_____
_____
_____
_____

Are OTAs allowed to use superficial thermal modalities in that state (i.e., hot packs, paraffin)? ☐ Yes   ☐ No
Are OTAs allowed to use advanced physical agent modalities in that state (i.e., ultrasound, electrical stimulation)
☐ Yes   ☐ No
What additional training, supervision, continuing education, or other criteria, if any, are required in that state in
order for an OTA to use physical agent modalities? _____
_____
_____

Are there other types of occupational therapy interventions in that state requiring additional training, supervision, continuing education, or other criteria (i.e., vision training, feeding, swallowing)? _____
_____
_____
_____
_____
_____

Learning Activity 3-3: National Certification

Information regarding national certification of occupational therapy practitioners can be found at the NBCOT website (www.nbcot.org). Realize that professional development/continuing education requirements for retaining NBCOT certification could differ from the amount or type of mandatory professional development/continuing education needed to maintain licensure in individual states. OTs and OTAs have a professional obligation to attain appropriate credentials, participate in on-going professional development activities, and have competency in skills necessary for ethical occupational therapy practice (AOTA, 2015a; 2015b; 2017). This learning activity will help you to become more knowledgeable about NBCOT initial certification and renewal requirements. You can also complete Learning Activity 3-4 in this chapter to create a professional development plan for your own continuing competence.

Instructions: Visit the NBCOT website to answer the following questions regarding OTA certification.

1. How is NBCOT certification different than state regulation?_____
_____
_____
_____

2. How does NBCOT certification help consumers of occupational therapy? _____
_____
_____
_____
_____

3. How many questions are on the certification exam?_____
4. What is the scoring scale for the certification exam? ____ to ____ , and the passing score is _____ .
5. How much time is allotted for the certification exam? _____
6. What is the cost to take the exam? _____
7. What is the physical address of the testing site where you plan to take the certification exam (www.prometric.com)? _____
8. Of the acceptable forms of identification listed on the NBCOT website, which two will you use for entry to the exam?
    1. _____
    2. _____
9. Can a felony conviction prevent an OTA from initial certification or occupational therapy practice? Explain briefly. _____
_____
_____
_____

10. The initial certification period is good for how many years? _____
11. What professional development or continuing education requirements must be completed to maintain national certification after the initial certification period?_____
_____
_____
_____

12. Review the Certification Renewal Activities Chart on the NBCOT website. List several of those activities you might choose to participate in to maintain certification following successful completion of the exam (Morreale & Amini, 2016). _____
_____
_____
_____

Learning Activity 3-4: Professional Development Plan

A professional development plan helps OTAs to achieve personal career goals and meet professional requirements for credentialing. There are various professional opportunities available to OTAs that you might consider, such as attaining an advanced academic degree or credentialing by professional organizations in areas relevant to OTA practice (e.g., assistive technology or seating and wheeled mobility; Morreale and Amini, 2016). Perhaps you see yourself eventually switching to a completely different occupational therapy practice area or aspire to be an occupational therapy educator, hold a managerial role, or become involved in clinical research. You may also decide you want to "give back" to the occupational therapy profession through volunteer activities which could include joining an AOTA committee, running for an elected occupational therapy office, supervising students, providing some pro bono services, participating in advocacy efforts for people with disabilities or victims of human trafficking, and so forth. (Morreale & Amini, 2016).

On-going professional development and clinical competency are some of the essential professional responsibilities you will have as an OTA (AOTA, 2015a, 2015b, 2017). You must also complete any mandated continuing education/professional development requirements related to occupational therapy licensure in the specific state in which you plan to work. NBCOT also delineates professional development requirements for practitioners desiring to maintain NBCOT certification for personal/professional reasons or, in some instances, as mandated by state regulation. Be cognizant of the fact that individual states could have different or additional professional development requirements than what is needed to maintain national certification.

As you begin the process of creating a professional development plan, think about where you would like to see yourself professionally a year from now, several years from now and, perhaps 5 or 10 years from now. Reflect on the areas of knowledge or specific skills you would like to obtain or improve upon that are relevant to your current and/or desired occupational therapy role(s). Contemplate any interest you might have regarding involvement in volunteer opportunities (e.g., special causes, pet projects, humanitarian efforts), clinical research projects, or specific ways in which you would like to promote or "give back" to the profession of occupational therapy (Morreale & Amini, 2016).

Instructions: Complete the Professional Development Plan presented on the following two pages by first identifying your professional goals. List the specific activities that will aid you in attaining the desired knowledge or skills you identified or allow you to "give back" to the profession. Determine the specific sequence of steps needed for goal-attainment and establish a timeline as when you plan to complete each of those methods and goals.

Adapted from Morreale, M. J., & Amini, D. (2016). *The occupational therapist's workbook for ensuring clinical competence.* SLACK Incorporated.

Professional Development Plan

1. List a projected area of practice and the professional/career role(s) where you would like to see yourself working in for each of the following time frames:

   a. 1 year from now: _____
   _____

   b. 2 to 3 years from now:_____
   _____

   c. 5 years from now: _____
   _____

   d. 10 years from now: _____
   _____

2. List several areas of knowledge or specific skills you would like to obtain or improve upon at this time.

   a. _____
   b. _____
   c. _____
   d. _____
   e. _____
   f. _____

3. List personal areas of interest for volunteerism, advocacy, clinical research projects, or to promote the profession of occupational therapy (i.e., supervise a Level I fieldwork student, volunteer for an AOTA or state occupational therapy association committee, write an article about occupational therapy, participate in a research study, advocate for people with mental illness).

   a. _____
   b. _____
   c. _____
   d. _____

   Then, for each of the items you listed, use the following format to help you create a plan for professional development to meet your goals.

Reproduced with permission from Morreale, M. J., & Amini, D. (2016). *The occupational therapist's workbook for ensuring clinical competence.* SLACK Incorporated.

Professional Development Plan (continued)

Personal Goal: List desired role, area of knowledge or specific skills you would like to obtain or improve upon; area of interest for advocacy, volunteerism, clinical research projects, or promoting the profession	Overall time frame to attain this goal	List the general methods you would choose for goal attainment (e.g., attend a workshop, participate in a journal club/study group, volunteer for a local Alzheimer's or victim's rights organization, find a mentor)	List specific steps for how each of these methods will be accomplished (e.g., locate potential workshops within a 50-mile home radius, complete application for a bachelor's or master's program, contact three peers to form a journal club or study group, join a state's OT association)	Indicate a time frame by which each step/method will have been completed (e.g., by the end of this week, within 30 days, within 2 months, by end of this year, second year)	Date actually completed; if not completed in designated time frame, indicate the reasons why

Adapted from Morreale, M. J., & Amini, D. (2016). *The occupational therapist's workbook for ensuring clinical competence.* SLACK Incorporated.

Learning Activity 3-5: American Occupational Therapy Association

Visit the AOTA website (www.aota.org) in order to complete the following questions.

1. What is AOTA's mission statement?

2. List the five pillars of Vision 2025.
    1.
    2.
    3.
    4.
    5.

3. List five reasons why AOTA is a valuable organization for occupational therapy practitioners.
    1.
    2.
    3.
    4.
    5.

4. How does AOTA benefit the general public?

5. List several ways in which AOTA membership can help to advance your career.

6. List the five subscriptions that are free with AOTA membership.
    1.
    2.
    3.
    4.
    5.

7. List the nine AOTA Special Interest Sections (SIS) in the order you feel would be the most beneficial to you personally:
    1.
    2.
    3.
    4.
    5.
    6.
    7.
    8.
    9.

8. List two personal and two professional discounts exclusively available to AOTA members that you might consider using.

    Personal Discounts: Professional Discounts:
    1.   1.
    2.   2.

9. What is the free social networking site designed by AOTA that members can utilize?

10. Define AOTPAC and explain briefly the purpose of this organization.

11. Define ACOTE and explain briefly the purpose of this organization

12. What is the cost and specific type of AOTA membership available to you if you were to join today?

13. Are you planning to become a member of AOTA at this time? If not, are you planning to join at a specific time in the future or have not yet decided? Indicate the reasons for your decision.

Worksheet 3-3

Cultural Sensitivity

1. Carl, a 45-year-old male, has multiple sclerosis and has been receiving outpatient occupational therapy. Today the OTA, Cindy, is meeting and working with him for the first time. Carl was accompanied by another male whom Carl introduced as his husband. Cindy has deep religious beliefs that oppose gay marriage, causing personal uneasiness. What should the OTA do?
   A. Explain to the client her discomfort with his lifestyle, but that she will try to do her best to help him
   B. Immediately speak to the supervising OT and refuse to treat the client
   C. Educate the client regarding the OTA's religious beliefs and offer to pray for him
   D. Set aside personal feelings and treat client and his partner with respect

2. Ali sustained a myocardial infarction and was admitted to an acute care hospital. Sarah, an OTA, is scheduled to teach him skilled bathing techniques today. When she gets to Ali's room, he tells her it is against his religion to have a female other than his wife help him with bathing. There are no male occupational therapy practitioners on staff. Which of the following is the best course of action for the OTA?
   A. Reassure Ali that she is a trained health professional and tell him not to worry
   B. Work on pertinent client factors necessary for bathing
   C. Ask a male nurse to teach Ali bathing techniques
   D. Document that the client refused occupational therapy today

3. Chava, a 65-year-old woman and homemaker, devoutly follows the Orthodox sect of Judaism. She is in a rehabilitation hospital following an exacerbation of chronic obstructive pulmonary disease (COPD). Her occupational therapy goals include increasing activity tolerance for home management. To enhance participation in meal preparation, the plan is for Chava to incorporate energy conservation techniques while preparing her own lunch today in occupational therapy. Of the following food choices, which is more culturally sensitive for an occupational therapy practitioner to offer Chava as a possible lunch choice, assuming there are no medical dietary restrictions?
   A. Cheeseburger
   B. Scrambled eggs and bacon
   C. Turkey and cheese sandwich
   D. Fresh fruit salad with cottage cheese

4. Parita is 78 years old and recently emigrated from India to the United States. Parita sustained a cerebrovascular accident last week that resulted in left hemiparesis. She is presently in a rehabilitation hospital where the clients are expected to wear regular clothes during the day. The occupational therapy intervention plan includes goals for independent transfers and safe functional ambulation for home management tasks. Parita is able to use a hemi-walker with minimal assistance, but the OTA notes the hemi-walker keeps getting caught in Parita's sari, her traditional clothing. The OTA discusses this safety hazard with the client and suggests alternate garments, but Parita refuses to wear clothing other than her traditional sari. Besides planning to try modifying or pinning the garments (if the client will allow this) and discussing this with the OT, which of the following is the OTA's best course of action?
   A. Document that Parita has poor safety awareness
   B. Document that Parita needs to use a narrow-based quad cane
   C. Document the safety hazard and client education provided
   D. Recommend discharge from occupational therapy

Worksheet 3-3 (continued)
Cultural Sensitivity

5. Martin is a 60-year-old male who recently had surgery to repair a torn rotator cuff. As part of the post-surgical protocol, the OTA is instructing Martin on a home program of range of motion exercises, which the surgeon wants Martin to perform several times daily. Martin informs the OTA he does not think he can perform the exercises during a 24-hour period each weekend because his faith requires rest on the Sabbath. Which of the following is the best course of action for the OTA?

    A. Educate Martin regarding the medical necessity of the exercises and insist that Martin perform his exercises daily over the weekend

    B. Educate Martin regarding the medical necessity of the exercises and suggest Martin discuss this with his religious leader

    C. Tell Martin he does not have to perform the exercises on the Sabbath

    D. Document that Martin is noncompliant

6. Howard, a 38-year-old devout follower of the Orthodox sect of Judaism, is receiving outpatient occupational therapy following a flexor tendon repair to his dominant right hand. Which of the following goals would probably not be suitable for Howard?

    A. Ability to hold a prayer book

    B. Ability to don a tallit during prayer ritual

    C. Ability to manipulate rosary beads during prayer ritual

    D. Ability to use tefillin during prayer ritual

7. Olivia is a 25-year-old Christian female who follows a vegan lifestyle. She was admitted to an inpatient behavioral health unit with a diagnosis of depression. The occupational therapy intervention plan includes having Olivia complete a project in crafts group to help improve her self-esteem. The OTA has decided to give Olivia a choice of two projects. Of the following activities, which would generally be more culturally sensitive to have Olivia choose from?

    A. A basket weaving project using bamboo reeds

    B. Egg decorating for upcoming Easter holiday

    C. A dream catcher project using branches and wool yarn

    D. A coin purse leather lacing project

8. Eva is a 65-year-old female of Haitian descent. She has been receiving outpatient occupational therapy for several weeks to address her severe chronic shoulder pain. Today when Eva arrives, she informs the OTA that her pain has recently subsided due to a religious healing service she attended in her community 2 days ago. What should the OTA's primary response be?

    A. Express happiness that the client's pain is better

    B. Ignore what the client said. Based on the client's condition, this sudden recovery defies logic and the OTA does not want to offend the client by telling her that

    C. Tell the client that this seems very unlikely and her improvement is really from the therapy she received

    D. Inform the OT that the client should have a psychological evaluation

Worksheet 3-3 (continued)
Cultural Sensitivity

9. Claire, a 56-year-old devout Catholic, is in a rehabilitation hospital following surgery for removal of a brain tumor. Today happens to be Good Friday. To prepare for Claire's upcoming discharge to home next week, the OT would like the OTA to assess Claire's safety for meal preparation tasks. To obtain the requisite items from the food service department for the session, which of the following items are more culturally sensitive for the OTA to offer Claire as a possible lunch choice today, assuming there are no medical dietary restrictions?
    A. Turkey sandwich
    B. Grilled cheese sandwich
    C. Canned chicken noodle soup
    D. Microwavable pepperoni pizza

10. Lin is a 30-year-old Asian male who immigrated to the United States 8 months ago. Following back surgery, he unknowingly became addicted to prescription painkillers when following the recommended dosage and was recently admitted to an inpatient chemical dependency program. The OT and OTA have observed Lin on the unit performing his hobbies of reading, playing Solitaire, and completing crossword puzzles. However, while leading an expressive group that Lin is attending for the first time, the OTA observes that Lin tends to be very quiet during group and does not make eye contact with the OTA. He barely interacts with the other clients and does not openly express his feelings. Which of the following is a possible fit for the OTA to document?
    A. That the client is depressed
    B. That the client's interpersonal behaviors may be influenced by his culture
    C. That the client is noncompliant with group process
    D. That the client has a poor prognosis

Worksheet 3-4
Cultural Sensitivity—More Practice

1. Tamara is a 22-year-old single parent of a 4-year-old boy with typical development and a 6-year-old girl, Jayla, who has Down syndrome and attends kindergarten. Jayla is receiving school-based occupational therapy and Tamara is observing today's session. Tamara is 5'4" and weighs 240 lb. Her children are at the top end of normal developmental ranges for weight. The OT and OTA have observed that the lunches Jayla brings to school are not healthy choices. Of the following statements, which is more appropriate for the OTA to express to Tamara during the session?

   A. You and your children should go on a diet.

   B. It concerns me that your children are overweight.

   C. Do you understand that your obesity will prevent you from taking care of your kids properly?

   D. Would you be open to having a dietician come talk to you about strategies for purchasing a variety of snacks and meals for the children?

2. Priya, a 22-year-old female from India, has been attending college in the United States. She has been receiving outpatient occupational therapy due to a hand injury resulting from a fall. During a session with the OTA, Priya mentions that her fiancé will soon be coming to the United States. The OTA asks how long they have been dating and Priya replies, "*Oh, I haven't met him yet in person, but we have been texting and calling each other for the past 2 months. Our families think we are a good match and have arranged for us to marry soon.*" This arouses the OTA's curiosity. Which of the following choices is a more suitable response from the OTA?

   A. I did not know arranged marriages still happen in this day and age.

   B. That seems like a very old-fashioned concept.

   C. Sounds like you have something great to look forward to.

   D. What if you do not like him? Do you have any choice about getting married?

3. Antonio and his family emigrated from Europe to the United States 3 months ago. His 14-month-old son sustained upper and lower limb fractures in a recent car accident and is receiving occupational therapy. In order to adhere to orthopedic precautions and improve motor development for activities of daily living (ADLs) and play, the OTA is teaching Antonio and his wife how to position the toddler properly. As the OTA asks Antonio to demonstrate holding the toddler for the tasks of diapering and bathing, Antonio refuses and states, "*It is the women's job to change the baby's diaper and bathe him. My wife always does that. You can't expect a man to do those things.*" Of the following choices, which is likely more suitable for the OTA to do at this time?

   A. Insist that Antonio participate in diapering and bathing tasks as they are part of the child's intervention plan

   B. Tell Antonio that fathers in the United States actively participate in diapering and bathing tasks so he should also

   C. Work with Antonio on other aspects of the child's care that he feels are acceptable for him to participate in

   D. Tell Antonio and his wife that he is sexist and that Antonio's help is needed with the baby

Worksheet 3-4 (continued)

Cultural Sensitivity—More Practice

4. Huan is a 91-year-old Chinese male living in his adult son and daughter-in-law's home, as traditional for their culture. Huan is diagnosed with end-stage dementia and is frail, bedridden, and dependent in ADLs. The family expresses that they desire to keep their beloved older family member in their home. Huan is beginning to develop Stage 1 pressure areas on his ankle and sacrum. In addition to skilled nursing to address skin integrity, the physician ordered home care occupational therapy to educate the family on bed mobility and positioning. When working with the family, which of the following is the OTA's best course of action?

   A. Provide the family education as ordered while communicating respect for their interest in keeping Huan at home.

   B. Insist that the family place the client in a nursing home to care for him better

   C. Recommend that Huan participate in an adult day care program

   D. Recommend physical therapy to improve Huan's mobility using a walker

5. Abraham, a 65-year-old male diagnosed with COPD, has been referred to outpatient occupational therapy following a short stay in a rehabilitation hospital. The OT has delegated today's session to the OTA, Sarah. Abraham is a devout follower of an Orthodox sect of Judaism and owns a small retail business. Sarah immediately recognizes him from shopping at his store. Which of the following is generally more suitable for Sarah to do when first greeting Abraham?

   A. Shake hands and introduce herself as his OTA

   B. Lightly touch his arm or back and introduce herself as his OTA

   C. Give him a slight side hug and introduce herself as his OTA

   D. Avoid physical contact and introduce herself as his OTA

Adapted from Morreale, M. J., & Amini, D. (2016). *The occupational therapist's workbook for ensuring clinical competence.* SLACK Incorporated.

Learning Activity 3-6: Improving Cultural Awareness

Interview someone who has different religious beliefs than you or has a different cultural or ethnic affiliation. Choose one or more of the categories in the following table and compare and contrast them for the two of you. Some possible topics to discuss are presented. Can you think of other questions you might ask to further improve cultural awareness? Each person should volunteer information based on their personal level of comfort for disclosure.

Category	Topics You Might Explore	My Religion, Culture, or Ethnicity Is: _____	Other Person's Religion, Culture, or Ethnicity Is: _____
Appearance and attire	Are there specific requirements or special types of clothing? What types of religious garments/accessories are worn (e.g., shawl, fringes, cross, turban)? Is modesty important? Are head coverings important? What are the attitudes toward body size, tattoos, piercings, make-up, hair styles? Are there gender differences?		
More-valued/ less-valued professions	What professions are revered in that culture (e.g., rabbi, doctor, teacher, master craftsman)? What professions are considered least desirable?		
Dating rituals/ courtship	How do people typically meet (e.g., arranged marriage, matchmaker, bars or clubs)? What is the length of a courtship/engagement? What is the level of physical contact allowed? Is family approval needed?		
Marriage rituals	Is the ceremony inside a house of worship? What is the type of ceremony? What is the attire/adornment worn by bride/ groom (e.g., color of dress, henna designs, headwear, tuxedo)? Besides the couple, who else is involved in the ceremony? What type of celebration follows the ceremony?		

Category	Topics You Might Explore	My Religion, Culture, or Ethnicity Is: _____	Other Person's Religion, Culture, or Ethnicity Is: _____
Rites of passage	Is there a special ceremony/celebration for transition to adulthood (e.g., Bar Mitzvah, Quinceañera, debutante ball)?		
Death rituals	Is there a specific time frame for burial?		
	What type of services (e.g., wake, Shiva, church service)?		
	Is there a special gathering following the burial or wake?		
	What is the disposition of the body (mausoleum, burial, scattering of ashes)?		
	What type of clothing is worn by deceased?		
	What type of clothing is worn by persons mourning/paying respect?		
	What type of burial container is used (e.g., pine box, ornate casket, urn)?		
	Is there belief in an afterlife?		
	Is there on-going visiting of the deceased's final resting place by survivors?		
Family roles	Who provides care for older relatives?		
	Are parents expected to live with married children?		
	Are there gender/family member roles and responsibilities (e.g., matriarch, patriarch, do the women work outside of home, do fathers change diapers)?		
	What are the styles of parenting (e.g., authoritarian, permissive, co-parenting)?		
Lifestyle and behaviors	What are the attitudes toward smoking, alcoholic beverages, and caffeine?		
	Are there dancing restrictions?		
	What are the attitudes toward television, the internet, movies, newspapers?		

Category	Topics You Might Explore	My Religion, Culture, or Ethnicity Is: _____	Other Person's Religion, Culture, or Ethnicity Is: _____
Lifestyles, health, and sickness	What are the attitudes toward sickness or disability (e.g., punishment from God, stoic nature)? Is there belief in natural, holistic, or alternative treatments? Is there belief in cures from spiritual or healing rituals?		
Foods	Are there special foods for meals, holidays, and celebrations? Are there dietary considerations (e.g., Kosher diet, specific meat products prohibited)? Are there religious rituals or special methods involving food?		
Religious beliefs and rituals	Is there belief in a higher power or deity? Are there specific rituals within a house of worship (e.g., kneeling, receiving Holy Communion)? Are there specific rituals outside of a house of worship (e.g., observing the Sabbath, lighting candles, saying the Rosary)? Is there a sense of community? What are the types of sacraments?		
Special holidays	What cultural, secular, or religious holidays are celebrated? Why and how are each of those holidays celebrated?		

Learning Activity 3-7: Exploring Other Cultures

Choose one or more of the following places to visit that involve a different cultural or religious affiliation than yours. This should be a place you typically do not go to and are generally unfamiliar with. After your visit, reflect on that experience and answer the following questions. Consider the customs that are well-documented in that culture and avoid stereotypes.

- Ethnic grocery store or market
- An authentic ethnic restaurant
- Different affiliation of worship
- Ethnic clothing store

- Established ethnic area of city (e.g., Chinatown, Little Italy)
- Cultural festival
- Other

1. Describe what you observed about the demeanor and behavior of the typical population in that venue. For example, did residents, customers or congregation members appear friendly, busy, devout, joyous, serious, and so forth, and why do you think they behaved that way? Was there a sense of fellowship or community there? Did you notice any significant gender differences?

2. How would you describe the interactions between workers or religious leaders and their customers/members there? For example, did relationships appear to be very casual, business-oriented, social, or caring, and so forth?

3. Compare and contrast what the typical workers, customers, and members were wearing to what you and your family normally wear.

4. Describe specific cultural aspects evident in that venue's environment, such as décor, smells, sounds, and so forth.

5. Identify several things you observed, tasted, or experienced there that were unfamiliar or not typical for you and describe how you felt about that.

6. Would you expect to go there again? Why or why not?

Worksheet 3-5

Attaining Service Competency

1. At her new job, an entry-level OTA is expected to perform transfer training with a specific client who requires maximum assistance. The OTA is unsure that she knows how to do this safely by herself. Which primary course of action should the OTA take?

    A. Ask the physical therapist or nursing staff to transfer the client

    B. Ask the OT for help

    C. Obtain more information on transfer techniques from textbooks and the internet

    D. Perform a different intervention

2. Today an OTA was delegated an outpatient client who had hand surgery 4 weeks ago. The surgical site is healed, and there are no surgical precautions at this time. The doctor's orders and OT's intervention plan indicate that the client needs to work on increasing grip strength and fine-motor skills in order to better manage ADLs and return to work. The OTA did not learn about that particular surgical procedure in school. Which of the following is the best course of action for the OTA before the client arrives several hours from now?

    A. Ask another occupational therapy practitioner to treat the client

    B. Tell the OT it is unethical for the OTA to treat this client

    C. Review client's chart and use resources to obtain more information regarding the client's diagnosis

    D. Reschedule the client for another day when the OTA's supervisor can be in the room at the same time to supervise

3. An OTA student is performing Level II fieldwork in an outpatient setting. To receive a passing grade at that site, students are expected to fabricate orthotic devices for various clients needing them. One of the clients coming to therapy tomorrow needs a wrist extension orthosis, and this intervention is delegated to the OTA student. However, the student has not made an orthosis since taking a skills class in school 6 months ago. Of the following choices, which is the best course of action for the OTA student?

    A. Make the orthosis on the client with the OT supervising

    B. Review an orthotic device textbook and videos

    C. Ask the OT to fabricate the client's orthosis, as OTAs are not allowed to fabricate orthotic devices

    D. Ask permission to make a similar orthotic device on an occupational therapy practitioner today

4. An OTA would like to learn more about sensory integration interventions for children with autism. Which of the following is the best method for the OTA to attain this information?

    A. Read evidence-based professional literature

    B. Attend professional seminars

    C. Ask a more experienced occupational therapy practitioner to mentor the OTA

    D. All of the above

5. An entry-level OTA just started a job at a school setting. When would it be most appropriate for the OTA to stop participating in professional development activities?

    A. When the OTA is fully competent in the current job

    B. When the OTA is no longer working as an OTA

    C. When the OTA has 10 years of clinical experience

    D. When the OTA has 5 years of clinical experience

Worksheet 3-5 (continued)

Attaining Service Competency

6. After attending 25 hours of occupational therapy seminars during a current NBCOT recertification cycle, a hospital-based OTA is on a tight budget and cannot afford any more professional seminars this year. To help accrue the remaining professional development units needed for NBCOT recertification, the OTA can choose from all except which of the following activities to complete?

    A. Develop a client satisfaction survey for the hospital's occupational therapy department
    B. Supervise Level I fieldwork students
    C. Publish an article in a local newspaper regarding the hospital's occupational therapy low-vision program
    D. Publish an article in an occupational therapy magazine that is not peer-reviewed

Learning Activity 3-8: Developing Professional Reasoning

During your fieldwork experience you are expected to teach energy conservation techniques for home management to a group of clients with COPD. Your supervisor tells you that an essential component of the client instruction is teaching them how to incorporate proper breathing techniques as the instrumental activities of daily living (IADLs) are performed. You have never worked with anyone with COPD and are not sure how to implement the task properly. The group is scheduled for 2 days from now. Consider how you will approach this dilemma and the possible outcomes.

Options to Address Problem	Potential Positive Outcomes if This Option Is Implemented	Potential Undesirable Outcomes if This Option is Implemented	Is This Option a Good Choice?
1. Tell your supervisor you are not competent to perform this task			
2. Ask your supervisor where you can get more information on this topic			
3. Ask your classmates or friends for help			
4. Try to remain calm and just "wing it" the day of the group			
5. Search for information resources			
Other options:			

What Relevant Resources Will You Use? (e.g., specific people to contact, book titles, websites, particular articles)	Action Plan for Each Resource (e.g., specific library databases, internet URLs, process for obtaining written materials/videos, contact phone numbers)
1.	
2.	
3.	
4.	
5.	

Worksheet 3-6

Evidence-Informed Practice

Occupational therapy practitioners use existing evidence and professional reasoning to make informed decisions regarding client care. A more current term that expands upon evidence-based practice is evidence-informed practice, which reflects not only the research but also clinical knowledge/expertise and patient expectations (Logan University, 2021). Evidence relevant to occupational therapy practice includes primary and secondary sources. Hierarchy of the levels of evidence is often depicted as a pyramid, with the highest level represented at the top (University of Notre Dame Australia, 2018). When reviewing information, practitioners should consider the data source and distinguish between peer-reviewed scholarly journals versus trade publications and popular magazines as these all differ significantly in intended audience, accountability, and content (Colorado State University, n.d.). OTs and OTAs should ensure that their clinical decisions are based on the best evidence that is available, including results from critically analyzed research, practitioner knowledge/expertise, and client preferences (Logan University, 2021; Morreale & Amini, 2016). Complete Worksheets 3-6 and 3-7 to test your understanding of basic research principles.

1. Which of the following situations would normally require that an occupational therapy practitioner consider the best available evidence when planning the intervention?
   A. For a client receiving radiation treatments at the wrist for bone cancer, implementing an ultrasound intervention per doctor's order to help reduce wrist pain and stiffness
   B. Deciding which brand of crayons to use with a child who is depressed
   C. Choosing to use a wheelchair with removable desk arms versus a wheelchair with non-removeable arm rests to transport a 45-year-old female client to therapy when both wheelchairs are available in the rehabilitation facility
   D. Suggesting that a special education teacher use a Samsung tablet versus an Apple iPad with a middle-school student diagnosed with autism spectrum disorder when both items are available in that setting

2. Which of the following situations would not typically necessitate that occupational therapy practitioners consider the best available evidence when planning the intervention?
   A. Having a client complete a Purdue Pegboard test to help the OT in determining the client's readiness to return to work
   B. Deciding whether to use a pen, pencil, or permanent marker when making a pattern for an orthotic device
   C. Suggesting mindfulness techniques and Tai Chi to help an adult client reduce anxiety
   D. Using a sensory approach when working on feeding and eating with a 5-year-old child with autism who has oral sensitivity

3. Which of the following publications is considered a trade magazine?
   A. *Advance for Occupational Therapy Practitioners*
   B. *American Journal of Occupational Therapy*
   C. *Time*
   D. *Psychology Today*

4. Which of the following choices is normally regarded as higher on the evidence pyramid?
   A. Cohort study
   B. Case report
   C. Systematic review
   D. Randomized controlled trial

Worksheet 3-6 (continued)
Evidence-Informed Practice

5. Which of the following types of evidence is not considered a primary source?
    A. Thesis
    B. Case report
    C. Randomized controlled trial
    D. Systematic review

Adapted from Morreale, M. J., & Amini, D. (2016). *The occupational therapist's workbook for ensuring clinical competence.* SLACK Incorporated.

Worksheet 3-7

Fundamentals of Research

Determine if the following statements are true (T) or false (F).

1. T ___   F ___   Newspaper articles are typically considered scholarly sources because they are reviewed by the editor before publication.

2. T ___   F ___   Randomized controlled trials are higher on the evidence pyramid than cohort studies and case reports.

3. T ___   F ___   Ways in which trade magazines differ from scholarly journals include factors such as glossy paper, colorized illustrations/pictures, and each issue beginning with page number one.

4. T ___   F ___   A systematic review is an individual research study that has a step-by-step process using a control group and experimental group.

5. T ___   F ___   The "gold standard" in medical research is the double-blind randomized control group pretest-posttest design.

6. T ___   F ___   A systematic review using quantitative methods to summarize results is a meta-analysis.

7. T ___   F ___   An example of a primary source is a systematic review.

8. T ___   F ___   Methods that collect and analyze data existing in non-numerical formats are used in a qualitative approach.

9. T ___   F ___   An example of a scholarly journal is *OT Practice*.

10. T ___   F ___   Diagnosis, age, cognitive status, and gender are examples of possible variables in qualitative and quantitative research.

11. T ___   F ___   Methods of data collection used in qualitative research often include interviews and review of artifacts.

12. T ___   F ___   In a statistical test, the fewer the participants, the more accurate the test outcome.

13. T ___   F ___   When a researcher includes more variables in a statistical test, a larger sample size is needed for accuracy.

14. T ___   F ___   In a statistical test, the less reliable an instrument is to measure a variable, the greater the sample size needed to ensure an accurate outcome.

15. T ___   F ___   Informed consent is normally not needed to become a study participant if the individual volunteers for that study

16. T ___   F ___   In experimental design studies, a random sampling of participants from a population or random assignment of participants to groups is always used.

17. T ___   F ___   In randomized controlled trials, the treatment group usually receives a placebo.

18. T ___   F ___   Double-blind refers to both the subjects and treatment providers not knowing which participants are part of the treatment group or control group.

Worksheet 3-7 (continued)

Fundamentals of Research

19. T ____ F ____ When performing qualitative research, data may be collected by observation and recorded as field notes.

20. T ____ F ____ The case study nonexperimental design involves only one participant and the gathered data can be numerical and non-numerical.

Learning Activity 3-9: Implementing Evidence-Informed Practice

Choose an occupational therapy topic you would like to learn more about from the following list. Narrow down your topic further by applying it to a specific relevant population (e.g., children with autism, well elderly, adults with Alzheimer's disease) or by choosing a more specific aspect of that category. Search the professional literature for five peer-reviewed research articles related to your topic. The articles must meet the following criteria:

- Have relevance to occupational therapy practice
- Published in peer-reviewed professional journals
- Published within the past 5 years
- The five articles in total must represent at least two different levels of the evidence

Include the citations for the five articles and identify the evidence level for each (e.g., case report, meta-analysis).

Possible topics:

- Animal assisted therapy/hippotherapy
- Hand skill development
- Upper extremity orthotic intervention
- Task-oriented approach
- Neurodevelopmental treatment (e.g., Brunnstrom, Bobath, Proprioceptive Neuromuscular Facilitation)
- ADL retraining
- Functional mobility training/fall prevention
- IADL retraining (e.g., meal preparation, home management)
- Driver rehabilitation

- Health and wellness (e.g., mindfulness, exercise, medication management)
- Facilitating leisure participation
- Sensory processing
- Visual perception
- Cognitive rehabilitation (e.g., Cognitive Orientation to Daily Occupational Performance [CO-OP], approaches to minimize unilateral neglect)
- Constraint-induced movement therapy
- Therapeutic use of computer or video games/Wii
- Caregiver training or perceptions

Topic chosen (include population and/or specific aspect):

Define your topic briefly:

List the five articles in the proper citation format used in your OTA program or facility (e.g., APA, MLA) and indicate the evidence level for each:

1. Evidence level:

    Citation:

2. Evidence level:

    Citation:

3. Evidence level:

    Citation:

4. Evidence level:

    Citation:

5. Evidence level:

    Citation:

Identify the areas of occupational therapy practice and/or populations that the information you found would be applicable to:

Explain how your topic relates to a client's occupational performance:

Do you feel this is a technique or procedure that you would use with clients? Why or why not?

List several alternatives to this technique/procedure that you might use with clients and discuss whether or not these would be a better choice.

Worksheet 3-8

Advocacy

Determine if the following statements are true (T) or false (F).

1. T ___   F ___   It is redundant to join a state occupational therapy association if you are already a member of AOTA.

2. T ___   F ___   Occupational therapy practitioners should advocate to help occupational therapy consumers receive the services they need.

3. T ___   F ___   An OTA student or OTA should join AOTA primarily to receive the journals.

4. T ___   F ___   An OTA cannot really do anything meaningful about changing a law that impacts occupational therapy.

5. T ___   F ___   OTA students are not able to meet with legislative staff regarding health care reform because students are not yet licensed professionals.

6. T ___   F ___   An OTA can demonstrate advocacy by joining AOTA.

7. T ___   F ___   Although advocacy is important to change laws, it does not impact reimbursement of occupational therapy.

8. T ___   F ___   Social media is not an effective method for advocacy because it is not a professional format.

9. T ___   F ___   Donating money is the most effective way to advocate.

10. T ___   F ___   One method to advocate for occupational therapy is by signing a petition.

11. T ___   F ___   It is very difficult for an OTA student or OTA to know what to write in a letter to legislators regarding current issues impacting occupational therapy.

12. T ___   F ___   Advocacy only affects federal issues.

13. T ___   F ___   The AOTA can contribute directly to political candidates.

14. T ___   F ___   Advocacy cannot impact state regulatory issues, such as occupational therapy scope of practice and continuing competency requirements, because state legislators create the laws.

15. T ___   F ___   An issue requiring occupational therapy advocacy is fair and equal access to health care.

Worksheet 3-9
Teamwork

1. Which of the following jobs is most important in a hospital?
    A. Nurse
    B. Housekeeper/janitor
    C. Occupational therapy practitioner
    D. Health information system manager

2. The desired goal of conflict resolution is primarily which one of the following?
    A. Getting a raise
    B. Meeting goals in a client's intervention plan
    C. Meeting yearly personal goals
    D. A win-win situation for all parties involved

3. The three rehabilitation department heads (physical therapy, occupational therapy, and speech therapy) are meeting to create a new mission statement for the rehabilitation department. On an average day, the physical therapy department provides 100 client sessions, the occupational therapy department provides 50, and the speech department provides 20. Which of the department heads should have the most say in what the mission statement should include?
    A. Physical therapy
    B. Occupational therapy
    C. Physical therapy and occupational therapy
    D. Physical therapy, occupational therapy, and speech therapy

4. An OTA and physical therapist assistant (PTA) are treating different clients at the same time in the rehabilitation gym. No other staff is present in the room. The OTA observes a client giving the PTA a hard time. The client is calling the PTA names and is complaining loudly about the care received. As the OTA is finishing up with the OTA's client, what primary course of action should the OTA take?
    A. Ask the PTA if there is anything the OTA can do to help
    B. Get the PTA's supervisor
    C. Do not interfere with the PTA and client interaction
    D. Tell the PTA's client that the negative behavior is not appropriate

5. During their daily supervision meeting, an OTA and OT collaborated about a certain client and determined the client needs supervision for safe functional ambulation at home. The OT asked the OTA to attend a team meeting later that day with that client's physical therapist, nurse, social worker, and physician to discuss the client's discharge plan. During the meeting, the physical therapist disagreed with the OTA that the client is unsafe. What should the OTA do first?
    A. Tell the team that the physical therapist is wrong
    B. Provide examples of the client's unsafe behavior
    C. Defer to the physical therapist because the physical therapist has more expertise regarding ambulation training
    D. Go get the OT

Learning Activity 3-10: Interprofessional Collaboration

Considering various practice settings, list several ways in which each of the following professional disciplines or support staff may directly impact an occupational therapy practitioner's role, function, or efficiency for safe and effective client care.

1. Social worker
   Example: *Orders the durable medical equipment that the OT or OTA recommends for client's home*

2. Food service staff
   Example: *Provides the food for occupational therapy meal preparation training*

3. Biomedical equipment technologist

4. Health records personnel

5. Physical therapist

6. Speech-language pathologist

7. Nursing staff

8. Housekeeper/janitor

9. Direct care worker

10. Teacher

11. Other:

12. Other:

Worksheet 3-10

Team Members

For each of the following practice settings indicated, list additional health team members who might collaborate to provide direct care/specialized services to clients or family/caregivers.

Early Intervention/School	*Behavioral Health Setting*
1. OT/OTA	1. OT/OTA
2.	2.
3.	3.
4.	4.
5.	5.
6.	6.
7.	7.
8.	8.
9.	9.
10.	10.
Home Care	*Rehabilitation Hospital*
1. OT/OTA	1. OT/OTA
2.	2.
3.	3.
4.	4.
5.	5.
6.	6.
7.	7.
8.	8.
9.	9.
10.	10.

Learning Activity 3-11: Exploring Areas of Practice

Use the AOTA website to explore opportunities for practitioners in the six primary areas of occupational therapy practice (AOTA, 2021b). When you have completed the following boxes, indicate which of the areas you might consider working in as an area of practice and explain why you chose it.

Practice Area	Identify Three Areas of Opportunity	Indicate Age Range Served	Type of Setting (e.g., school, client's home)	Kinds of Interventions (e.g., groups, environmental modifications, consultation)
Children and youth	1. 2. 3.			
Health and wellness	1. 2. 3.			
Mental health	1. 2. 3.			
Productive aging	1. 2. 3.			

Rehabilitation and disability	1. 2. 3.			
Work and industry	1. 2. 3.			

Learning Activity 3-12: Defining Neglect, Abuse, and Human Trafficking

Health care practitioners may encounter clients or other individuals who are apparent victims of domestic violence, child or elder abuse, neglect, or, perhaps, even human trafficking. Many government agencies and nonprofit organizations have been created to disseminate information about these transgressions and aid victims. For example, the National Center on Elder Abuse, part of the U. S. Department of Health and Human Services (USDHHS), provides information on its website (https://ncea.acl.gov/) to help health care workers and members of the public to recognize signs of adult/elder abuse and how to report it. Helpful resources regarding the topic of child abuse and neglect can be found at The Child Welfare Information Gateway website, a service of the Children's Bureau at the USDHHS (www.childwelfare.gov). Resources and training regarding the problem of human trafficking are also available through a variety of resources, such as the USDHHS Office on Trafficking in Persons (OTIP) (www.acf.hhs.gov/otip).

OTs and OTAs must have an understanding of pertinent laws and always keep abreast of changes in occupational therapy licensure regulations in the states in which they are providing occupational therapy services. For example, the Florida Department of Health recently mandated that to maintain licensure in that state, occupational therapy practitioners (and certain other health providers) must complete specified training from approved continuing education providers regarding the issue of human trafficking (Florida Department of Health, 2021).

When encountering possible victims of neglect, abuse, or human trafficking, OTs and OTAs in all practice settings are obliged to adhere to ethical standards, follow facility/agency policies and procedures, and abide by applicable federal and state laws delineating any mandatory reporting requirements. It is essential that practitioners recognize the possible danger signs in persons who may be victims of crimes and take appropriate action.

Define the following terms:

Active neglect:

Passive neglect:

Physical abuse:

Psychological/emotional abuse:

Financial exploitation:

Sexual abuse:

Human trafficking:

Abandonment:

Domestic violence:

Learning Activity 3-13: Identifying Risk Factors for Neglect and Abuse

1. List several agencies or organizations that health care workers or members of the public can contact to report suspected neglect/abuse of adults/elders and children in your geographical area:

   Adults/elders:

   Children:

2. Identify several community risk factors that can contribute to neglect/abuse of children and/or adults.

3. List 10 possible factors or characteristics in parents/guardians/caregivers that may contribute to maltreatment of children and/or adults.

   1.

   2.

   3.

   4.

   5.

   6.

   7.

   8.

   9.

   10.

4. Identify various signs/symptoms of *neglect* that an OT practitioner might observe in an individual.

Learning Activity 3-14: Recognizing Signs of Abuse

For each of the following scenarios, indicate the kind of neglect and/or abuse you believe is happening, if any, and explain the appropriate actions that an OTA might take in that situation.

1. You are an OTA working in a school setting. One of the students on your caseload is Caleb, a second-grader diagnosed with cerebral palsy. He was referred to occupational therapy to work on increasing independence in managing his clothing for toileting. Today you are working with him in the restroom and you notice several large bruises on his buttocks and the front of his left thigh. When you question Caleb about these bruises, he hesitates for a few seconds, looks away, and says he fell at home. You have some doubts as to whether he is telling the truth, but you also know he is sometimes unsteady when ambulating and has fallen in the past.

    Type of concern: _____ What do you do?

2. You are an OTA working at an outpatient clinic with Marissa, an 18-year-old recovering from left ulna and radius fractures. Once her cast was removed last week, she was referred to occupational therapy and evaluated. Marissa reported her fractures were caused by "falling on an icy sidewalk." The OT has delegated today's intervention to you and is presently attending a meeting on another floor. Marissa has been accompanied to therapy by Lou, a reported "friend" who looks about 50-years-old. Today you notice that Marissa has a black eye and a bruised, swollen cheek. There is no mention of this in the OT evaluation, so you ask Marissa about these facial bruises and Lou gives her a stern look. Marissa does not answer and looks down at the floor but Lou states that Marissa is "clumsy and walked into a pole." During the session Lou gets up to go to the restroom and you overhear him whisper to Marissa, "*Just keep your mouth shut while I'm gone a minute.*" When Lou is out of earshot, you question Marissa further about her facial injuries and forearm fractures. She begins to tell you, "*Look, he gives me a place to live with the other girls plus some spending money as long as I do my job. I can't talk about it—I already said too much. Be quiet—I see he's coming back now.*"

    Type of concern: _____ What do you do?

3. You are an OTA working at an assisted living facility with Miriam, a 75-year-old female recovering from hip surgery. Miriam has intact functional cognition but needs some temporary help with dressing, bathing, and home management due to physical limitations from the hip surgery. Prior to her surgery Miriam was independent and lived alone in a private house with stairs. Now she is temporarily residing at the assisted living facility until she can regain her independence, return home safely, and resume driving. She is expected to make a full recovery. Miriam is widowed and has only one child, a son who lives 1,000 miles away.

    Today, while you are working with Miriam in her room, she begins to cry and tells you her son just sold her house without her permission. She also reports she checked her bank account recently and some money in her checking account is missing. She "thinks" her son has taken the money. Miriam states, "*Sometimes my son drinks too much and takes too many pain pills*" and "*He's got a lot of financial problems because he lost his job this year.*" Miriam also says you are the first person she has trusted to tell all this information to.

    Type of concern: _____ What do you do?

Morreale, M. J. (2022). *Developing clinical competence: A workbook for the OTA* (2nd ed.). SLACK Incorporated.

4. You are an OTA working in home care. One of your clients, Betty, is a 78-year-old female with moderate-stage Alzheimer's disease. She is incontinent, requires moderate assistance to transfer, and needs assistance with all self-care. Betty lives at home with her 83-year-old husband, Larry, who is her primary caregiver. They have been married for 55 years but have no living children. Larry is devoted to his wife and has stated, "*I will never, ever put the love of my life in a nursing home. My sweetie belongs here at home with me. It is not always easy, but we manage okay.*" An aide has been coming on Mondays, mostly to give Betty a shower and do some housekeeping chores.

    Today, Friday, you arrive at the home and discover that Larry has been sick for the past 3 days with flu-like symptoms. He has been sleeping on the couch during this time and is very weak. You see that Betty is in bed with sheets wet from urine. You also observe that she is wearing a nightgown and adult diaper that are both soaked through with urine and feces. Because Betty's diaper has half slipped off, you notice she is developing a red rash in her perineal area.

    Type of concern: _____ What do you do?

5. You are working in a group home with Alex who has an intellectual disability and limited verbal skills. Today you notice several red marks on his right arm that look like cigarette burns. You try to ask Alex what happened, but he only replies with, "*I bad, I very bad*" and tries to hide behind the door. You ask the worker on duty about the marks on Alex's arm but the worker shrugs and says, "*Maybe Alex has some bug bites on his arm from being outdoors. He probably just scratched them too hard.*"

    Type of concern: _____ What do you do?

Answers to Worksheets

Worksheet 3-1: Roles and Responsibilities

An OTA performs occupational therapy services under the supervision of an OT (AOTA, 2015b, 2020b). The OTA collaborates with the OT to perform delegated tasks for which the OTA has service competency, are within the scope of ethical OT practice, and adhere to federal, state, and facility guidelines (AOTA, 2015b, 2020a, 2020b). The following answers are based on AOTA's *Guidelines for Supervision, Roles, and Responsibilities During the Delivery of Occupational Therapy Services* (AOTA, 2020b); *Scope of Practice* (AOTA, 2014); and *Standards of Practice for Occupational Therapy* (AOTA, 2015b). Additional pertinent references are noted in the chart as appropriate.

	Task	OT	OTA
1.	Instruct client in a home exercise program	*	*
2.	Develop the occupational therapy intervention plan	*	
3.	Determine if a client performs a cooking task safely	*	*
4.	Gait training *This is typically the role of physical therapy, although occupational therapy can support function (AOTA, 2021c).*		
5.	Teach positioning techniques to a parent of a child with cerebral palsy	*	*
6.	Upgrade an exercise program *Based on the intervention plan*	*	*
7.	Determine discharge from occupational therapy	*	
8.	Respond to a referral to occupational therapy	*	
9.	Implement occupational therapy interventions	*	*
10.	Teach one-handed shoe-tying	*	*
11.	Complete the occupational therapy initial evaluation report independently	*	
12.	Administer a standardized assessment	*	*
13.	Interpret initial evaluation results	*	
14.	Fabricate an orthosis	*	*
15.	Customize a resident's wheelchair with specialized inserts	*	*
16.	Administer superficial thermal modalities as the sole client intervention during a session *A physical agent modality is not considered occupational therapy unless it is followed up by additional therapeutic intervention to improve function (AOTA, 2018c).*		
17.	Document occupational therapy treatment (AOTA, 2015b)	*	*
18.	Provide intervention to a home care client	*	*
19.	Instruct client in workplace ergonomics	*	*
20.	Provide specialized instruction in self-care	*	*

	Task	OT	OTA
21.	Help a student put on boots for recess *Anyone can help a child don boots. However, if the occupational therapy practitioner was implementing the occupational therapy intervention plan, such as teaching self-care skills, or working on client factors, such as bilateral integration or balance, then that would be considered skilled occupational therapy (Morreale & Borcherding, 2017).*		
22.	Develop goals for an Individualized Education Program (IEP)	*	
23.	Assess transfer skills	*	*
24.	Provide occupational therapy in a neonatal intensive care unit (AOTA, 2018b)	*	
25.	Attain certification in hand therapy (Hand Therapy Certification Commission, 2018)	*	
26.	Attain AOTA board certification in pediatrics (AOTA, 2021a)	*	
27.	Use evidence-informed practice	*	*
28.	Make recommendations to a teacher regarding compensatory techniques for a student receiving occupational therapy services	*	*
29.	Delegate aspects of an occupational therapy initial evaluation	*	
30.	Write short-term goals in a treatment note as a sub-step toward implementing an established intervention plan	*	*
31.	Update a client's intervention plan	*	
32.	Write a discharge report independently	*	
33.	Adapt an ADL device to improve a client's self-care performance	*	*
34.	Assess range of motion using a goniometer	*	*
35.	Teach nursing staff how to apply a client's orthotic device	*	*
36.	Provide a handout on cardiac precautions *Anyone can give a client a brochure or handout. This is not considered skilled occupational therapy unless followed up by skilled instruction or practice (Morreale & Borcherding, 2017).*		
37.	Supervise a rehabilitation aide	*	*
38.	Supervise a volunteer in the occupational therapy department	*	*
39.	Supervise a Level I OTA student (Accreditation Council for Occupational Therapy Education [ACOTE], 2018)	*	*
40.	Supervise a Level II OTA student (ACOTE, 2018)	*	*
41.	Supervise a Level I OT student (ACOTE, 2018)	*	*
42.	Supervise a Level II OT student (ACOTE, 2018)	*	
43.	Lead an occupational therapy group in a behavioral health setting	*	*
44.	Observe a child color a picture *Simply watching someone do an activity is not skilled occupational therapy. However, if the OT was assessing the child's performance skills, such as balance, coordination, or safety, then that could be considered a skilled service (Morreale & Borcherding, 2017).*		
45.	Recommend durable medical equipment upon client's discharge home	*	*

	Task	OT	OTA
46.	Assess a client's orientation to person, place, and time	*	*
47.	Inform nursing staff about a client's report of pain	*	*
48.	Provide an inservice to the rehabilitation staff about an evidence-informed practice article	*	*
49.	Assess vital signs	*	*
50.	Attend a team meeting to discuss a client's care and progress *In certain instances, some settings or payers may require that an OT also be present*	*	*

Worksheet 3-2: Supervision

1. C. Steve has mutual responsibility to ensure that he receives appropriate supervision levels (AOTA, 2020b). He should go through the proper chain of command and discuss his concerns with his supervising OT first. The OT may not be aware that Steve has those concerns. If Steve and his OT supervisor are not able to come to a satisfactory arrangement, he might then seek help from the rehabilitation director. While Steve could ask his colleagues about their level of supervision, their needs may not be relevant to Steve's and it could also be perceived negatively as complaining or gossiping. Thus, it is best to first speak to the OT directly.

2. A. It is not ethical for Huma to perform those assessments as they clearly require supervision based on Huma's student status, lack of knowledge, and inexperience (AOTA, 2020a, 2020b). As Huma has already discussed her concerns with the fieldwork educator without a satisfactory resolution, the next step is to ask her academic fieldwork coordinator to intervene. As a student, it would not be appropriate in this instance to go over her supervisor's head and speak to the rehabilitation director before contacting the academic fieldwork coordinator.

3. D. An OTA cannot ethically perform a delegated task that the OTA believes will cause harm to the client (AOTA, 2015b, 2020a). As the OTA was not able to resolve the situation with the OT, the next step is for the OTA to seek help from the OT's supervisor. Walking off the job is not a productive solution.

4. C. It is not ethical for the OTA to delegate a skilled occupational therapy task to an aide. However, an aide can provide a client with a form to fill out that the OTA will review with the client later. All the other answers require professional judgment and knowledge and are not appropriate for the aide to perform (AOTA, 2020b; Morreale & Borcherding, 2017).

5. A. It is not appropriate for a volunteer to review client charts as this would violate confidentiality. Teaching a client how to use adaptive equipment is skilled intervention that is not appropriate to delegate to a volunteer or aide (AOTA, 2020b). However, it can be appropriate for a volunteer to assist with preparing equipment, in this case cutting out pieces of hook and loop fastener that the occupational therapy practitioner can apply to orthoses.

Worksheet 3-3: Cultural Sensitivity

1. D. As a health professional, an OTA should respect the sociocultural background and personal factors of the client and not discriminate based on Carl's sexual orientation (AOTA, 2015b, 2020a, 2020c; Davis & Rosee, 2015, Robins, 2006). An OTA is also expected to educate family/significant others as needed to facilitate the discharge process (AOTA, 2015b). The OTA can have personal religious values or beliefs but must always demonstrate cultural sensitivity, set aside personal judgment or bias, and treat the client with dignity and respect. It would be disrespectful, uncomfortable, and embarrassing for the client and partner in this situation for the OTA to discuss personal beliefs or to offer to "pray for their redemption". The OTA should also discuss any ethical conflicts or concerns with the OT to become more culturally sensitive.

2. B. It is important to respect the client's cultural and religious beliefs and not insist that the client perform tasks that violate his morals (AOTA, 2015b, 2020a, 2020c; Royeen & Crabtree, 2006). If there is no male occupational therapy practitioner on staff that could work on bathing with this client, the OTA might instead work on the relevant skills needed for bathing, such as range of motion, activity tolerance, or balance. While it is not appropriate to ask another discipline to provide skilled occupational therapy, collaboration with other team members is helpful. However, the OT and OTA might also determine if training the client's wife for this task or having

the client's wife present in the room would make a difference in allowing an occupational therapy practitioner to work on bathing with this client.

3. D. When implementing meal preparation interventions, it is appropriate for an OTA to discuss food choices with the client ahead of time, as the client may have allergies, food preferences and/or cultural considerations. Observant followers of the Orthodox sect of Judaism normally follow Kosher guidelines, which prohibit pork products and the consumption of meat and dairy products together at meals. Also realize that special plates, utensils, and food preparation methods may be needed to adhere to Kosher requirements (Chabad-Lubavitch Media Center, 2020d). More information about practices of the Jewish faith can be found using the search feature at www.Chabad.org.

4. C. It is important to respect Parita's deep-rooted cultural beliefs and consider the traditional clothing that Parita will wear upon discharge from the facility (AOTA, 2015b, 2020a, 2020c). However, it is still important to note the safety hazard and document any client education provided along with the need for supervision or assistance. Perhaps the garment can be pinned or modified to minimize the hazard. The OTA (or OT) should also discuss the concern with a physical therapist practitioner who has expertise to assess what other mobility devices might be appropriate and safer for Parita to use.

5. B. It is important to respect the client's cultural and religious beliefs and not insist that the client perform tasks that violate his faith (AOTA, 2015b, 2020a, 2020c; Royeen & Crabtree, 2006). In this case, the OTA should recommend that the client discuss the medical necessity of the exercises with his religious leader, as there may be special dispensation for activities needed to improve an individual's health.

6. C. Rosary beads are prayer beads associated with Catholicism, not Judaism. Tefillin is a leather item containing parchment scrolls and Bible passages that adult Jewish men secure on their arm during weekday morning prayers (Chabad-Lubavitch Media Center, 2020b). A, B, and D are incorporated into Jewish rituals for males which include wearing a prayer shawl with fringes (tallit) and skull cap head covering called a yarmulke or kippah (Chabad-Lubavitch Media Center, 2020a, 2020c). More information about practices of the Jewish faith can be found using the search feature at www.Chabad.org.

7. A. A vegan does not eat or use animal products, so plant-based craft materials are the most culturally sensitive (Merriam-Webster, 2020). B, C, and D would not be good choices for this client as they consist of animal-based products (wool, eggs, and leather). String and cord are also safety concerns.

8. A. A primary goal for clients with severe pain is to manage the pain for improved quality of life and occupational performance. In this case, the client's perception is that she now has markedly decreased pain, which is the desired outcome. The OTA should respect the client's cultural belief regarding a healing service or other cultural remedies (Royeen & Crabtree, 2006). It would not be useful to disagree or argue with this client. Of course, appropriate intervention would be needed for any cultural practices that are truly harmful.

9. B. For Catholics, Good Friday is a holy day requiring abstinence from meat and fasting for adults (of certain ages). However, limited food consumption is allowed and exceptions may be made for a person's health (ThoughtCo, 2020).

10. B. As this client's communication style may be culturally influenced, an OTA must be careful not to jump to other conclusions (Asher, 2006; Davis & Rosee, 2015). The OTA's observations should be discussed with the OT and other team members. Perhaps alternate communication methods, such as a journal entry or art project, may be more appropriate for this client to express his emotions more easily.

Worksheet 3-4: Cultural Sensitivity—More Practice

Resource: Black, 2017

1. D. OTAs should always try to establish good rapport with clients and significant others. In this case it is best to gently, and in a non-judgmental manner, discuss possible services that could be beneficial. Using a strong term with negative connotations such as "obese" might cause the child's mother to feel insecure, untrusting, or become defensive. The OTA should not insinuate that the client cannot be a good mother due to her size. Answer B is not correct as the children have not yet exceeded normal weight ranges.

Morreale, M. J. (2022). *Developing clinical competence: A workbook for the OTA* (2nd ed.). SLACK Incorporated.

2. C. Answers A and B may cause embarrassment for the client. Answer D is also not very culturally sensitive or tactful. Answer C is a positive response that shows respect for the client's cultural beliefs.

3. C. It is important for practitioners to respect the client's cultural beliefs, such as gender roles (AOTA, 2020c; Royeen & Crabree, 2006). Of course, any cultural practices that are truly harmful to the client or others would need to be addressed. The OTA might discuss with the child's father the extra stress that a child's disability can create and suggest that his wife may need extra help. Calling him sexist is judgmental, inappropriate, and would not be a helpful approach.

4. A. It is very clear that this family does not want to place their loved older family member in a skilled nursing facility as this would go against their cultural beliefs. The OTA could encourage the family to discuss concerns that they may have with their ability to care for Huan so that appropriate strategies can potentially be recommended. The team should strive to provide appropriate resources and support to enable this client to remain at home safely for as long as medically possible. Due to Huan's medical status, it is not feasible for him attend an adult day care program outside of the home or perform ambulation.

5. D. Actions that may violate this client's religious boundaries include physical contact that is taboo such as hugs, social touching, or shaking hands with an unrelated member of the opposite sex (Davis & Rosee, 2015).

Adapted from Morreale, M. J., & Amini, D. (2016). The occupational therapist's workbook for ensuring clinical competence. SLACK Incorporated.

Worksheet 3-5: Attaining Service Competency

1. B. The OTA should seek supervision and help from her OT supervisor to ensure the client's safety (AOTA, 2015b, 2020b). While the OTA could perform a different intervention or ask other disciplines to perform the transfer, competence in transfers is an essential function of this OTA's job. The OTA needs to learn how to perform transfers safely and, thus, needs to discuss this with the OT. The OTA must also follow the facility's policies and procedures for maximum assistance transfers, such as possibly requiring the use of a mechanical lift or two people to perform the transfer (Morreale & Amini, 2016).

2. C. The OTA should be able to perform the intervention without the OT directly present (if allowed by state and other regulatory agencies) as there are no surgical precautions, the interventions are basic and very clear, and the client outcome appears stable. The OTA should review the client's health documentation in the chart and utilize resources to obtain information about the diagnosis. However, the OTA should contact the OT if the OTA has further significant concerns or questions—rather than proceeding with treatment.

3. D. As orthotic device fabrication is a conventional occupational therapy intervention (AOTA, 2014), this task may be delegated to an OTA with service competency if allowed by that state's practice act and other regulatory agencies. Because of the student's inexperience and length of time that has passed since skills class, the primary course of action should be for the student to practice making an orthosis with an occupational therapy practitioner at that site before attempting to fabricate one on a client (under the direct supervision of the fieldwork educator). Of course, the student can also review a textbook and utilize internet resources as additional learning tools.

4. D. Utilizing a variety of resources will be the most useful for learning.

5. B. Health care, including occupational therapy, is always evolving as new evidence emerges, society changes, and new laws are passed. An occupational therapy practitioner has a responsibility for on-going professional development while practicing occupational therapy (AOTA, 2015a, 2017).

6. A. NBCOT provides an extensive listing of activities that may be used to meet professional development requirements for recertification (NBCOT, 2020). Answer A does not meet the NBCOT criteria presently.

Worksheet 3-6: Evidence-Informed Practice

1. A. *The two wheelchairs are simply used as a means of transport to the therapy session and will not usually impact the efficiency or efficacy of therapy itself. Both technology devices are available and essentially equivalent technology so deciding to use one over the other can normally be based on practitioner preference alone* (Morreale & Amini, 2016).

2. B.

3. A. *Answer B is a scholarly journal and C, D are popular magazines (University of Colorado, n.d.).*
4. C (University of Notre Dame, Australia, 2018)
5. D (University of Notre Dame, Australia, 2018)

Worksheet 3-7: Fundamentals of Research

1. F. Newspaper articles are typically considered scholarly sources because they are reviewed by the editor before publication. (University of Colorado, n.d.)

2. T. Randomized controlled trials are higher on the evidence pyramid than cohort studies and case reports. (University of Notre Dame, Australia, 2018)

3. T. Ways in which trade magazines differ from scholarly journals include factors such as glossy paper, colorized illustrations/pictures, and each issue beginning with page number one. (University of Colorado, n.d.)

4. F. A systematic review is an individual research study that has a step-by-step process using a control group and experimental group. (University of Notre Dame, Australia, 2018)

5. T. The "gold standard" in medical research is the double-blind randomized control group pretest-posttest design. (Bell, 2015)

6. T. A systematic review using quantitative methods to summarize results is a meta-analysis. (University of Notre Dame, Australia, 2018)

7. F. An example of a primary source is a systematic review. *A systematic review is a secondary source.* (University of Notre Dame, Australia, 2018)

8. T. Methods that collect and analyze data existing in non-numerical formats are used in a qualitative approach. (Bell, 2015)

9. F. An example of a scholarly journal is *OT Practice. This is a trade magazine.* (University of Colorado, n.d.)

10. T. Diagnosis, age, cognitive status, and gender are examples of possible variables in qualitative and quantitative research. (Bell, 2015)

11. T. Methods of data collection used in qualitative research often include interviews and review of artifacts. (Bell, 2015)

12. F. In a statistical test, the fewer the participants, the more accurate the test outcome. (Bell, 2015)

13. T. When a researcher includes more variables in a statistical test, a larger sample size is needed for accuracy. (Bell, 2015)

14. T. In a statistical test, the less reliable an instrument is to measure a variable, the greater the sample size needed to ensure an accurate outcome. (Bell, 2015)

15. F. Informed consent is normally not needed to become a study participant if the individual volunteers for that study (Bell, 2015)

16. T. In experimental design studies, a random sampling of participants from a population or random assignment of participants to groups is always used. (Bell, 2015)

17. F. In randomized controlled trials, the treatment group usually receives a placebo. *The control group receives the placebo* (Bell, 2015)

18. T. Double-blind refers to both the subjects and treatment providers not knowing which participants are part of the treatment group or control group. (Bell, 2015)

19. T. When performing qualitative research, data may be collected by observation and recorded as field notes. (Bell, 2015)

20. T. The case study nonexperimental design involves only one participant, and the gathered data can be numerical and non-numerical. (Bell, 2015)

Worksheet 3-8: Advocacy

The AOTA website (www.aota.org) contains an Advocacy and Policy section that explains the role and functions of the American Occupational Therapy Association Political Action Committee (AOTPAC) and delineates current state and federal issues and proposed legislation affecting occupational therapy. AOTA has a Regulatory Affairs Department that advocates for federal issues such as reimbursement, and a State Affairs Group that deals with regulatory and legislative issues for all states (AOTA, 2021d). The AOTA's Legislative Action Center (part of the Advocacy and Policy section) describes AOTA's advocacy efforts and suggests ways that individuals can get involved (AOTA, n.d., 2021e).

1. F. It is redundant to join a state occupational therapy association if you are already a member of AOTA.

    State associations collaborate with AOTA to address that area's state and local issues affecting occupational therapy. Both have unique member benefits, resources, and networking opportunities.

2. T. Occupational therapy practitioners should advocate to help occupational therapy consumers receive the services they need.

    The principle of justice is addressed in the Code of Ethics *(AOTA, 2020a).*

3. F. An OTA student or OTA should join AOTA primarily to receive the journals.

    Although the journals are a very useful benefit, membership includes other important benefits such as advocacy, professional and career resources, social media platform, discounts, and so forth.

4. F. An OTA cannot really do anything meaningful about changing a law that impacts occupational therapy.

    The AOTA website lists a variety of ways that occupational therapy practitioners can help influence public policy (AOTA, n.d., 2021e).

5. F. OTA students are not able to meet with legislative staff regarding health care reform because students are not yet licensed professionals.

    Students can participate in AOTA's Capitol Hill Day or, as constituents, can contact their elected representatives (AOTA, n.d., 2021e).

6. T. An OTA can demonstrate advocacy by joining AOTA.

    Membership dollars help support advocacy efforts.

7. F. Although advocacy is important to change laws, it does not impact reimbursement of occupational therapy.

    Legislation such as the Individuals with Disabilities Education Act, Medicaid, and Medicare regulations (e.g., Prospective Payment System, Medicare B therapy cap) directly impact health care access and/or reimbursement of occupational therapy services. Advocacy can influence public policy and help make a difference in how individual lawmakers vote.

8. F. Social media is not an effective method for advocacy because it is not a professional format.

    Social media can spread the word regarding important issues. Also, online petitions can be used to increase awareness and support.

9. F. Donating money is the most effective way to advocate.

    Monetary donations certainly help support advocacy activities. However, other ways to help include volunteering, writing letters, calling elected representatives, meeting with legislative staff, and networking with other professionals and organizations. The AOTA Legislative Action Center, in the Advocacy and Policy section of the AOTA website, delineates current issues and ways that individuals and groups can advocate (AOTA, n.d., 2021e).

10. T. One method to advocate for occupational therapy is by signing a petition.

Petitions can increase awareness and let elected officials know what issues are important to constituents.

11. F. It is very difficult for an OTA student or OTA to know what to write in a letter to legislators regarding current issues impacting occupational therapy.

The AOTA Legislative Action Center has sample letters that OTAs may use as a template and send out to legislators regarding specific current issues affecting occupational therapy (AOTA, 2021e).

12. F. Advocacy only affects federal issues.

Advocacy can also influence local and state policy issues. State occupational therapy associations collaborate with the AOTA to advocate for issues such as state occupational therapy licensure laws, access to health care, rights of people with disabilities, and reimbursement for covered health services in that state (e.g., Medicaid, workers' compensation, Early Intervention).

13. F. The AOTA can contribute directly to political candidates.

Funds must be contributed through a political action committee. The American Occupational Therapy Political Action Committee (AOTPAC) is a non-profit, non-partisan, voluntary unincorporated committee made up of AOTA members. (AOTPAC, 2020).

14. F. Advocacy cannot impact state regulatory issues, such as occupational therapy scope of practice and continuing competency requirements, because state legislators create the laws.

Advocacy can influence state policy issues and how individual lawmakers vote. State occupational therapy associations collaborate with the AOTA to advocate for issues such as a state's OT licensure regulations, access to health care, rights of people with disabilities, and so forth.

15. T. An issue requiring occupational therapy advocacy is fair and equal access to health care.

The principle of justice is addressed in the AOTA 2020 Occupational Therapy Code of Ethics *(AOTA, 2020a).*

Worksheet 3-9: Teamwork

Resource: Davis & Rosee, 2015

1. This is really a trick question, as every job is extremely important in health care. Besides the direct client services that health professionals provide, other employees such as support staff, cleaning staff, food service workers, health information technology personnel, and other disciplines are essential for keeping clients safe, equipment working properly, and the facility running smoothly. Think about what would happen if bathrooms, medical devices, and operating rooms were not cleaned; the electronic documentation system was not working; food was not prepared; or the facility could not send bills to insurance companies for care implemented.

2. D. When several parties do not agree initially on an issue, the best result is a win-win situation in which the parties have negotiated and each feels satisfied with the final outcome or compromise. OTAs often encounter workplace situations that require peaceful, practical solutions. Some issues that may cause conflict include compensation and benefits, productivity levels, frequency and amount of supervision, a client's care plan, personality conflicts with colleagues or clients, vacation schedules, office space, and so forth.

3. D. If the mission statement represents the entire rehabilitation department, the three department heads should have equal input.

4. A. The best course of action is to first ask the PTA if the PTA needs any help with anything. The PTA can then decide if the OTA can intervene in some way or if the situation warrants contacting the physical therapy supervisor. The client may have cognitive problems or a history of violence that the PTA knows about, but the OTA does not. Of course, if the OTA believes that the PTA or anyone else is in imminent danger, then the OTA should take immediate action according to the facility's policies and procedures for handling emergencies or security issues.

5. B. It is not productive to criticize or embarrass the team member. The OTA should tactfully provide specific examples of the client's unsafe behavior so that the team can understand the client's need for supervision. It is important to do what is in the client's best interest. In this case, if the OTA knows the client is truly unsafe, the OTA has an obligation to speak up.

Worksheet 3-10: Team Members

The team members listed below may not be present in every setting or you might find that other disciplines are also necessary for client care.

Early Intervention/School	Behavioral Health Setting
1. OT/OTA 2. Physical therapist/PTA 3. Speech therapist 4. Child development specialist 5. School nurse 6. Teacher/special educator 7. Teacher's aide 8. Psychologist 9. Blind mobility specialist 10. Social worker/guidance counselor 11. Adaptive physical education teacher 12. Vocational rehabilitation counselor	1. OT/OTA 2. Psychiatrist 3. Nurse 4. Social worker 5. Recreation therapist 6. Dance therapist 7. Music therapist 8. Art therapist 9. Direct care worker 10. Dietician 11. Pharmacist 12. Rehabilitation counselor
Home Care	**Rehabilitation Hospital**
1. OT/OTA 2. Physical therapist/PTA 3. Speech therapist 4. Physician/physician's assistant 5. Nurse 6. Home health aide 7. Social worker 8. Dietician 9. Clergy 10. Respiratory therapist 11. Pharmacist	1. OT/OTA 2. Physical therapist/PTA 3. Speech therapist 4. Audiologist 5. Nurse 6. Physician/physician's assistant 7. Certified nursing assistant 8. Social worker 9. Rehabilitation counselor 10. Orthotist/prosthetist 11. Respiratory therapist 12. Recreation therapist 13. Assistive technology specialist 14. Exercise physiologist 15. Dietician 16. Pharmacist 17. Clergy

References

Accreditation Council for Occupational Therapy Education. (2018). 2018 Accreditation council for occupational therapy education (ACOTE) standards and interpretive guide (effective July 31, 2020). *American Journal of Occupational Therapy, 72*(Suppl. 2), 7212410005. https://doi.org/10.5014/ajot.2018.72S217

American Occupational Therapy Association. (n.d.). *Advocacy resources.* CQ-Roll Call. https://cqrcengage.com/aota/file/pM5q8zQHAWO/Advocacy-Resources-Handout-Web.pdf

American Occupational Therapy Association. (2014). Scope of practice. *American Journal of Occupational Therapy, 68*(Suppl. 3). https: //doi.org./10.5014/ajot.2014.686S04

American Occupational Therapy Association. (2015a). Standards for continuing competence. *American Journal of Occupational Therapy, 69*(Suppl. 3), 6913410055. http://dx.doi.org/10.5014/ajot.2015.696S16

American Occupational Therapy Association. (2015b). Standards of practice for occupational therapy. *American Journal of Occupational Therapy, 69*(Suppl. 3), 6913410057. http://dx.doi.org/10.5014/ajot.2015.696S06

American Occupational Therapy Association. (2017). Continuing professional development in occupational therapy. *American Journal of Occupational Therapy, 71*(Suppl. 2), 7112410017. https// doi.org/10.5014/ ajot.2017.716S13

American Occupational Therapy Association. (2018a). Guidelines for documentation of occupational therapy. *American Journal of Occupational Therapy, 72*(Suppl. 2), 7212410010. https:// doi.org/ 10.5014/ajot.2018.72S203

American Occupational Therapy Association. (2018b). Occupational therapy's role in the neonatal intensive care unit. *American Journal of Occupational Therapy, 72*(Suppl. 2), 7212410020. https://doi.org/10.5014/ ajot.2018.72S204

American Occupational Therapy Association. (2018c). Physical agent and mechanical modalities. *American Journal of Occupational Therapy, 72*(Suppl. 2), 7212410055. https://. doi.org/ 10.5014/ajot.2018.72S220

American Occupational Therapy Association. (2020a). AOTA 2020 occupational therapy code of ethics. *American Journal of Occupational Therapy, 74*(Suppl. 3), 7413410005. https://doi.org/10.5014/ajot.2020.74S3006

American Occupational Therapy Association. (2020b). Guidelines for supervision, roles, and responsibilities during the delivery of occupational therapy services. *American Journal of Occupational Therapy, 74*(Suppl. 3), 7413410020. https:// doi.org/10.5014/ajot.2020.74S3004

American Occupational Therapy Association. (2020c). Occupational therapy practice framework: Domain and process (4th ed.). *American Journal of Occupational Therapy, 74*(Suppl. 2), 7412410010. https://doi.org/10.5014/ajot.2020.74S2001

American Occupational Therapy Association. (2021a). *AOTA's advanced certification program.* Retrieved May 12, 2021, from https://www.aota.org/Education-Careers/Advance-Career/Board-Specialty-Certifications-Exam.aspx

American Occupational Therapy Association. (2021b). *Practice.* Retrieved May 12, 2021, from https://www.aota.org/ Practice.aspx

American Occupational Therapy Association. (2021c). *Scope of practice q & a: Gait assessment for falls risk.* Retrieved May 12, 2021, from https://www.aota.org/Practice/Manage/Scope-of-Practice-QA/gait.aspx

American Occupational Therapy Association. (2021d). *State policy.* Retrieved May 12, 2021, from https://www.aota.org/ Advocacy-Policy/State-Policy.aspx

American Occupational Therapy Association. (2021e). *Take action.* Retrieved May 12, 2021, from https://www.aota.org/ Advocacy-Policy/Congressional-Affairs/Take-Action.aspx

American Occupational Therapy Political Action Committee. (2021). *AOTPAC frequently asked questions.* American Occupational Therapy Association. Retrieved May 12, 2021, from https://www.aota.org/advocacy-policy/aotpac/fact.aspx

Asher, A. (2006). Asian americans. In M. Royeen & J. L. Crabtree (Eds.), *Culture in rehabilitation: From competency to proficiency* (pp. 151-180). Pearson Education.

Bell, S. (2015). Understanding research. In K. Sladyk & R. Ryan (Eds.), *Ryan's occupational therapy assistant: Principles, practice issues, and techniques* (5th ed., pp. 556-570). SLACK Incorporated.

Black, R. M. (2017). Cultural impact on occupation. In K. Jacobs & N. MacRae (Eds.), *Occupational therapy essentials for clinical competence.* (3rd ed., pp. 13-28). SLACK Incorporated.

Chabad-Lubavitch Media Center. (2020a). *Tallit (prayer shawl).* Chabad.org. Retrieved March 10, 2020, from https://www. chabad.org/search/keyword_cdo/kid/16013/oq/Tallit%20(Prayer%20Shawl)/jewish/Tallit-Prayer-Shawl.htm

Chabad-Lubavitch Media Center. (2020b). *Tefillin.* Chabad.org. Retrieved March 10, 2020, from https://www.chabad.org/ search/keyword_cdo/kid/1543/oq/Tefillin/jewish/Tefillin.htm

Chabad-Lubavitch Media Center. (2020c). *The kippah (Yarmulke).* Chabad.org. Retrieved March 10, 2020, from https:// www.chabad.org/library/article_cdo/aid/3913641/jewish/The-Kippah-Yarmulke.htm

Chabad-Lubavitch Media Center. (2020d). *What is kosher?* Chabad.org. Retrieved March 10, 2020, from https://www. chabad.org/library/article_cdo/aid/113425/jewish/What-Is-Kosher.htm

Colorado State University. (n.d.). *Introduction to scholarly vs trade vs popular journals.* Retrieved June 22, 2021, from https://libguides.colostate.edu/howtodo/scholarlyvspopular

Davis, L., & Rosee, M. (2015). *Occupational therapy student to clinician: Making the transition.* SLACK Incorporated.

Florida Department of Health. (2021). *Florida board of occupational therapy: Renewal information.* Florida Board of Occupational Therapy. https://floridasoccupationaltherapy.gov/renewals/#tab-ce

Hand Therapy Certification Commission. (2018). *Eligibility requirements.* https://www.htcc.org/certify/test-information/eligibility-requirements

Logan University (2021). *Evidence informed practice: Home.* Retrieved June 22, 2021, from https://libguides.logan.edu/eip

Merriam-Webster. (2020). *Definition of vegan.* www.merriam-webster.com/dictionary/vegan

Morreale, M. J., & Amini, D. (2016). *The occupational therapist's workbook for ensuring clinical competence.* SLACK Incorporated.

Morreale, M. J., & Borcherding, S. (2017). *The OTA's guide to documentation* (4th ed.). SLACK Incorporated.

National Board for Certification in Occupational Therapy. (2020). *NBCOT certification renewal activities chart.* https://www.nbcot.org/-/media/NBCOT/PDFs/Renewal_Activity_Chart.ashx?la=en&hash=1B1765963E596B6BF27064B05197B2DA48157E8A

Robins, S. (2006). Understanding sexual minorities. In M. Royeen & J. L. Crabtree (Eds.), *Culture in rehabilitation: From competency to proficiency* (pp. 357-376). Pearson Education.

Royeen, M., & Crabtree, J. L. (Eds.). (2006). *Culture in rehabilitation: From competency to proficiency.* Pearson Education.

ThoughtCo. (2020, August 26). *Can catholics eat meat on good friday?* LearnReligions. Retrieved May 12, 2021, from https://www.learnreligions.com/eat-meat-on-good-friday-542169

University of Notre Dame Australia. (2018). *Levels of evidence.* https://library.nd.edu.au/researchers/systematicreviews/evidence

Applying Fundamental Principles

The worksheets and learning activities presented in this chapter are designed to test your knowledge and understanding of fundamental aspects of occupational therapy practice such as, infection control basics, American Occupational Therapy Association (AOTA) Official Documents (2021), and application of language and principles of the *Occupational Therapy Practice Framework: Domain and Process, Fourth Edition* (*OTPF—4*; AOTA, 2020c). Other essential skills addressed in this chapter include grading and adapting, occupational analysis, and the appropriate handling of unpredictable or challenging clinical situations. Answers to worksheet exercises are provided at the end of the chapter.

Contents

Morreale, M. J. *Developing Clinical Competence:*
A Workbook for the OTA, Second Edition (pp. 165-204).
© 2022 SLACK Incorporated.

Learning Activity 4-1: Basics of Infection Control

The Centers for Disease Control and Prevention (CDC; www.cdc.gov) and World Health Organization (WHO; www.who.int) websites contain useful information for health care providers and members of the public to learn about different kinds of pathogens and how they are transmitted. These organizations strive to curb the spread of illnesses/communicable diseases for individuals and populations by creating protocols for best health practices. Detailed guidelines for health care workers are provided on the CDC and WHO websites to help ensure client and worker safety. Safe practices entail adhering to established infection control procedures, for example, performing proper hand hygiene and using personal protective equipment (PPE) appropriately (CDC, 2020; Siegel et al., 2019; WHO, 2009, 2020).

Explain briefly the following ways in which pathogens can be transmitted and provide two examples of each:

Direct contact transmission:

Examples:

1.

2.

Indirect contact transmission:

Examples:

1.

2.

Droplet transmission:

Examples:

1.

2.

Airborne transmission:

Examples:

1.

2.

Define the following acronyms and terms:

Health care-associated infection:

MRSA:

C.difficile:

VRE:

Epidemic:

Pandemic:

Explain the term PPE and list five examples of PPE that an occupational therapy assistant (OTA) might use in clinical practice:

1.

2.

3.

4.

5.

Worksheet 4-1

Using Standard Precautions

1. An OTA is working at an inpatient setting and providing intervention at bedside. Of the following choices, which is normally more suitable for an OTA to do?
   A. Use a facility-approved alcohol-based hand rub upon entering the client's room and ask the client to wear gloves
   B. When entering the room, rinse hands under water before treating the client
   C. Use gloves to save time by eliminating need for handwashing or use of alcohol-based hand rub
   D. Use a facility-approved alcohol-based hand rub before and after intervention

2. An OTA performing handwashing with soap and water in a health setting should normally do all except which of the following?
   A. Use a washcloth to rub soap thoroughly in between fingers
   B. Dry hands with a single-use paper towel
   C. Always apply a pea-sized amount of soap
   D. Use clean non-dominant hand to turn off the faucet

3. Which of the following statements is correct?
   A. It is preferable to use an alcohol-based hand rub rather than soap and water when hands are visibly soiled or after using the toilet
   B. When using an alcohol-based hand rub, hands should be rubbed together for 7 to 8 seconds then any excess gel wiped off using a paper towel
   C. When wearing gloves for client care, avoid saving gloves for reuse later with the same client even if that would reduce costs
   D. When washing hands, it is preferable to mix an alcohol-based hand rub together with soap and water

4. To enable safe feeding and eating, an OTA is working on head and upper body positioning with a young child who drools excessively and gags. Of the following choices, which would generally be more suitable for the OTA to use as PPE?
   A. Gloves and surgical mask
   B. Respirator and lab coat
   C. Sterile disposable gown, booties, and goggles
   D. Disposable emesis basin

5. Which of the following conditions is spread through an airborne route?
   A. Group A *streptococcus*
   B. *Staphylococcus aureus*
   C. Pertussis
   D. Tuberculosis

6. What is the primary route of transmission for measles and chickenpox?
   A. Airborne
   B. Droplet
   C. Direct contact
   D. Indirect contact

Worksheet 4-1 (continued)

Using Standard Precautions

7. Which of the following is an example of possible indirect contact transmission of pathogens?
   A. A needlestick injury
   B. Shared toys
   C. Getting coughed on
   D. A worker's cut bare hand having accidental contact with client's urine

8. An OTA is implementing cognitive interventions with a client in acute care who has tuberculosis. Which of the following PPE is more suitable for the OTA to use during intervention?
   A. Surgical mask
   B. Lab coat
   C. Respirator
   D. Face shield

9. Of the following choices, which should an OTA normally do first when accidentally exposed to a blood-borne pathogen?
   A. Fill out an incident report
   B. Put Bacitracin or Neosporin on the exposed site
   C. Wash the exposed area
   D. Go get the occupational therapist (OT) or rehabilitation supervisor

10. When removing gloves used as PPE, an OTA should do all except which of the following?
    A. Wash hands after removal
    B. Avoid touching the forearm during removal
    C. Remove gloves by pulling first at the fingertips
    D. Throw gloves away

Learning Activity 4-2: Official Documents of the American Occupational Therapy Association

The AOTA develops official documents that delineate the values, beliefs, and standards of the association regarding specific subjects and are valuable resources guiding occupational therapy practice (AOTA, 2021). Some of these documents are created to address broad occupational therapy principles, such as ethics, whereas others have a greater focus on certain populations or practice settings (e.g., neonatal intensive care or domestic violence victims). Some of the documents relate to more specific clinical aspects of care (e.g., wound management, physical agent modalities, feeding). The Official Documents can be found in the practice section of the AOTA website (www.aota.org) and are published in the *American Journal of Occupational Therapy* (AJOT).

Choose one of the following six primary areas of practice that you would like to work in:

1. _____ Children and youth

2. _____ Mental health

3. _____ Productive aging

4. _____ Rehabilitation and disability

5. _____ Work and industry

6. _____ Health and wellness

Refer to the list of AOTA Official Documents to answer the following questions.

1. Which of the AOTA *Position Statements* are applicable to your chosen practice area?

2. Which of the AOTA *Guidance Documents* are applicable to your chosen practice area?

3. Which of the AOTA *Professional Standards* are applicable to your chosen practice area?

4. Which of the AOTA *Societal Statements* are applicable to your chosen practice area?

Worksheet 4-2

Using American Occupational Therapy Association Official Documents

1. The *OTPF—4* was developed, in part, to be consistent with terminology used in which WHO document?
   A. International Classification of Functioning, Disability and Health (ICF)
   B. International Classification of Diseases (ICD)
   C. Health Insurance Portability and Accountability Act (HIPAA)
   D. Current Procedural Terminology (CPT)

2. Carol is an OTA who is reentering practice after a long absence. Due to all the changes in health care, Carol is unsure if AOTA guidelines now allow for an initial evaluation to be delegated to an OTA. Besides reviewing that state's licensure laws and regulations, which of the following documents delineates the specific OT and OTA practice responsibilities and better outlines aspects of the occupational therapy process appropriate for delegation to an OTA?
   A. *AOTA 2020 Occupational Therapy Code of Ethics*
   B. *Standards of Practice for Occupational Therapy*
   C. *Occupational Therapy Practice Framework*
   D. *Guidelines for Documentation of Occupational Therapy*

3. An OTA is unsure as to whether there is an obligation to treat a client whose lifestyle choices conflict with the OTA's religious or personal beliefs. Of the following document choices, which is likely more suitable to help with making this decision?
   A. *Guidelines for Supervision, Roles, and Responsibilities During the Delivery of Occupational Therapy Services*
   B. *Standards for Continuing Competence*
   C. *Scope of Practice*
   D. *AOTA 2020 Occupational Therapy Code of Ethics*

4. Which of the following choices is an AOTA Official Document that is not categorized as a Position Statement?
   A. *Scope of Practice*
   B. *Obesity and Occupational Therapy*
   C. *The Practice of Occupational Therapy in Feeding, Eating, and Swallowing*
   D. *Occupational Therapy and Complementary Health Approaches and Integrative Health*

5. Which of the following practice settings or interventions is not specifically mentioned in the title of an AOTA Position Statement?
   A. Wound management
   B. Medication management
   C. Primary care
   D. Feeding and eating

6. Of the following choices, which document better describes the array of services that occupational therapy practitioners provide?
   A. *Standards of Practice for Occupational Therapy*
   B. *Guidelines for Supervision, Roles and, Responsibilities During the Delivery of Occupational Therapy Services*
   C. *Scope of Practice*
   D. *Standards for Continuing Competence*

Worksheet 4-2 (continued)

Using American Occupational Therapy Association Official Documents

7. An OTA is developing a professional development plan involving five essential criteria (e.g., knowledge, critical reasoning, interpersonal skills, performance skills, ethical practice) to assess, retain, and document continuing competence. Although all the following document choices are relevant, which is more clearly represented in this scenario?
   A. *Standards of Practice for Occupational Therapy*
   B. *Guidelines for Supervision, Roles, and Responsibilities During the Delivery of Occupational Therapy Services*
   C. *AOTA 2020 Occupational Therapy Code of Ethics*
   D. *Standards for Continuing Competence*

8. An OTA taught a client with back pain how to use a long shoehorn and reachers yesterday. The OTA is unsure as to whether it is proper to ask the rehabilitation aide to practice this same task with the client today. In addition to reviewing that state's relevant licensure laws and regulations, the OTA would like to use an AOTA document that provides specific criteria for delegating client-related tasks. Which of the following choices is a better fit for this?
   A. *Guidelines for Supervision, Roles, and Responsibilities During the Delivery of Occupational Therapy Services*
   B. *Scope of Practice*
   C. *Accreditation Council for Occupational Therapy Education Standards*
   D. *Standards of Practice for Occupational Therapy*

9. An OTA is tasked with gathering some AOTA resources for an OT manager who is developing a new occupational therapy evaluation form for home care clients. Which of the following documents is less of a fit than the others for use in creating this evaluation form?
   A. *Occupational Therapy Practice Framework: Domain and Process, Fourth Edition*
   B. *Accreditation Council for Occupational Therapy Education Standards and Interpretive Guide*
   C. *Guidelines for Documentation of Occupational Therapy*
   D. *Scope of Practice*

10. An OT working in an outpatient setting is deciding whether to delegate certain physical agent modality interventions to the OTA. Of the following documents, which would generally be less of a fit in helping the therapist make this decision?
    A. *Guidelines for Supervision, Roles, and Responsibilities During the Delivery of Occupational Therapy Services*
    B. *Physical Agents and Mechanical Modalities*
    C. *Standards of Practice for Occupational Therapy*
    D. *Value of Occupational Therapy Assistant Education to the Profession*

Adapted from Morreale, M. J., & Amini, D. (2016). *The occupational therapist's workbook for ensuring clinical competence.* SLACK Incorporated.

Worksheet 4-3

Occupational Therapy Practice Framework

A person's daily activities can be classified as the various occupations delineated in the *OTPF—4* (AOTA, 2020c). However, some activities may not fit neatly into a single *OTPF—4* category, depending on the perspective of the individual or population's interests and needs (AOTA, 2020c). For example, making bread may be classified as an instrumental activity of daily living (IADL; meal preparation), a leisure activity for someone whose hobby is baking, or may be considered social participation or volunteer work if a group is making Challah bread for a religious service or a fundraising event.

Indicate which area(s) of occupation that each of the listed items belong to, according to your personal interests, values, and roles.

Client Activity	ADLs	IADLs	Health Management	Play	Leisure	Work	Education	Rest and Sleep	Social Participation
Baking muffins									
Cleaning contact lenses									
Taking the train to get to a job									
Donning an orthosis									
Playing hopscotch with others									
Attending religious services									
Making a collage for an occupational therapy class assignment									
Watching television to fall asleep									
Feeding the household cat or dog									
Listening to music									
Preparing a résumé									
Walking to the dinner table									
Taking a nap									

Worksheet 4-3 (continued)

Occupational Therapy Practice Framework

Client Activity	ADLs	IADLs	Health Management	Play	Leisure	Work	Education	Rest and Sleep	Social Participation
Babysitting a younger sibling									
Organizing school papers into folders									
Volunteering at a hospital gift shop									
Attending a bridal shower or bachelor party									
Paying bills									
Getting to next class on time									
Knitting a sweater to wear									
Using contraception									
Setting an alarm clock									
Reading emails									
Taking vitamins									
Sewing a button back on a shirt									
Planting flowers in the yard									
Writing a performance review for a staff member									
Navigating a wheelchair in the home									

Worksheet 4-3 (continued)

Occupational Therapy Practice Framework

Client Activity	ADLs	IADLs	Health Management	Play	Leisure	Work	Education	Rest and Sleep	Social Participation
Dressing a doll									
Exercising at the gym									
Calling 911 when smelling smoke									
Eating lunch with colleagues									
Getting a manicure									
Ironing a shirt									
Reading an evidence-based article									
Building a sandcastle with others									
Driving to a dentist appointment									
Going to the library									
Helping out at a food pantry									
Checking your blood pressure or glucose levels									

Learning Activity 4-3: *Occupational Therapy Practice Framework*—More Practice

Identify 10 activities not already listed in Worksheet 4-3 that you personally do in a typical day or week. Indicate which area(s) of occupation (AOTA, 2020c) that each of the listed items belong to, according to your personal interests, values, and roles.

My Typical Daily or Weekly Activities	ADLs	IADLs	Health Management	Play	Leisure	Work	Education	Rest and Sleep	Social Participation
1.									
2.									
3.									
4.									
5.									
6.									
7.									
8.									
9.									
10.									

Adapted from Morreale, M. J., & Amini, D. (2016). *The occupational therapist's workbook for ensuring clinical competence.* SLACK Incorporated.

Now choose a religious, secular, or cultural holiday you celebrate. List five activities that you personally do related to that holiday. Indicate which area(s) of occupation that each of the listed items belong to, according to your personal interests, values, and roles.

A holiday I celebrate is: _____

My Holiday-Related Activities	ADLs	IADLs	Health Management	Play	Leisure	Work	Education	Rest and Sleep	Social Participation
1.									
2.									
3.									
4.									
5.									

Worksheet 4-4

Differentiating Client Factors and Performance Skills

For each of the following sentences, indicate whether it represents a client factor (F) or performance skill (S) according to the *OTPF—4* (AOTA, 2020c). Remember that conditions arise from deficiencies in underlying structures and functions and may affect occupational performance.

1. _____ The client who had shoulder surgery achieved left arm abduction to 160 degrees.

2. _____ The resident is able to manipulate knitting needles with both hands.

3. _____ The client has intact short-term memory.

4. _____ The client admitted to the acute psychiatric unit today has signs and symptoms consistent with severe depression.

5. _____ The client has a pain level of "7" today per the 10-point visual analog scale.

6. _____ The client demonstrates good dynamic standing balance when pulling up his pants.

7. _____ The student remained calm when another student bumped into him.

8. _____ The client sitting in the power wheelchair has poor lymphatic drainage causing 1+ edema in his right leg.

9. _____ The client has a below-knee amputation.

10. _____ The child playing hopscotch is able to hop on one leg four times without falling.

11. _____ During a family intervention, the client stated agreement with need to attend sobriety meetings.

12. _____ The infant demonstrates a positive Babinski sign.

13. _____ The client at risk for thrombosis is using an intermittent compression pump on her legs when lying in her hospital bed.

14. _____ The client with autism is exhibiting tactile defensiveness during art class.

15. _____ The client achieved a right grip strength of 100 lb when using a dynamometer.

Worksheet 4-4 (continued)

Differentiating Client Factors and Performance Skills

16. _____ The child with asthma has difficulty using her inhaler properly.

17. _____ The client would benefit from paraffin to help loosen stiff finger joints.

18. _____ Because of increased tone in the client's fingers, the OT pre-molded the orthotic device on her own hand to prevent difficulty when making a resting pan orthosis.

19. _____ The resident can roll from side to side using bed rails.

20. _____ The client has the condition of Bell's palsy, which is creating difficulty with her ability to coordinate chewing.

Worksheet 4-5

Differentiating Client Factors and Performance Skills—
More Practice

For each of the following sentences, indicate whether it represents a client factor (F) or performance skill (S) according to the *OTPF—4* (AOTA, 2020c). Remember that conditions arise from deficiencies in underlying structures and functions and may affect occupational performance.

1. _____ The student uses a static tripod grasp when writing.

2. _____ The client needed to rest after standing to cook at the stove.

3. _____ The client with schizophrenia hears voices in his head.

4. _____ The client was able to tear open the package of potato chips.

5. _____ The client lying in bed has unilateral neglect.

6. _____ The client's resting blood pressure of 160/95 resulted in the OT contacting the client's physician.

7. _____ The client demonstrates an improvement in muscle strength from Fair to Good for left elbow flexion.

8. _____ The client is able to don and doff his protective fracture brace independently.

9. _____ The client is able to carry a 10-lb grocery bag from her car to the kitchen.

10. _____ The client is unable to cut her toenails because she has difficulty bending.

11. _____ The client's scaphoid fracture needed 6 months to heal completely.

12. _____ The client's gray hair and wrinkles make her appear older than she really is.

13. _____ The resident cannot push up with his arms to perform a sliding board transfer.

14. _____ The client is incontinent of urine secondary to a prolapsed bladder.

15. _____ The client with chemical dependency endures the side effects of withdrawal.

Worksheet 4-5 (continued)

Differentiating Client Factors and Performance Skills— More Practice

16. _____ The client's loss of protective sensation in his feet is a safety concern due to his diabetes.

17. _____ The child with dyspraxia did not fall today while running in gym class.

18. _____ The resident asked for a calendar to help her remember her therapy appointments.

19. _____ The client diagnosed with an anxiety disorder chooses not to attend occupational therapy group today.

20. _____ The client with a nut allergy cannot be exposed to peanut butter.

Worksheet 4-6

Habits, Rituals, Routines, and Roles

For each of the following activities, indicate whether it is a habit, ritual, routine, or role, according to the *OTPF—4* (AOTA, 2020c).

1. _____ Always decorating the tree on Christmas Eve.

2. _____ A family has a tradition of making s'mores over the fire whenever camping.

3. _____ Flossing every time after brushing teeth.

4. _____ Taking care of the family pet before leaving for work

5. _____ Saying a prayer when lighting candles on the Sabbath.

6. _____ Reading a bedtime story after the child's nightly bath and tucking him into bed.

7. _____ A daughter who is caring for an older parent with dementia.

8. _____ Smoking a cigarette right after dinner.

9. _____ Buckling a seat belt before driving.

10. _____ Shaking hands when meeting someone new.

11. _____ The woman who enjoys gardening is known as having a "green thumb."

12. _____ Identifying as a Roman Catholic and joining the church choir.

13. _____ The young musician is proficient at playing a piano.

14. _____ Kissing your spouse when they come home from work.

15. _____ An avid Bingo player.

16. _____ Making breakfast and packing your child's lunch before driving him to school.

Worksheet 4-6 (continued)

Habits, Rituals, Routines, and Roles

17. _____ Completing your shift as a volunteer firefighter.

18. _____ A mother helping the teacher by accompanying the child's class on a field trip.

19. _____ Saying prayers at the gravesite on the 1-year anniversary of the deceased's date of death.

20. _____ Hanging up your coat when you come home.

Worksheet 4-7

Grading and Adapting

For each of the statements following, indicate if the intervention is an example of grading (G) or adapting (A).

1. _____ In order to manage clothing without assistance during toileting at school, the OTA suggested that the student use elastic waist pants rather than pants with fastenings.

2. _____ During yesterday's intervention session, the OTA asked a client diagnosed with social anxiety to make a phone call to a pizzeria to ask the cost of a large pizza. Today they went to the pizzeria together so that the client could place an order for two slices of pizza.

3. _____ The OTA had the child use a button board with smaller buttons than previously to work on three-point pinch.

4. _____ The OTA attached a brake extension to a wheelchair for the client with left hemiplegia.

5. _____ An OTA is working on home management skills with a client diagnosed with traumatic brain injury. Last week the OTA asked the client to bake prepared refrigerated dough cookies, and today the OTA had the client attempt to make cookies using a boxed mix.

6. _____ The OTA suggested that the child with hand weakness practice handwriting for 5 minutes daily this week and 10 minutes daily next week.

7. _____ The OTA taught the client to use a calendar to remember appointments.

8. _____ To help improve decision-making skills, the OTA gave the client diagnosed with depression a choice of only two craft projects yesterday and a choice of three projects today.

9. _____ The OTA instructed the client with chronic obstructive pulmonary disease to sit during ironing when the client returns home.

10. _____ The OTA had the client with bilateral integration problems roll out dough with a rolling pin during last week's session. Today the OTA had the client mix dough ingredients with her dominant hand while holding onto a bowl with the non-dominant hand.

11. _____ The OT asked the OTA to attach a zipper pull to the student's backpack.

12. _____ The OT told the toddler's parents that the child could now eat semi-soft foods in addition to puréed food.

Worksheet 4-7 (continued)
Grading and Adapting

13. _____ The OT asked the OTA to discontinue the client's forearm-based thumb spica orthosis today and issue a hand-based thumb spica orthosis instead.

14. _____ The OTA instructed the caregiver to purchase an electric tea kettle with an automatic shut off for the client with early-stage dementia.

15. _____ The OTA instructed the client in use of a pill organizer to aid in remembering to take medication properly.

16. _____ The OT determined that the OTA could initiate light therapy putty exercises today with the client diagnosed with a metacarpal fracture.

17. _____ The OTA worked on the client's wheelchair mobility by having him navigate his manual wheelchair outdoors today.

18. _____ The OTA asked the teacher to allow the first-grade student to eat raisins or granola at his desk to minimize fidgeting during class.

19. _____ The OTA gave the client with schizophrenia a structured leisure worksheet because the client could not come up with three desired leisure tasks when initially asked.

20. _____ As the client with multiple sclerosis could not tolerate gardening outdoors due to the heat and humidity, the OTA instructed the family to set up an indoor windowsill garden.

Adapted from Morreale, M. J., & Amini, D. (2016). *The occupational therapist's workbook for ensuring clinical competence.* SLACK Incorporated.

Worksheet 4-8

Grading and Adapting—Making Coffee

List ways to grade and adapt the occupation of making coffee by indicating various modifications for the activity demands designated at the top of each column.

Activity Demand: Task Material—Coffee	Activity Demand: Required Action of Opening Coffee Container	Activity Demand: Required Action of Measuring Coffee	Activity Demand: Required Action of Heating the Water/Brewing Coffee
Example: Instant coffee	Example: Can of coffee requiring use of a can opener	Example: Use a measuring spoon	Example: Boil water in teakettle using stove

Worksheet 4-9

Grading and Adapting—Laundry

List the sequence of steps to wash clothes and various ways to grade and adapt each of those steps.

Sequence of Steps to Perform the Occupation of Laundry	Grade/Adapt Task Methods	Grade/Adapt Task Materials
Example: Carry a laundry basket full of clothes to washer	Example: Place dirty clothes directly in machine when getting changed	Example: Use a rolling laundry cart Use a laundry bag

Learning Activity 4-4: Occupational Analysis— Preparing Breakfast (Traumatic Brain Injury)

Your client is a 35-year-old female recovering from a traumatic brain injury. She has difficulty performing IADLs (e.g., meal preparation, laundry) due to deficits in organization, problem solving, and safety. However, this client does not have any impairment in range of motion, strength, or endurance.

For the occupation of preparing breakfast, put the following items in order of preparation difficulty from easier to harder for this client scenario. Indicate the activity demands that make each task easier or harder. Compare your answers for this exercise to your answers for Learning Activity 4-5. Is your order of difficulty the same or different?

A. Scrambled eggs and bacon
B. Frozen breakfast sandwich
C. Cereal and milk
D. Smoothie (made from scratch)
E. Hard-boiled eggs
F. Frozen waffles
G. Toast
H. Pancakes (using a mix)
I. Yogurt
J. Fresh fruit salad (apple, grapes, melon)

List Tasks in Order of Difficulty From Easier to Harder	Activity Demands
1.	
2.	
3.	
4.	
5.	
6.	
7.	
8.	
9.	
10.	

Learning Activity 4-5: Occupational Analysis— Preparing Breakfast (Rheumatoid Arthritis)

Your client is a 65-year-old female with severe rheumatoid arthritis. She has difficulty with home management and self-care tasks due to multiple joint contractures in both hands and inability to make a full fist or perform tip pinch.

For the occupation of preparing breakfast, put the following food choices in order of preparation difficulty from easier to harder for this client scenario. Indicate the activity demands that make each task easier or harder. Compare your answers for this exercise to your answers for Learning Activity 4-4. Is your order of difficulty the same or different?

- A. Scrambled eggs and bacon
- B. Frozen breakfast sandwich
- C. Cereal and milk
- D. Smoothie (made from scratch)
- E. Hard-boiled eggs
- F. Frozen waffles
- G. Toast
- H. Pancakes (using a mix)
- I. Yogurt
- J. Fresh fruit salad (apple, grapes, melon)

List Tasks in Order of Difficulty From Easier to Harder	Activity Demands
1.	
2.	
3.	
4.	
5.	
6.	
7.	
8.	
9.	
10.	

Handling Situations Appropriately

An OTA must perform all professional duties competently. This includes communicating effectively, implementing appropriate interventions skillfully, documenting client care accurately, and completing departmental tasks capably within acceptable time frames. In addition, an OTA must "expect the unexpected" and be prepared to handle unpredictable or challenging situations that may arise during the workday. It is essential that practitioners demonstrate good professional reasoning and respond expeditiously when faced with emergency situations, difficult client behaviors, safety issues, unusual occurrences, and ethical problems (AOTA, 2015a, 2015b, 2020a). As you complete Learning Activities 4-6 and 4-7, consider the suggestions in the table below for managing atypical or challenging situations.

Handling Situations Appropriately
• Remain calm
• Exercise prudence
• Obtain help as needed
• Use good professional reasoning
• Demonstrate professionalism and sensitivity
• Incorporate therapeutic use of self
• Maintain client dignity
• Show empathy
• Do what is in the best interest of the client
• Make safety a priority
• Know relevant emergency procedures and undergo training for first aid/cardiopulmonary resuscitation (CPR)
• Utilize proper infection control techniques
• Understand liability issues
• Keep current with legislation influencing occupational therapy practice
• Complete documentation requirements
• Adhere to facility policies and procedures
• Follow-up as needed
• Notify your supervisor and appropriate others according to facility policy and relevant laws
• Implement preventative measures
• Learn from the experience
• Maintain healthy habits and manage your own stress level for optimal work performance

Learning Activity 4-6: Handling Situations Appropriately

Indicate how you would respond appropriately with professionalism and sensitivity to the following actual clinical situations that various occupational therapy practitioners have encountered (identifying details have been changed). Consider what you would say to the clients, the immediate action you would take, and any follow-up that may be required.

1. Marge, a 75-year-old client in a skilled nursing facility, is 10 days status post pinning for a right femoral neck fracture. When you arrive at her room to bring her to therapy, Marge is lying in bed. Marge states that she just fell out of bed but was able to get back in bed by herself. She starts to cry and states, *"I should not have told you I fell. I'm okay now. Please do not tell anyone what happened or they will put a restraint on me."*

2. You are transferring a client from the hospital bed to a chair. The client is wearing only a hospital gown and is a little groggy from just waking up. As you are providing moderate assistance to transfer the client from sit to stand, the client suddenly becomes incontinent of feces, most of which lands directly on your shoe. The client does not appear to realize what just happened.

3. There are several clients present in the therapy room. As they are performing their exercises, they are making small talk and joking around. As the conversation turns to the topic of an upcoming election, the clients get into a very heated discussion and begin yelling at each other and using profanity.

4. A man receiving occupational therapy following a carpal tunnel release has been carrying a briefcase to each session. He typically asks for copies of his treatment notes and evaluations and places them in the briefcase. One day, when his intervention session has ended and the OTA is leaving the clinic to go to the occupational therapy office, the client calls the OTA back and says, "Look what I forgot to leave in my car." He then pulls out a handgun from the briefcase and turns it over several times to allow the OTA a good look.

5. A man is sent to occupational therapy directly from the physician's office for fabrication of a volar resting pan orthosis. The client had surgery 2 days ago to repair a lacerated extensor indicis tendon and had his surgical dressing removed moments ago. The OT realizes this appointment is urgent and squeezes the client into the therapist's busy, full work schedule today. However, the OT only has enough time to fabricate the orthosis and provide minimal instruction until the next day when the client will be scheduled for a full evaluation and follow-up orthotic check. The man is fitted with the orthotic device and told not to remove it until he sees the OT tomorrow. However, the client does not show up the next day for his appointment. The OT calls to reschedule, but the client misses each appointment. Finally, after 2 weeks the client reappears without an appointment and complains to the OTA in the front office that his hand smells. The OT is in a meeting, so the OTA removes the orthosis carefully and observes that the client's volar hand is severely macerated, and the orthosis is soggy and odorous. When asked why this is, the client reported that he followed the OT's instruction not to remove his orthosis until he was seen back in therapy. In the meantime, the client had bathed everyday with the orthosis on, not removing it to dry his skin.

6. You are working in a skilled nursing facility with Harold, a 78-year-old client diagnosed with moderate stage Alzheimer's disease and a recent shoulder fracture. When you enter Harold's room to bring him to therapy, you discover that Harold has completely disrobed and is wandering around the room.

7. An OT working in an outpatient clinic fabricated a finger orthosis 2 days ago for a client. Today an OTA has been delegated this client for a follow-up orthotic check. When the client arrives, he reports that he accidentally flushed the orthosis down the toilet yesterday when washing his hands after toileting.

8. You are working in an outpatient clinic with a client who has a neurological condition. You transfer the client to the mat table to work on upper extremity exercises with the client positioned in supine. As the client initiates the exercises, you suddenly notice that the client was incontinent of urine, resulting in his pants and the mat getting wet. The client does not mention what just occurred.

9. You are a female OTA providing home care services to a young male client with a diagnosis of traumatic brain injury. Today you are alone in his basement apartment working with him on a dressing activity. Suddenly, the client reaches and grabs your breast.

10. You are working in an outpatient therapy clinic. One day you are sitting at a table with a client who is performing fine-motor activities. All of a sudden you notice that your client is slumped over and appears to be turning blue.

Debbie Amini, EdD, OTR/L, FAOTA has contributed significantly to this learning activity.

Learning Activity 4-7: Handling Situations Appropriately— More Practice

Indicate how you would respond appropriately with professionalism and sensitivity to the following actual clinical situations that various occupational therapy practitioners have encountered (identifying details have been changed). Consider what you would say to the clients, the immediate action you would take, and any follow-up that may be required.

1. Joe, a 55-year-old male client, has undergone hand surgery and is receiving outpatient occupational therapy. He has an outgoing personality, likes to make people laugh, and enjoys being the center of attention. Today there are five other middle-aged clients in the therapy clinic. Joe begins to loudly tell a joke that has sexual overtones.

2. A client is receiving outpatient occupational therapy following a shoulder fracture. The client has deep religious beliefs and always brings a holy book to read in the clinic waiting room and during his hot pack treatments. Today the client inquiries about the OTA's religious affiliation, which is very different than that of the client. The client states that the OTA is misguided and begins to proselytize. The client then asks the OTA to look at a passage in the holy book.

3. An OTA is working with Stanley, a 75-year-old male who exhibits left hemiplegia and severe left neglect. As the OTA is walking past Stanley's hospital room, Stanley calls out excitedly for the OTA to come into his room right now. The OTA goes in his room and observes that Stanley is beaming. Stanley begins lifting his unaffected right arm and leg up and down vigorously while saying, *"Look, look—it's a miracle! I can now move my arm and leg!"*

4. An OTA working in a skilled nursing facility has been delegated a client who is diagnosed with chronic obstructive pulmonary disease. Today the client makes several derogatory remarks regarding the supervising OT's ethnicity (or religion) and then states, *"Do I have to work with that OT? I would prefer to just work with you."*

5. An OTA working in home care has been delegated a client, Eva, who is recovering from a hip fracture. Eva lives with her spouse and presently requires contact guard assistance to ambulate with a walker. As the OTA arrives at the client's home and is ringing the doorbell, the OTA can see Eva through the glass door panels. The OTA then observes that, as Eva starts to get up out of her chair unattended, she trips and falls to the floor. The client did not lose consciousness and calls out for help.

Answers to Worksheets

Worksheet 4-1: Using Standard Precautions

***Note that in a pandemic or local health emergency situation, the use of extra and/or different types of PPE may be required along with enhanced, stricter protocols for worker and client health and safety.

Additional resource: Fairchild et al., 2018

1. D. (CDC, 2020; WHO, 2009)
2. B. Enough soap should be applied to cover all surfaces of hand. After rubbing and rinsing, a single-use towel should be used to dry hands and turn off faucet (WHO, 2009).
3. C. Soap and water should be used after toileting and in situations when hands are visibly soiled (WHO, 2009). When using an alcohol-based hand-rub, hands should be rubbed together until dry. Health care workers should remove gloves after each patient and reusing gloves is not recommended (CDC, 2020; WHO, 2009, 2021).
4. A. A lab coat is not considered PPE (Siegel et al., 2019)
5. D. The other three choices are transmitted through droplet (Siegel et al., 2019)
6. A. (Siegel et al., 2019)
7. B. The other choices are examples of direct contact transmission. Indirect contact transmission means there is a contaminated intermediate person or object through which the infectious agent is transferred, for example a worker's hands or patient-care device (Siegel et al., 2019)
8. C. A lab coat is not considered PPE. A fitted respirator is indicated for airborne precautions rather than a surgical mask or face shield. (Siegel et al., 2019)
9. C.
10. C. A non-sterile glove should be removed by pinching it at the wrist level (without touching forearm skin) and peeling it away from hand thus, turning glove inside out (WHO, 2009)

Worksheet 4-2: Using American Occupational Therapy Association Official Documents

1. A. The *OTPF—4* was created, in part, to be consistent with the terminology used by the WHO's International Classification of Functioning, Disability and Health (AOTA, 2020c).
2. B. This document sets forth specific clinical practice requirements for OTs and OTAs in the areas of evaluation, intervention, and outcomes (AOTA, 2015b).
3. D. This document delineates occupational therapy core values such as equality, altruism, client dignity, and guiding principles which include beneficence, veracity, justice, and so forth (AOTA, 2020a).
4. C.
5. D.
6. C. This document describes the general, wide variety of services that OTs and OTAs provide. Answers A, B, and D address other aspects of practice (AOTA, 2014).
7. D. (AOTA, 2015a) This document specifically describes the five essential criteria noted.
8. A. This document delineates specific guidelines for the kinds of tasks that may or may not be delegated ethically to an aide (AOTA, 2020b).
9. B. The Accreditation Council for Occupational Therapy Education Standards delineate the criteria for all levels of OT and OTA academic programs (Accreditation Council for Occupational Therapy Education, 2018).
10. D.

Worksheet 4-3: *Occupational Therapy Practice Framework*

Some items fit neatly into one category, whereas other activities may be placed into several different categories depending on the particular context and one's personal values, interests, or roles (AOTA, 2020c). For example, reading email can be a work-related task, a leisurely way to pass time, or considered a means of social communication. Thus, your classifications could be slightly different than the following ones.

Client Activity	ADLs	IADLs	Health Management	Play	Leisure	Work	Education	Rest and Sleep	Social Participation
Baking muffins		*			*				
Cleaning contact lenses			*						
Taking the train to get to a job		*							
Donning an orthosis	*								
Playing hopscotch with others				*					
Attending religious services		*							
Making a collage for an occupational therapy class assignment							*		
Watching television to fall asleep					*			*	
Feeding the household cat or dog		*							
Listening to music					*				
Preparing a résumé						*			
Walking to the dinner table	*								
Taking a nap			*					*	
Babysitting a younger sibling		*				*			
Organizing school papers into folders							*		

Client Activity	ADLs	IADLs	Health Management	Play	Leisure	Work	Education	Rest and Sleep	Social Participation
Volunteering at a hospital gift shop						*			*
Attending a bridal shower or bachelor party									*
Paying bills		*							
Getting to next class on time							*		
Knitting a sweater to wear					*				
Using contraception			*						
Setting an alarm clock								*	
Reading emails					*	*			*
Taking vitamins			*						
Sewing a button back on a shirt		*							
Planting flowers in the yard		*			*				
Writing a performance review for a staff member						*			
Navigating a wheelchair in the home	*								
Dressing a doll				*					
Exercising at the gym			*		*				
Calling 911 when smelling smoke		*							
Eating lunch with colleagues					*	*			*
Getting a manicure	*				*				*

Client Activity	ADLs	IADLs	Health Management	Play	Leisure	Work	Education	Rest and Sleep	Social Participation
Ironing a shirt		*							
Reading an evidence-based article						*	*		
Building a sandcastle with others				*					*
Driving to a dentist appointment		*	*						
Going to the library					*		*		
Helping out at a food pantry						*			*
Checking your blood pressure or glucose levels			*						

Worksheet 4-4: Differentiating Client Factors and Performance Skills

According to the *OTPF—4* (AOTA, 2020c), client factors are what the client *has* (e.g., anatomical/physiological structures and functions, beliefs) whereas performance skills (motor, social interaction, and process skills) are what the client *does* (i.e., observable actions). For example, ROM and strength are client factors which affect motor performance skills such as reaching to put cans in a cabinet or bending to tie shoes. As another example, having vocal nodules or brain lesions may affect communication skills such as ability to modulate voice, talk on the telephone, or say a prayer. Realize that some things that are observable such as Bell's palsy or edema may be considered *conditions*, not client factors. Conditions typically arise from deficiencies in underlying structures and functions such as impaired facial nerves, brain lesions, impaired sensory processing, or poor lymphatic drainage and can affect occupational performance.

1. F. The client who had shoulder surgery achieved left arm abduction to 160 degrees.
2. S. The resident is able to manipulate knitting needles with both hands.
3. F. The client has intact short-term memory.
4. F. The client admitted to the acute psychiatric unit today has signs and symptoms consistent with severe depression.
5. F. The client has a pain level of "7" today per the 10-point visual analog scale.
6. S. The client demonstrates good dynamic standing balance when pulling up his pants.
7. S. The student remained calm when another student bumped into him.
8. F. The client sitting in the power wheelchair has poor lymphatic drainage causing 1+ edema in his right leg.
9. F. The client has a below-knee amputation.

10. S. The child playing hopscotch is able to hop on one leg four times without falling.

11. S. During a family intervention, the client stated agreement with need to attend sobriety meetings.

12. F. The infant demonstrates a positive Babinski sign.

13. F. The client at risk for thrombosis is using an intermittent compression pump on her legs when lying in her hospital bed.

14. F. The client with autism is exhibiting tactile defensiveness during art class.

15. F. The client achieved a right grip strength of 100 lb when using a dynamometer.

16. S. The child with asthma has difficulty using her inhaler properly.

17. F. The client would benefit from paraffin to help loosen stiff finger joints.

18. F. Because of increased tone in the client's fingers, the OT pre-molded the orthotic device on her own hand to prevent difficulty when making a resting pan orthosis.

19. S. The resident can roll from side to side using bed rails.

20. S. The client has the condition of Bell's palsy, which is creating difficulty with her ability to coordinate chewing.

Reproduced with permission from Morreale, M. J., & Amini, D. (2016). *The occupational therapist's workbook for ensuring clinical competence.* SLACK Incorporated.

Worksheet 4-5: Differentiating Client Factors and Performance Skills— More Practice

According to the *OTPF—4* (AOTA, 2020c), client factors are what the client *has* (e.g., anatomical/physiological structures and functions, beliefs) whereas performance skills (motor, social interaction, and process skills) are what the client *does* (i.e., observable actions). For example, the client factors of sensation and vision affect motor skills such as putting a key in a lock or cutting vegetables safely. As another example, the client factors of self-concept and emotional regulation affect process skills such as desire to live and waiting one's turn patiently. Realize that some things that are observable or measurable such as pain or edema may be considered *conditions*, not client factors. Conditions such as depression, hypertension, allergies, frequent colds, or fracture non-union may arise due to deficiencies in underlying structures or functions such as chemical imbalance, impaired cardiac function, blocked vessels, or a poor immune system and may affect occupational performance.

1. S. The student uses a static tripod grasp when writing.

2. S. The client needed to rest after standing to cook at the stove.

3. F. The client with schizophrenia hears voices in his head.

4. S. The client was able to tear open the package of potato chips.

5. F. The client lying in bed has unilateral neglect.

6. F. The client's resting blood pressure of 160/95 resulted in the OT contacting the client's physician.

7. F. The client demonstrates an improvement in muscle strength from Fair to Good for left elbow flexion.

8. S. The client is able to don and doff his protective fracture brace independently.

9. S. The client is able to carry a 10-lb grocery bag from her car to the kitchen.

10. S. The client is unable to cut her toenails because she has difficulty bending.

11. F. The client's scaphoid fracture needed 6 months to heal completely.

12. F. The client's gray hair and wrinkles make her appear older than she really is.

13. S. The resident cannot push up with his arms to perform a sliding board transfer.

14. F. The client is incontinent of urine secondary to a prolapsed bladder.

15. S. The client with chemical dependency endures the side effects of withdrawal.

16. F. The client's loss of protective sensation in his feet is a safety concern due to his diabetes.

17. S. The child with dyspraxia did not fall today while running in gym class.

18. S. The resident asked for a calendar to help her remember her therapy appointments.

19. S. The client diagnosed with an anxiety disorder chooses not to attend occupational therapy group today.

20. F. The client with a nut allergy cannot be exposed to peanut butter.

Worksheet 4-6: Habits, Rituals, Routines, and Roles

For each of the following activities, indicate if it is a habit, ritual, routine, or role.

1. Ritual. Always decorating the tree on Christmas Eve.

2. Ritual. A family has a tradition of making s'mores over the fire whenever camping.

3. Habit. Flossing every time after brushing teeth.

4. Routine. Taking care of the family pet before leaving for work

5. Ritual. Saying a prayer when lighting candles on the Sabbath.

6. Routine. Reading a bedtime story after the child's nightly bath and tucking him into bed.

7. Role. A daughter who is caring for an older parent with dementia.

8. Habit. Smoking a cigarette right after dinner.

9. Habit. Buckling a seat belt before driving.

10. Ritual. Shaking hands when meeting someone new.

11. Role. The woman who enjoys gardening is known as having a "green thumb."

12. Role. Identifying as a Roman Catholic and joining the church choir.

13. Role. The young musician is proficient at playing a piano.

14. Habit. Kissing your spouse when they come home from work.

15. Role. An avid Bingo player.

16. Routine. Making breakfast and packing your child's lunch before driving him to school.

17. Role. Completing your shift as a volunteer firefighter.

18. Role. A mother helping the teacher by accompanying the child's class on a field trip.

19. Ritual. Saying prayers at the gravesite on the 1-year anniversary of the deceased's date of death.

20. Habit. Hanging up your coat when you come home.

Reproduced with permission from Morreale, M. J., & Amini, D. (2016). *The occupational therapist's workbook for ensuring clinical competence.* SLACK Incorporated.

Worksheet 4-7: Grading and Adapting

For each of the statements following, indicate if the intervention is an example of grading (G) or adapting (A).

1. A. In order to manage clothing without assistance during toileting at school, the OTA suggested that the student use elastic waist pants rather than pants with fastenings.

2. G. During yesterday's intervention session, the OTA asked a client diagnosed with social anxiety to make a phone call to a pizzeria to ask the cost of a large pizza. Today they went to the pizzeria together so that the client could place an order for two slices of pizza.

3. G. The OTA had the child use a button board with smaller buttons than previously to work on three-point pinch.

4. A. The OTA attached a brake extension to a wheelchair for the client with left hemiplegia.

5. G. An OTA is working on home management skills with a client diagnosed with traumatic brain injury. Last week the OTA asked the client to bake prepared refrigerated dough cookies, and today the OTA had the client attempt to make cookies using a boxed mix.

6. G. The OTA suggested that the child with hand weakness practice handwriting for 5 minutes daily this week and 10 minutes daily next week.

7. A. The OTA taught the client to use a calendar to remember appointments.

8. G. To help improve decision-making skills, the OTA gave the client diagnosed with depression a choice of only two craft projects yesterday and a choice of three projects today.

9. A. The OTA instructed the client with chronic obstructive pulmonary disease to sit during ironing when the client returns home.

10. G. The OTA had the client with bilateral integration problems roll out dough with a rolling pin during last week's session. Today the OTA had the client mix dough ingredients with her dominant hand while holding onto a bowl with the non-dominant hand.

11. A. The OT asked the OTA to attach a zipper pull to the student's backpack.

12. G. The OT told the toddler's parents that the child could now eat semi-soft foods in addition to puréed food.

13. G. The OT asked the OTA to discontinue the client's forearm-based thumb spica orthosis today and issue a hand-based thumb spica orthosis instead.

14. A. The OTA instructed the caregiver to purchase an electric tea kettle with an automatic shut off for the client with early-stage dementia.

15. A. The OTA instructed the client in use of a pill organizer to aid in remembering to take medication properly.

16. G. The OT determined that the OTA could initiate light therapy putty exercises today with the client diagnosed with a metacarpal fracture.

17. G. The OTA worked on the client's wheelchair mobility by having him navigate his manual wheelchair outdoors today.

18. A. The OTA asked the teacher to allow the first-grade student to eat raisins or granola at his desk to minimize fidgeting during class.

19. A. The OTA gave the client with schizophrenia a structured leisure worksheet because the client could not come up with three desired leisure tasks when initially asked.

20. A. As the client with multiple sclerosis could not tolerate gardening outdoors due to the heat and humidity, the OTA instructed the family to set up an indoor windowsill garden.

Adapted from Morreale, M. J., & Amini, D. (2016). *The occupational therapist's workbook for ensuring clinical competence.* SLACK Incorporated.

Worksheet 4-8: Grading and Adapting—Making Coffee

Here are some suggestions although you may come up with others. Consider which modifications are needed due to motor difficulties versus cognitive impairment.

Activity Demand: Task Material—Coffee	Activity Demand: Required Action of Opening Coffee Container	Activity Demand: Required Action of Measuring Coffee	Activity Demand: Required Action of Heating the Water/Brewing Coffee
Example: Instant coffee	*Example: Can of coffee requiring use of a can opener*	*Example: Use a measuring spoon*	*Example: Boil water in teakettle using stove*
Whole coffee beans	Jar with lid	Single-serve instant coffee packet	Microwave water
Coffee "teabags"	Tear off pouch	Pods/K-cups	Electric kettle/hot pot with/without automatic shut-off
Specific type of coffee (decaffeinated versus regular, espresso-type coffee, flavored)	Cut pouch with scissors	Premeasured drip coffee package	Automatic drip coffee maker with/without automatic shut-off
	Box/carton (pods)		
	Screw cap/bottle top		

Activity Demand: Task Material—Coffee	Activity Demand: Required Action of Opening Coffee Container	Activity Demand: Required Action of Measuring Coffee	Activity Demand: Required Action of Heating the Water/Brewing Coffee
Bottle of liquid iced coffee Ground coffee	Can of coffee with a metal/foil pull-off lid Can of coffee with a plastic lid Place coffee in another container or bag Carafe/thermos (containing hot coffee	Have family member pre-measure and place in plastic bags or containers	Programmable machine family member can preset Espresso/cappuccino machine K-cup machine Electric percolator Stovetop glass percolator Stovetop metal percolator (espresso) French press

Worksheet 4-9: Grading and Adapting—Laundry

List the sequence of steps to wash clothes and ways to grade and adapt each step. You may come up with other suggestions. An OT practitioner determines which methods are needed to grade and/or adapt specific activity demands for a client's particular situation.

Sequence of Steps to Perform the Occupation of Laundry	Grade/Adapt Task Methods	Grade/Adapt Task Materials
Example: Carry a laundry basket full of clothes to washer	Example: Place dirty clothes directly in machine when getting changed	Example: Use a rolling laundry cart Use a laundry bag
Check pockets before putting clothes in laundry basket Sort items (by color, materials delicate, hand-wash) Open machine lid/door and put appropriate amount of items in machine Open detergent containers and measure detergent, fabric softener, bleach (pour into cap, use scoop measure) Put detergent, bleach, softener in proper machine dispensers and close lid Set proper cycles temp, delicate/heavy-duty, fabric softener, extra rinse and turn machine on Remember to take clothes out of machine	Post visual reminders Post list of instructions Sit instead of stand Take clothes to dry cleaner Use a laundry service Use a hamper or basket to determine correct amount of laundry to put in machine Use premeasured detergent or pods Use markings on caps Label dispensers clearly Post list of instructions	Wear clothing without pockets Use a divided laundry cart Use a reacher Use a front-loading versus a top-loading machine Use a coin-operated machine Premeasured detergent/pods Use dispenser type bottle Laundry detergent sheets Powder versus liquid Dryer sheets

Sequence of Steps to Perform the Occupation of Laundry	Grade/Adapt Task Methods	Grade/Adapt Task Materials
Put clothes in dryer and set time/setting on dryer Remember to take clothes out of machine and put away	Sit instead of stand Take clothes to dry cleaner Use a laundry service Use a hamper or basket to determine correct amount of laundry to put in machine Use premeasured detergent or pods Use markings on caps Label dispensers clearly Post list of instructions Label cycles clearly Designate a consistent day and time to do laundry Stay by machine to perform other tasks Sit instead of stand Hang up clothes instead Post list of instructions Store clothing close to washer and dryer Use a timer	Use a different measuring device Purchase single-use items from laundromat vending machine Use small-sized containers Pod or detergent sheet versus liquid or powder Use an "all-in-one" product Use small-sized containers Use machine with more or less buttons or cycles Pre-programmed cycles Push buttons, digital panel, or a dial Clothesline, drying rack Machine with an audible signal

References

Accreditation Council for Occupational Therapy Education. (2018). 2018 Accreditation Council for Occupational Therapy Education (ACOTE) standards and interpretive guide (effective July 31, 2020). *American Journal of Occupational Therapy, 72*(Suppl. 2), 7212410005. https://doi.org/10.5014/ajot.2018.72S217

American Occupational Therapy Association. (2014). Scope of practice. *American Journal of Occupational Therapy, 68*(Suppl. 3). https://doi.org/10.5014/ajot.2014.686S04

American Occupational Therapy Association. (2015a). Standards for continuing competence. *American Journal of Occupational Therapy, 69*(Suppl. 3), 6913410055. http://dx.doi.org/10.5014/ajot.2015.696S16

American Occupational Therapy Association. (2015b). Standards of practice for occupational therapy. *American Journal of Occupational Therapy, 69*(Suppl. 3), 6913410057. http://dx.doi.org/10.5014/ajot.2015.696S06

American Occupational Therapy Association. (2020a). AOTA 2020 occupational therapy code of ethics. *American Journal of Occupational Therapy, 74*(Suppl. 3), 7413410005. https://doi.org/10.5014/ajot.2020.74S3006

American Occupational Therapy Association. (2020b). Guidelines for supervision, roles, and responsibilities during the delivery of occupational therapy services. *American Journal of Occupational Therapy, 74*(Suppl. 3), 7413410020. https://doi.org/10.5014/ajot.2020.74S3004

American Occupational Therapy Association. (2020c). Occupational therapy practice framework: Domain and process (4th ed.). *American Journal of Occupational Therapy, 74*(Suppl. 2), 7412410010. https://doi.org/10.5014/ajot.2020.74S2001

American Occupational Therapy Association. (2021). *Official documents & policies approved by the representative assembly.* https://www.aota.org/Practice/Manage/Official.aspx

Centers for Disease Control and Prevention. (2020). *Hand hygiene guidance.* Retrieved May 12, 2021, from https://www.cdc.gov/handhygiene/providers/guideline.html

Fairchild, S. L., O'Shea, R. K., & Washington, R. D. (2018). *Pierson and Fairchild's principles & techniques of patient care*

(6th ed.). Elsevier Incorporated.

Morreale, M. J., & Amini, D. (2016). *The occupational therapist's workbook for ensuring clinical competence.* SLACK Incorporated.

Siegel J. D., Rhinehart, E., Jackson, M., Chiarello, L., and the Healthcare Infection Control Practices Advisory Committee. (2019). *2007 guideline for isolation precautions: Preventing transmission of infectious agents in healthcare settings.* https://www.cdc.gov/infectioncontrol/guidelines/isolation/index.html

World Health Organization. (2009). *WHO guidelines on hand hygiene in health care: A summary.* https://www.who.int/publications/i/item/9789241597906-summary

World Health Organization. (2021). *Infection prevention and control.* Retrieved May 12, 2021, from https://www.who.int/infection-prevention/en/

CHAPTER 5

Incorporating Occupations and Activities

Occupational therapy practitioners use a variety of methods and interventions to promote occupational performance and role competence, maintain health and wellness, and improve quality of life (American Occupational Therapy Association [AOTA], 2020). Depending on the client's unique circumstances, the intervention plan may include approaches such as developing or remediating underlying client factors and performance skills; modifying the task, environment, or performance patterns; or compensating for lost function (AOTA, 2020). Although methods and tasks can be an important part of a client's intervention plan to support occupation, these interventions should supplement, but never replace, activities and occupations (AOTA, 2020). Occupational therapy practitioners must use a holistic approach that incorporates meaningful "real-life" interventions that address or support the client's therapeutic goals for occupational engagement (AOTA, 2020). Activities and occupations are emphasized in this chapter, along with select methods and tasks that also contribute to occupational performance (e.g., client/family education and training, provision of adaptive/durable medical equipment [DME], therapeutic exercises). Note that space limitations allow for only select initial evaluation data to be presented here. A "real" evaluation would include more complete information, such as the specific aspects of occupations needing assistance and the various factors, contexts, or performance skills hindering or supporting occupational performance. Answers to worksheet exercises are provided at the end of the chapter.

Contents

Morreale, M. J. *Developing Clinical Competence:*
A Workbook for the OTA, Second Edition (pp. 205-244).
© 2022 SLACK Incorporated.

Worksheet 5-1

Teaching-Learning Process—Total Hip Replacement

Elaine, a client in acute care, is a 65-year-old female who had left total hip replacement surgery (posterolateral approach) 2 days ago. She presently has partial–weight-bearing status for her affected leg, and her secondary diagnoses include hypertension and hyperlipidemia. Elaine was evaluated by the occupational therapist (OT) yesterday and received preliminary instruction in total hip precautions. Upon reviewing the initial evaluation report, the occupational therapy assistant (OTA) sees that the client's upper extremity function and cognition are intact, but the client requires moderate assistance to transfer using a walker. The expected discharge plan is for Elaine to go to a short-term rehabilitation facility 3 days from now and then eventually return home. Today the OTA was delegated the task of teaching the client lower body dressing techniques. Consider the process for implementing this intervention session, such as equipment/supplies needed, methods of instruction, and sequence of steps that the OTA should use for the occupation of dressing.

1. Where will the session take place?

2. What is the anticipated length of session?

3. What equipment/supplies will the OTA need to bring to the session?

4. What are several things the OTA should do prior to entering the client's room?

5. List the general sequence of steps delineating how the session should be implemented:
   A. Perform hand hygiene and use _____ as indicated.

   B. Introduce self as an OTA and first explain…

   C.

   D.

   E.

   F.

   G.

   H.

   I.

In what ways, if any, would you implement the intervention session any differently if the client was 90 years old with mild dementia?

Learning Activity 5-1: Teaching-Learning Process—
Carpal Tunnel Syndrome

Your client, Ben, is a 35-year-old software developer diagnosed with carpal tunnel syndrome in his dominant right hand. He is otherwise in good health. Ben was evaluated by the OT at an outpatient clinic 3 days ago. Here is some information taken from the initial evaluation report:

- *Chief complaint*: Ben reports he has been experiencing decreased hand strength and increased pain, numbness, and tingling in his right thumb, index, and long fingers for the past 4 months.
- *Pain*: Client reports right hand pain as 7/10 with activity, 5/10 at rest.
- *Sensation*: Right hand: Two-point discrimination: 8-mm index and long fingers, 5-mm ring and small fingers. Phalen's test is positive, eliciting numbness/tingling at 15 seconds.
- *Active range of motion (AROM)*: Both upper extremities within normal limits (WNL).
- *Activities of daily living (ADLs)/Instrumental activities of daily living (IADLs)*: Ben's symptoms are creating difficulty with sleeping, job performance, his daily exercise routine at the gym, and yard maintenance.

Strength	Right Hand	Left Hand
Grip	78 lb	98 lb
3-point pinch	20 lb	28 lb
Lateral pinch	28 lb	30 lb
Tip pinch	17 lb	22 lb

After completing Ben's evaluation, the OT fabricated and issued a volar wrist immobilization orthosis for Ben to wear at work, nighttime, and during heavy tasks. Today Ben has his first follow-up appointment, and the OTA will be working with Ben to start teaching him median nerve gliding exercises, tendon gliding exercises, and ergonomics for work. Consider the process for implementing these interventions, such as equipment/supplies needed, specific methods of instruction, and typical sequence of steps that the OTA should follow. Incorporate several activities needed for Ben's desired level of job performance.

1. Where will the session take place?
2. What is the anticipated length of session?
3. What equipment/supplies will the OTA need to gather for the therapy session?
4. Use resources to locate specific instructions/pictures for the nerve and tendon gliding exercises and ergonomic recommendations that Ben will need to be instructed on.
5. The OTA has collaborated with the OT and reviewed Ben's chart. List the general sequence of how the OTA should implement all of Ben's interventions for today, including several activities needed for his job:
   A. Perform hand hygiene
   B. Introduce OTA and explain...
   C.
   D.
   E.
   F.
   G.
   H.
   I.
   J.
6. How do the tendon and nerve gliding exercises relate to Ben's occupational performance?

Worksheet 5-2

Cerebrovascular Accident Interventions

Marvin, a 62-year-old male diagnosed with a left cerebrovascular accident (CVA), was admitted to a subacute rehabilitation facility today. Marvin retired from his postal worker job 2 years ago, divorced his wife last year, and lived alone independently prior to his stroke. Here is some information taken from Marvin's occupational therapy initial evaluation report:

- *Upper extremity status*:
  - Hand dominance: Right
  - Range of motion (ROM): Passive range of motion (PROM) WNL both upper extremities
  - Strength: Right upper extremity (RUE) flaccid, left upper extremity (LUE) within functional limits (WFL)
  - Sensation: Has intact protective sensation RUE but absent light touch; LUE WNL
- *Communication*: Exhibits dysarthria but understands and follows three-step verbal commands.
- *Balance and mobility*: Weakness noted in trunk and right lower extremity. Dynamic sitting and standing balance are fair. While seated in wheelchair, client tends to lean to the right and slide forward with a posterior pelvic tilt. He requires moderate assistance to ambulate using mobility device.
- *ADLs*: Requires moderate assistance for self-care and transfers.

Marvin does not have any other significant underlying medical conditions that would impact his rehabilitation program. In collaboration with the OT, which of the following equipment, adaptive devices, or modalities are likely appropriate for an OTA to use with Marvin at this time to address his primary deficits? Assume that interventions would include not only the provision of a particular piece of equipment or DME, but actual instruction and practice in its use. Indicate Y (yes) or N (no) for each item.

1. _____ Rocker knife

2. _____ Non-slip matting

3. _____ Built-up utensils

4. _____ Plate guard

5. _____ Walker

6. _____ Power wheelchair

7. _____ Electric razor

8. _____ Sock aid

9. _____ Therapy putty

Worksheet 5-2 (continued)
Cerebrovascular Accident Interventions

10. _____ Exercise bands

11. _____ Pulleys

12. _____ Vest restraint

13. _____ Wheelchair arm support

14. _____ Soap-on-a-rope

15. _____ Wash mitt

16. _____ Soap/shampoo dispenser

17. _____ Long-handled sponge

18. _____ Tub seat/bench

19. _____ Hot pack to right shoulder

20. _____ Paraffin to right hand

21. _____ Constraint-induced movement therapy

22. _____ Teach self-ROM

23. _____ Lapboard

24. _____ Large pegboard

25. _____ Nine-Hole Peg Test

Worksheet 5-3

Total Hip Replacement Interventions

Anna is a 74-year-old female who had left total hip replacement surgery (posterolateral approach) 5 days ago due to degenerative joint disease that was causing severe left hip pain. She was admitted to a skilled nursing facility yesterday for short-term rehabilitation, with an expected discharge plan to return home in 2 weeks. Anna's medical history includes hypertension, Type 2 diabetes, and Vitamin B_{12} deficiency. Anna was a teacher who retired at age 62. She never married and has lived alone independently in senior housing for the past 9 years. Per physician's orders, Anna has toe-touch weight-bearing status for left lower extremity and presently requires moderate assistance to transfer and ambulate short distances with a mobility aid. She is unable to perform lower body dressing and bathing due to her total hip precautions. Both upper extremities exhibit good ROM and muscle strength of fair plus.

The intervention plan for Anna includes goals for modified independence in lower body bathing, dressing, and transfers, and to increase upper extremity muscle strength by half a muscle grade to support ADL independence. In collaboration with the OT, which of the following equipment, adaptive devices, or techniques are likely appropriate for an OTA to use with Anna at this time to address her primary deficits? Assume that interventions would include not only the provision of a particular piece of equipment or DME, but actual instruction and practice in its use. Mark Y (yes) or N (no) for each item.

1. _____ Raised toilet seat

2. _____ Adduction cushion

3. _____ Built-up utensils

4. _____ Commode

5. _____ Crossing legs to tie shoes

6. _____ Walker

7. _____ Power wheelchair

8. _____ Long-handled shoehorn

9. _____ Sock aid

10. _____ Hot pack to left hip

11. _____ Paraffin to left hand

12. _____ Teach stair climbing with crutches

Worksheet 5-3 (continued)
Total Hip Replacement Interventions

13. _____ Wheelchair arm support

14. _____ Exercise bands

15. _____ Quad cane

16. _____ Elastic shoelaces

17. _____ Wedge cushion for wheelchair

18. _____ Reacher

19. _____ Long-handled sponge

20. _____ Tub seat/bench

21. _____ Leg lifter

22. _____ Constraint-induced movement therapy

23. _____ Sliding board

24. _____ Buttonhook

25. _____ Hospital bed for home

Worksheet 5-4

Improving Basic and Instrumental Activities of Daily Living Occupations

1. An OTA is working with a client, Harriet, on functional ambulation in the kitchen so that Harriet can prepare meals safely. Harriet is recovering from a left femur fracture, has partial–weight-bearing status, and uses a walker slowly. Which of the following is a correct sequence for using the walker?
   A. Advance walker, then weak leg, then strong leg
   B. Advance weak leg, then walker, then strong leg
   C. Advance walker, then strong leg, then weak leg
   D. Advance strong leg, then weak leg, then walker

2. A client admitted to an inpatient rehabilitation hospital has a diagnosis of bilateral below-knee amputations and is not a candidate for prostheses. He is independent in sliding board transfers, but his wheelchair will not be able to fit through his bathroom doorway at his small, ranch-style home, where he lives with his wife. Which of the following is more suitable for the OTA to instruct the client in use of to enable him to perform toileting independently at home?
   A. Raised toilet seat and grab bar
   B. Commode
   C. Power mobility scooter
   D. Platform walker

3. An OTA is working on transfer training with a client who uses a walker and is diagnosed with Parkinson's disease. When having the client transfer from a chair to a standing position, the OTA should instruct the client to do which of the following?
   A. Keep client's knees close together
   B. Hold onto a transfer belt around the OTA's waist
   C. Lean forward over client's center of gravity
   D. Have client use his arms to push up from walker

4. A client in acute care is diagnosed with a right CVA. His LUE is flaccid and he exhibits fair dynamic standing balance, left neglect, and impulsivity. One of the client's goals is to achieve independence in shaving. Which of the following interventions is more suitable to facilitate the client's shaving performance?
   A. Sitting on edge of bed using a bedside table (with mirror) and a disposable safety razor
   B. Standing at sink using electric razor
   C. Sitting in a chair at the sink using electric razor
   D. Sitting in a chair at the sink using a disposable safety razor

5. A client diagnosed with amyotrophic lateral sclerosis is working with an OTA to improve self-feeding skills. The client has good trunk control but exhibits weakness of the intrinsic hand muscles and oral musculature. In general, to better facilitate feeding skills, the OTA should place the client in which of the following positions?
   A. Sitting in a chair and using an electronic feeding device
   B. Sitting in a chair with chin slightly tucked
   C. Sitting in a chair with neck hyperextended
   D. Sitting in a chair with client's pelvis in a posterior tilt

Worksheet 5-4 (continued)

Improving Basic and Instrumental Activities of Daily Living Occupations

6. A 5-year-old child with a developmental delay is having difficulty donning a coat due to motor planning difficulties with bringing the coat around her back. Which primary method is likely more suitable to help the child become independent in donning her coat?
    A. Use an over-the-head method to don coat
    B. Use mirroring technique
    C. Write down step-by-step instructions
    D. Use a larger size coat

7. An OTA is teaching energy conservation techniques to a female client who has a diagnosis of chronic obstructive pulmonary disease (COPD). The client uses portable oxygen and fatigues easily but can ambulate short distances using a wheeled walker. Of the following recommendations, which would be more suitable for homemaking?
    A. Use a barbecue grill instead of having to bend when using the oven broiler
    B. Use a tub seat when bathing
    C. Exhale before picking up a laundry basket, then inhale while placing it on top of dryer
    D. Use a flat sheet rather than a tightly fitted sheet

8. An OTA is working with a client who is diagnosed with a complete C4 spinal cord injury. Assuming the OTA is competent in all of the following tasks, which of the following would generally be a less suitable occupational therapy intervention for this client?
    A. Instruct client in use of a mouthstick to operate computer keyboard
    B. Instruct client in functional mobility using a sip-and-puff wheelchair
    C. Instruct client in use of environmental controls to operate television
    D. Instruct client in use of hand controls for driving

9. An OTA is working with a male client who is diagnosed with a complete C6 spinal cord injury. Which of the following would generally be a less suitable occupational therapy intervention for this client?
    A. Instruct client in use of a buttonhook
    B. Instruct client in adaptive shaving techniques
    C. Instruct client in use of a wrist-driven hinge orthosis for feeding
    D. Instruct client in wheelchair push-ups to relieve pressure while sitting

10. An OTA is working with a client who is diagnosed with a complete C7-C8 spinal cord injury. Which of the following would generally be a less suitable occupational therapy intervention for this client?
    A. Instruct client in light meal preparation
    B. Instruct client in functional mobility using a power wheelchair
    C. Instruct client in wheelchair push-ups to relieve pressure while sitting
    D. Instruct client in use of a padded bench/chair for bathing

Worksheet 5-5

Total Knee Replacement Interventions

Harvey is a 70-year-old male who had right total knee replacement surgery 3 days ago and was subsequently admitted to a subacute rehabilitation facility yesterday. Harvey lives with his wife in senior housing with elevator access. Prior to admission, he worked part-time as a sales clerk in a home improvement store and was independent in all ADLs, including driving. Expected discharge to home is in 1 week. Here is some information taken from Harvey's occupational therapy evaluation report:

- *Weight-bearing status*: Weight-bearing as tolerated right lower extremity.
- *ROM*: Both upper extremities WFL, right knee extension lacks 10 degrees and flexion is limited to 75 degrees.
- *Strength*: Both upper extremities WFL.
- *Pain*: Right knee pain reported as 4/10 at rest and 7/10 when standing with walker.
- *Functional mobility and transfers*: Client needs minimal assistance sit ⟷ stand and contact guard assistance and increased time to ambulate using a walker.
- *Activity tolerance*: Activity tolerance for standing is limited to approximately 5 minutes due to post-surgical knee pain and stiffness.
- *ADLs*: Requires minimal assistance for lower body bathing; moderate assistance to place underwear and pants over right foot and to don right sock and shoe.

In collaboration with the OT, which of the following equipment, adaptive devices, or interventions are likely appropriate for an OTA to use with Harvey at this time to address his deficits? Assume that interventions would include not only the provision of a particular piece of equipment or DME, but actual instruction and practice in its use. Mark Y (yes) or N (no) for each item.

1. _____ Raised toilet seat

2. _____ Tub seat/bench

3. _____ Pillow under right knee when lying in bed

4. _____ Buttonhook

5. _____ Long-handled shoehorn

6. _____ Commode

7. _____ Hot pack to right knee

8. _____ Elastic shoelaces

9. _____ Sock aid

Worksheet 5-5 (continued)
Total Knee Replacement Interventions

10. _____ Reacher

11. _____ Beanbag toss activity while seated on mat

12. _____ Ambulation using parallel bars

13. _____ Squatting exercises to increase knee ROM

14. _____ Using ambulation device while obtaining items from refrigerator

15. _____ Standing to make a sandwich

16. _____ Power wheelchair mobility training

17. _____ Pegboard activity

18. _____ Cone stacking activity with wrist weights

19. _____ Standing at bathroom sink to shave with electric razor

20. _____ Ambulating up and down the hallway

Worksheet 5-6

Activities as Interventions—Using a Menu

Occupational therapy practitioners work with clients who have brain injuries, intellectual and developmental disabilities, mental health conditions, and problems with social interaction. It is beneficial to incorporate activities and occupations during therapy sessions as an effective means to increase the client's occupational performance. For this exercise, determine 10 ways in which a menu can be used in occupational therapy to improve specific mental functions, process skills, or social interaction skills needed for various occupations, either by role playing (using a take-out menu or the menu on a restaurant website) or going to the on-site cafeteria or another eating establishment in the community. List the occupation category, client factor/performance skill being addressed, along with the specific intervention task and methods of implementation. Two examples are provided.

Occupation	Client Factor/Performance Skill to Be Addressed	Specific Intervention Activity	Method (i.e., role play, menu choices, educate client)
IADL—Financial management	Improve calculation skills	Select an appetizer, entrée, and dessert that total less than $20.00 before tax and tip	Choose items from menu Teach math skills
Health management	Demonstrate healthy food choices Improve problem solving	Choose an entrée and side dish that are not deep fried	Choose items from menu Educate client regarding healthy versus unhealthy foods and emotional eating (e.g., comfort foods)

Learning Activity 5-2: Activities as Interventions— Using a Newspaper

Occupational therapy practitioners work with clients who have brain injuries, intellectual and developmental disabilities, mental health conditions, or problems with social interaction. It is beneficial to incorporate activities and occupations during therapy sessions as an effective means to increase the client's occupational performance. For this exercise, determine 10 ways in which a newspaper can be used in occupational therapy to improve specific mental functions or process skills needed for various occupations. For each of your tasks, determine how it might change the task demands if you were to use a "real" newspaper instead of a web-based newspaper. List the occupation category, client factor/performance skill being addressed, along with the specific intervention activity. Two examples are provided.

Occupation	Client Factor/Performance Skill to Be Addressed	Specific Intervention Activity	A "Real" Newspaper Versus a Web-Based Newspaper
Leisure participation	Improve scanning/visual field awareness	Scan page to find television schedule for a specific time of day	A "real" newspaper that is open provides a much larger area for scanning
IADL—Community mobility	Improve problem solving and topographical orientation	Read a restaurant review and then figure out directions to get there	A web-based newspaper may have a link for directions to the restaurant

Learning Activity 5-3: Activities as Interventions—
Using a Food Circular

Occupational therapy practitioners work with clients who have brain injuries, intellectual and developmental disabilities, mental health conditions, or problems with social interaction. It is beneficial to incorporate activities and occupations during therapy sessions as an effective means to increase the client's occupational performance. For this exercise, determine 10 ways in which a food sale circular can be used in occupational therapy to improve specific mental functions, process skills, or social interaction skills needed for occupational performance. List the occupation category, client factor/performance skill being addressed, along with the specific intervention activity. Two examples are provided.

Occupation	Client Factor/Performance Skill to Be Addressed	Specific Intervention Activity
IADL—Shopping and financial management	Improve categorization skills	Match a stack of coupons to items that are listed in the food circular
IADL—Shopping Social participation	Improve assertiveness skills	Request a rain check for an advertised sale item that is not in stock

Morreale, M. J. (2022). Developing clinical competence: A workbook for the OTA (2nd ed.). SLACK Incorporated.

Worksheet 5-7

Improving Basic and Instrumental Activities Daily Living Occupations—More Practice

1. A client diagnosed with dysphagia has dietary restrictions that allow only thickened liquids and puréed foods. The client also exhibits fair plus upper extremity muscle strength and weak grasp. Which of the following methods is a possible choice when teaching this client feeding skills?
    A. Position client sitting in a chair and using a straw to sip plain apple juice
    B. Position client sitting in a chair and using a large-handled spoon to eat pudding
    C. Position client sitting in a chair and holding a spoon with universal cuff to eat soft scrambled eggs
    D. Position client sitting in a chair and using a chin tuck and two-handled lightweight cup when sipping black coffee containing artificial sweetener

2. An OTA is working in a rehabilitation hospital with a 72-year-old client who sustained a right CVA 2 weeks ago. The client has subluxation at the glenohumeral joint and is beginning to demonstrate some limited motor return, but only for left scapula and glenohumeral motions. The client also requires moderate assistance to transfer to the bed, wheelchair, and toilet. Of the following devices, which is a possible choice for the OTA to use at this time to address the client's upper extremity deficits?
    A. Airplane splint
    B. Arm trough
    C. Pulleys
    D. Therapy putty

3. An OTA is working with a 52-year-old client who exhibits left upper and lower extremity hemiplegia. The client requires assistance for self-care tasks and is presently unable to perform functional ambulation independently. Which of the following devices is not suitable for the OTA to recommend at this time?
    A. Plate guard
    B. Hand-held shower head
    C. Rolling walker
    D. Buttonhook

4. An OTA is working with a client who has a diagnosis of right macular degeneration. To help compensate for deficits associated with this condition, which of the following devices is a possible choice for the OTA to recommend?
    A. Hearing aid
    B. Magnifying glass
    C. Sock assist
    D. Forearm-based thumb spica orthosis

5. An OTA is working with an older adult who lives alone. The client is diagnosed with a vestibular problem that is creating safety concerns. To help compensate for deficits associated with this condition, which of the following is more suitable for the OTA to do?
    A. Recommend client use a tub seat when bathing
    B. Recommend use of a personal sound amplifier device
    C. Recommend client use towel bar for stability when transferring on and off toilet
    D. Recommend client pull up from walker when transferring sit to stand

Worksheet 5-7 (continued)

Improving Basic and Instrumental Activities Daily Living Occupations—More Practice

6. An OTA is working with an older adult who lives alone and is diagnosed with bilateral presbycusis. To help compensate for deficits associated with this condition, which of the following devices is a possible choice for the OTA to recommend?
   A. Reacher
   B. Elevated toilet seat
   C. Large-print books
   D. Telephone amplifier

7. An OTA is working with a male client who has severe COPD and sustained a Colles fracture of his dominant right arm. The client's cast was removed 1 week ago and he has difficulty grasping and manipulating objects. Of the following interventions, which is more suitable for the OTA to implement at this time to improve the client's hand function?
   A. Exercising with pulleys
   B. Fluidotherapy
   C. Buttoning a shirt
   D. Sanding and staining a wood birdhouse

8. An OTA's primary role in hospice care is which of the following?
   A. Teach bed mobility and transfers
   B. Fabricate orthotic devices and teach proper positioning
   C. Implement interventions to support occupational engagement
   D. Improve upper body strength

9. A 32-year-old client with a hand amputation has an upper limb prosthesis classified as a passive terminal device. During prosthetic training, which of the following is more suitable for the OTA to have the client do with the prosthetic hand?
   A. Perform sensory activities to help distinguish hot and cold water
   B. Perform sensory activities to help distinguish sharp from dull objects
   C. Attempt to use it as a gross assist
   D. Test the battery before attempting a functional task

10. A 45-year-old client with a below-elbow amputation is learning how to use a body-powered prosthesis. During prosthetic training, which of the following is more suitable for an OTA to have the client do with the prosthetic hand?
    A. Attempt to pick up a plastic cup
    B. For desensitization, pick blocks out of a container filled with uncooked rice
    C. Practice isolated finger motion for buttoning a shirt
    D. Perform activities to promote stereognosis

Worksheet 5-8

Fracture Interventions

Abe is 64-year-old male who is a retired police officer. He sustained multiple closed fractures in his dominant right hand due to a recent motor vehicle accident in which he was a passenger. The cast was removed 2 days ago, and Abe was referred to outpatient occupational therapy. The physician's orders state: "OT for RUE P/AROM, PAMs PRN, and ADL/IADL retraining; 2 to 3 times weekly for 4 weeks."

Here is some information taken from Abe's evaluation report that the OT completed yesterday.

- *Medical history*: Parkinson's disease (4 years), degenerative joint disease left hip, and history of kidney stones.
- *Prior level of function*: Lives with wife in a garden apartment. Prior to injury client was independent in ADLs and IADLs except for driving, which he stopped doing 1 year ago due to Parkinson's effects.
- *Edema*: None noted RUE.
- *Pain*: Right hand reported as 5/10.
- *Sensation*: Intact.
- *Upper extremity ROM*:
  ◦ Bilateral resting tremors noted
  ◦ LUE: WNL
  ◦ RUE: Shoulder and elbow WNL
  ◦ Right forearm pronation 0/76, supination 0/54
  ◦ Right wrist flexion 0/42, extension 0/32, ulnar deviation 0/10, radial deviation 0/8
  ◦ Client presents with moderate stiffness in right hand, inability to flex fingers to touch palm, opposition only to index finger
- *Functional mobility and transfers*: Client able to perform functional ambulation and transfers independently with slightly increased time. Reports pain in left hip (5/10) when standing more than a few minutes.
- *ADLs/IADLs*: Since his injury, client reports difficulty performing activities requiring grasp or fine-motor skills, such as managing clothing fastenings, shaving, brushing teeth, eating, writing, and performing home maintenance.

The intervention plan for Abe includes goals to increase right wrist and hand ROM/strength to enable modified independence in ADL. In collaboration with the OT, which of the following equipment, adaptive devices, or adapted techniques might be appropriate for an OTA to use with Abe during the first week of therapy to address his primary deficits? Assume that interventions would include not only the provision of a particular piece of equipment or DME, but actual instruction and practice in its use. Mark Y (yes) or N (no) for each item.

1. _____ Built-up pen

2. _____ Pegboard

3. _____ Built-up utensils

4. _____ Arm push-ups while sitting on mat

5. _____ Universal cuff

Worksheet 5-8 (continued)
Fracture Interventions

6.   _____ Paraffin to right hand

7.   _____ Sock aid

8.   _____ Retrograde massage

9.   _____ Vigorous stretching to increase wrist and finger ROM

10. _____ Elastic shoelaces

11. _____ Metacarpophalangeal (MP) extension resting orthosis

12. _____ Wash mitt

13. _____ Practice transfers using a raised toilet seat

14. _____ Sensory retraining

15. _____ Towel scrunching with fingers

16. _____ Shoes with Velcro closures

17. _____ Hot pack to wrist and fingers

18. _____ Hot pack to left hip

19. _____ Pulleys

20. _____ Walker

Worksheet 5-9

Chronic Obstructive Pulmonary Disease Interventions

Frank is a 72-year-old male residing with his wife, who has dementia, in an assisted living facility. He recently experienced an exacerbation of COPD, was admitted to an acute care hospital for 3 days, and then transferred to a rehabilitation hospital where he is presently. Frank worked as a painter but retired at age 58 due to respiratory ailments. In addition to the medications needed to address his respiratory problems, Frank has been taking Coumadin (warfarin) since being diagnosed with atrial fibrillation 2 years ago. Prior to this recent hospitalization, Frank was able to drive, manage ADLs with increased time, and perform functional ambulation independently (short distances) but used a rollator whenever leaving his room, such as going to the dining room with his wife for all meals or going out into the community. At the rehabilitation hospital Frank is now on portable oxygen. He needs minimal assistance to perform transfers, moderate assistance to complete lower body bathing and dressing, and cannot stand for more than 2 minutes without shortness of breath. Upper extremity ROM is WNL.

In collaboration with the OT, which of the following equipment, adaptive devices, or interventions are likely suitable for an OTA to use with Frank to improve performance skills and client factors for occupational performance and enable return to his residence? Assume that interventions would include not only the provision of a particular piece of equipment or DME, but actual instruction and practice in its use. Mark Y (yes) or N (no) for each item.

1. _____ Raised toilet seat

2. _____ One-arm-drive wheelchair

3. _____ Instruction in joint protection

4. _____ Buttonhook

5. _____ Sanding and painting wood

6. _____ Commode

7. _____ Hot pack to shoulders

8. _____ Disposable safety razor

9. _____ Exercise bands

10. _____ Reacher

11. _____ Ergonomics for yard work

12. _____ Standing while playing a game

Worksheet 5-9 (continued)

Chronic Obstructive Pulmonary Disease Interventions

13. _____ Energy conservation for doing laundry

14. _____ Using ambulation device while getting clothes from dresser

15. _____ Standing to cook at stove

16. _____ Pursed lip breathing

17. _____ Long-handled shoehorn

18. _____ Sawing and staining wood to make a picture frame

19. _____ Teaching stair climbing

20. _____ Shampoo and soap dispenser in shower

Worksheet 5-10

Meal Preparation Adaptations

Carmen is a 65-year-old homemaker who sustained a left CVA 2 weeks ago and is receiving home care services following short-term hospitalization. She lives with her husband in a private home and was fully independent in all ADLs prior to this illness. At the present time, Carmen's cognitive abilities appear to be intact, but she exhibits Broca's aphasia and right hemiparesis. Her dominant RUE is beginning to exhibit minimal motor return but is essentially nonfunctional except for some gross stabilization of objects. The client also demonstrates modified independence for functional ambulation using a hemi-walker. However, Carmen is unsafe when bending to reach for objects in lower kitchen/bathroom cabinets or floor. Her activity tolerance for safe standing is approximately 4 to 5 minutes. In each of the boxes below, list several suggestions indicating how the following breakfast tasks can be adapted to help enable safe and independent performance.

Adaptive Equipment and Compensatory Methods	Scrambled Eggs	Bacon	Fresh Fruit Salad (e.g., apple, grapes, pear, strawberries)	Pancakes
Required tools/equipment (list adaptive equipment or compensatory methods)	Example: Use a nonstick pan for easier clean up			
Required supplies (food items)	Example: Use a cooking spray to grease pan			
Required actions and timing	Example: Sit, rather than stand, at stove			

Worksheet 5-11

Supported Employment

Joe is a 20-year-old male with Down syndrome. He attends a supported employment program with the goal for him to work in a supermarket packing groceries. Joe does not have any physical limitations that would hinder his job performance. However, he does exhibit difficulty with time management and transitioning between activities. Joe needs to learn how to perform his job functions correctly, including interacting appropriately with customers. Consider the activity demands for a grocery packing job. Use a professional format to list six goals for Joe that relate to his employment and reflect the following categories listed.

Example: *Joe will be able to complete grocery packing for three customers without asking when he can take a break, within 1 month.*

1. Time management

2. Activity transition

3. Social interaction

4. Packing groceries (specific aspect)

5. Packing groceries (specific aspect)

6. Packing groceries (specific aspect)

Morreale, M. J. (2022). *Developing clinical competence: A workbook for the OTA* (2nd ed.). SLACK Incorporated.

Worksheet 5-12

Creative Problem Solving

One of the most important skills of an occupational therapy practitioner is the ability to creatively problem solve all challenging situations. To help you practice this skill, fill in the blanks after each scenario. It is important to remember that each client is unique and has individual circumstances. A therapist must always use professional reasoning to determine which interventions are appropriate and safe to use with a "real" client.

1. As part of a home visit, you are addressing self-feeding skills with a client diagnosed with CVA. The client needs a solution to keep the plate from sliding on the table, but you did not bring any non-slip matting (e.g., Dycem) with you. List four items commonly found in a home that you may be able to substitute at this time.

    a. _____

    b. _____

    c. _____

    d. _____

2. You are working in an outpatient setting with a client diagnosed with Parkinson's disease. As the client has balance deficits, you recommend that the client use a tub seat for safety while bathing. The client tells you he cannot afford to purchase a tub seat. Besides possibly helping the client to obtain financial assistance or donated/borrowed equipment, what other practical solutions could you offer for this problem?

    a. _____

    b. _____

3. You are working with an outpatient client who is diagnosed with rheumatoid arthritis. She has decreased ROM in both shoulders and impaired fine motor skills. The client takes great pride in her appearance but reports difficulty putting on and removing jewelry. What are some practical suggestions you can offer for this occupation?

    a. _____

    b. _____

    c. _____

    d. _____

    e. _____

    f. _____

Worksheet 5-12 (continued)

Creative Problem Solving

4. You have issued an orthotic device that has a complex set of straps to position the client's extremity properly. Besides verbal and written instructions and actual practice, what can you do to make it easier for the client to apply the correct sequence and position of the straps?

   a. _____

   b. _____

   c. _____

   d. _____

5. You are working in a hospital with a client who will be going home with an indwelling catheter in place. The client needs instruction in lower body dressing and managing clothing for toileting. He plans to remain at home until the catheter is removed next week. What recommendations could you offer?

   a. _____

   b. _____

   c. _____

   d. _____

   e. _____

Answers to Worksheets

The worksheet answers include interventions that are possible choices for the scenarios presented but may not be suitable for all clients with that specific condition. A client situation may also warrant other types of interventions or devices that are not included here.

Worksheet 5-1: Teaching-Learning Process—Total Hip Replacement

Each intervention session may vary in terms of specific tasks performed and the order implemented depending on the client's medical status, level of function, doctor's orders, time frames, client activity tolerance, and so forth, but here are some suggestions:

1. Where will the session take place? *Client's hospital room*

2. What is the anticipated length of session? *Fifteen to forty-five minutes depending on client's activity tolerance, practitioner caseload, other disciplines needing access to client, and so forth.*

3. What equipment/supplies will the OTA need to bring for the session? *Possible items include:*
   - *Documentation materials (e.g., laptop/hand-held device, paper, pen, documentation forms)*
   - *Adaptive equipment: sock aid, reacher, dressing stick, long-handled shoehorn, elastic laces*
   - *Gloves/personal protective equipment for potential contact with blood or body fluids*
   - *Written client education materials*
   - *Ensure walker is in room*
   - *Hospital scrubs for dressing practice if client does not have street clothes in room*
   - *As needed, stethoscope or other equipment to assess vital signs*

4. What are several things the OTA should do prior to entering the client's room?
   - *Collaborate with OT and review the occupational therapy evaluation report and intervention plan*
   - *Establish OTA's schedule and coordinate time frames with physical therapy/other disciplines as needed*
   - *Check client's chart for changes in medical status and any new orders. Review nursing, physical therapy documentation along with information from other disciplines as indicated*
   - *Obtain any further knowledge needed regarding this diagnosis or client's condition*
   - *Carefully consider any precautions/contraindications and safety concerns for this client, as well as pertinent infection control issues*
   - *Double check that this is the correct room and correct patient (e.g., check wrist band, verbally ask client)*

5. List the general steps of how the session should be implemented
   - *Perform hand hygiene and use personal protective equipment as indicated*
   - *Introduce OTA and explain purpose of session (refer back to Chapter 1 for communication tips)*
   - *Note any devices hooked up to client requiring caution during treatment such as a catheter, monitor, or intravenous line*
   - *Take vital signs if part of protocol or as indicated during session*
   - *Review general total hip precautions and determine client understanding and carryover*
   - *Ensure bed brakes are locked and adjust bed rail as needed. Explain transfer procedure then transfer client safely to a sitting position (on edge of bed or into a chair depending on client's status and intervention plan) adhering to total hip precautions and using walker and safe client footwear if performing stand-pivot transfer.*
   - *Explain/demonstrate use of adaptive devices for lower body dressing, one at a time*
   - *Following each explanation/demonstration, have client practice use of adaptive equipment to don lower body clothing/scrubs while adhering to precautions and providing assistance as needed. Incorporate use of walker and provide contact guard/physical assist when client stands to pull up clothing.*
   - *Provide opportunities for problem solving and client feedback*
   - *Determine if client needs to practice using any of the devices a second time this session (or future sessions), or if clothing needs to be removed and hospital gown put back on*
   - *Client may also don upper body clothing if indicated*
   - *Transfer client back to bed or determine if client should remain sitting in chair*

- *Make sure equipment is properly placed and client is comfortable, safe, and can reach the call button*
- *Dispose of any personal protective equipment or used linens properly*
- *Wash hands*
- *Document according to facility time frame*

Changes in the teaching-learning process for a 90-year-old client with mild dementia would depend on various factors, such as the client's prior level of function. Depending on the expected discharge plan, lower body dressing may or may not be a priority for this client (e.g., lived alone independently versus resided in a nursing home). If the client also had age-related hearing loss or visual impairment, you would ensure that hearing aids and glasses are in place and possibly use large-print educational materials. As short-term memory impairment and slower processing would likely be evident, this client may require repeated directions, written instructions, visual aids, greater task breakdown, or additional opportunities to practice new skills. More rest breaks may also be needed due to client's advanced age.

Worksheet 5-2: Cerebrovascular Accident Interventions

Resources: Gillen, 2011, 2018; Logigian, 2015

1. Y. Rocker knife
2. Y. Non-slip matting
3. N. Built-up utensils

   Client is unable to use flaccid right hand presently and should not need built-up utensils for his unaffected left hand.
4. Y. Plate guard
5. N. Walker

   This requires use of two hands, and client cannot grip walker with a flaccid hand. Physical therapy will determine when a hemi-walker or other mobility aid is appropriate for client to use.
6. N. Power wheelchair

   Client should be able to operate a manual wheelchair using his left arm and leg or a one-arm-drive wheelchair.
7. Y. Electric razor
8. N. Sock aid

   Client cannot use right hand, so it would be difficult to use this device one-handed. It would probably be more suitable to teach one-handed compensatory techniques
9. N. Therapy putty

   Client cannot use this with a flaccid right hand.
10. N. Exercise bands

    Cannot use with a flaccid RUE. LUE strength is already WFL.
11. N. Pulleys

    Using pulleys for PROM to a flaccid RUE might overstretch joint tissue/cause harm to shoulder.
12. N. Vest restraint

    Restraining the client with a vest restraint is not appropriate. If Marvin is demonstrating poor posture in chair, other less restrictive alternatives should be tried, such as client education, verbal reminders, lateral cushions/supports, a seatbelt or lapboard (if client has ability to remove), and so forth.
13. Y. Wheelchair arm support
14. Y. Soap-on-a-rope
15. Y. Wash mitt
16. Y. Soap/shampoo dispenser

17. Y. Long-handled sponge

18. Y. Tub seat/bench

19. N. Hot pack to right shoulder

    Not indicated for a flaccid extremity with no pain or PROM deficits. Also, cardiovascular status may not be stable.

20. N. Paraffin to right hand

    Not indicated for a flaccid extremity with no pain or PROM deficits. Also, cardiovascular status may not be stable.

21. N. Constraint-induced movement therapy

    Client does not have the requisite motor skills in his involved arm for this intervention as the arm is flaccid. Constraining the strong arm would not allow the client to perform any functional tasks at this time.

22. Y. Teach self-ROM

23. N. Lapboard

    This could be considered a restraint if the client is not able to remove it himself. Other alternatives might be considered first, such as a side-arm support or pillow.

24. N. Large pegboard

    Clients involved arms is flaccid, and this task would not be useful for the uninvolved arm. If the client had perceptual deficits it could possibly be used with the unaffected arm to work on specific perceptual skills, although a functional task would be more appropriate.

25. N. Nine-Hole Peg Test

    Client does not have any motor function in his involved dominant RUE, so this test would not be a useful measure at this time.

Worksheet 5-3: Total Hip Replacement Interventions

Resources: Coppard & Padilla, 2019; Gower & Bowker, 2015; Murphy & Lawson, 2018

1. Y. Raised toilet seat

2. N. Adduction cushion

    Client needs an abduction cushion.

3. N. Built-up utensils

    No difficulties with grasp noted

4. Y. Commode

5. N. Crossing legs to tie shoes

    Contraindicated to adduct hip due to surgical precautions.

6. Y. Walker

    Generally, the physical therapist would determine if this device is appropriate for gait training at this time. However, occupational therapy can support functional mobility and safety for occupational performance.

7. N. Power wheelchair

    If a wheelchair is needed, a manual wheelchair is normally used following hip replacement surgery.

8. Y. Long-handled shoehorn

9. Y. Sock aid

10. N. Hot pack to left hip

    A hot pack is not indicated for acute post-surgical conditions, but a cold pack might be appropriate for pain and swelling. State regulation and facility policy delineate the disciplines that may implement specific physical agents.

11. N. Paraffin to left hand

Not indicated for client's condition as no ROM deficits are noted.

12. N. Teach stair climbing with crutches

Teaching stair climbing is typically the role of the physical therapist, although occupational therapy can support function. Crutches are not an appropriate mobility device for this client due to her age and functional level.

13. N. Wheelchair arm support

Client does not have unilateral neglect or ROM deficits.

14. Y. Exercise bands

Increasing upper body strength may be beneficial for walker use.

15. N. Quad cane

Cannot use with toe-touch weight-bearing status.

16. Y. Elastic shoelaces

17. N. Wedge cushion for wheelchair

This would provide excessive hip flexion. However, an elevated seat cushion would be appropriate.

18. Y. Reacher

19. Y. Long-handled sponge

20. Y. Tub seat/bench

21. Y. Leg lifte

Useful to help lift involved lower limb when transferring to a tub bench or bed.

22. N. Constraint-induced movement therapy

This technique is useful for clients with neurological conditions (e.g., stroke) to improve upper limb function (Gillen, 2011, 2018). Client does not have neurological impairment and has good voluntary motion in both upper extremities.

23. N. Sliding board

Instruction in stand-pivot transfers is a more appropriate method for this client and condition.

24. N. Buttonhook

Client has full AROM in both upper extremities and no coordination deficits are noted.

25. N. Hospital bed for home

Client has potential for good bed mobility and does not have another co-morbid condition that would warrant use of a hospital bed, such as respiratory problems.

Worksheet 5-4: Improving Basic and Instrumental Activities of Daily Living Occupations

Resources: Coppard & Padilla, 2019; Gower & Bowker, 2015; Murphy & Lawson, 2018

1. A. (Fairchild et al., 2018)

2. B. The client should be able to transfer independently onto the commode using a sliding board. A raised toilet seat is not useful in this instance as the client cannot enter the bathroom. Using a platform walker is not feasible. A power mobility scooter may not fit through the door or, most likely, will not be able to get close enough to the toilet for a sliding board transfer. Another option is for the client and spouse to arrange for architectural changes in the home to allow for bathroom wheelchair access.

3. C. The client's knees should be apart to provide a wider base of support. A transfer belt could be placed around the client's waist, but not the OTA's. A walker is unstable as a device to push up from, so this would be unsafe. The client needs to lean forward ("nose over toes") to facilitate rising from chair.

4. C. An electric razor is safer than a disposable safety razor that has sharp blades. As the client has unilateral neglect and impulsivity, he needs to focus all his attention on the task at hand to best perform shaving. Standing would be more distracting in this case, as the client would have to work to maintain his balance. However, realize there are instances when an occupational therapy practitioner would work on balance (or other client factors) and ADL performance simultaneously, depending on the desired outcome for that session.

5. B. Clients should be as upright as possible when feeding. Neck hyperextension could hinder swallowing and be unsafe. Specialized swallowing techniques or alternate neck positions may be needed for some clients (Morawski et al., 2019). If weakness is only evident in the hand intrinsic muscles, the client should be able to manage self-feeding with a universal cuff or adapted utensils.

6. A. The better strategy would be to teach an easier method, which in this case is over-the-head. While demonstration and written instructions could possibly help, they are not the best option. A larger coat would still require the same sequence of motor planning.

7. D. Using a flat sheet as a bottom sheet entails less effort than using a tightly fitted sheet. While a tub seat is useful, it is not related to homemaking. It is contraindicated to use open flames (barbecue grill) around oxygen. The client should inhale before exertion and exhale during the exertion.

8. D. Driving is not feasible at this level, whereas the other interventions are appropriate (Bashar & Hughes, 2018; Fike et al., 2015; Spinal Cord Injury Information Pages, 2020).

9. D. The triceps are not innervated at this level, although the client may be able to shift sideways to relieve pressure. Using a buttonhook and razor are feasible options but may require set up and use of a holder or a tenodesis grasp wrist-driven hinge orthosis (Bashar & Hughes, 2018; Fike et al., 2015; Spinal Cord Injury Information Pages, 2020).

10. B. It is appropriate for a client at this level to use a manual wheelchair. The client should also be able to perform many functional tasks, such as light meal preparation and bathing. As the triceps are innervated at this level, the client should be instructed in wheelchair push-ups to help relieve pressure while sitting (Bashar & Hughes, 2018; Fike et al., 2015; Spinal Cord Injury Information Pages, 2020).

Worksheet 5-5: Total Knee Replacement Interventions

Resources: Coppard & Padilla, 2019; Murphy & Lawson, 2018

1. Y. Raised toilet seat

    Could be useful to aid in transfers.

2. Y. Tub seat/bench

3. N. Pillow under right knee when lying in bed

    A pillow under the affected knee can contribute to a knee flexion contracture, which is undesirable.

4. N. Buttonhook

    There are no upper extremity deficits noted.

5. Y. Long-handled shoehorn

6. Y. Commode

7. N. Hot pack to right knee

    A hot pack is not indicated for acute post-surgical conditions, but a cold pack might be appropriate for pain and swelling. State regulation and facility policy delineate the disciplines that may implement specific physical agents.

8. Y. Elastic shoelaces

9. Y. Sock aid

    Could possibly be useful but may not be needed.

10. Y. Reacher

11. N. Beanbag toss activity while seated on mat

    Sitting balance is not a problem.

12. N. Ambulation using parallel bars

    This is typically a physical therapy intervention. However, occupational therapy can support functional ambulation for ADL performance (AOTA, 2020).

13. N. Squatting exercises to increase knee ROM

    This is typically a physical therapy intervention. Also, knee may be unstable postoperatively.

14. Y. Using ambulation device while obtaining items from refrigerator

    Realize that while activity tolerance for standing is an important goal for this client and condition, this activity may increase pain. The occupational therapy practitioner must decide if the client would benefit more from a compensatory method, such as using a wheelchair, or determine if the client needs to work through the pain, depending on physician orders and the client's particular situation.

15. Y. Standing to make a sandwich

    Realize that while activity tolerance for standing is an important goal for this client and condition, this activity may increase pain. The occupational therapy practitioner must decide if the client would benefit more from a compensatory method, such as sitting on a chair at the kitchen counter or determine if the client needs to work through the pain, depending on physician orders and the client's particular situation.

16. N. Power wheelchair mobility training

    Power wheelchair is not indicated.

17. N. Pegboard activity

    No fine-motor deficits noted.

18. N. Cone stacking activity with wrist weights

    Could possibly use to increase endurance, but strength is already WFL and client has other ADL priorities. Can use while standing to work on improving standing tolerance but functional activities/occupations should be incorporated instead whenever possible.

19. Y. Standing at bathroom sink to shave with electric razor

    Realize that while activity tolerance for standing is an important goal for this client and condition, this activity may increase pain. The occupational therapy practitioner must decide if the client would benefit more from a compensatory method, such as sitting in a chair at the sink, or determine if the client needs to work through the pain, depending on physician orders and the client's particular situation.

20. N. Ambulating up and down the hallway

    Ambulation training is typically a physical therapy intervention, although occupational therapy can support functional mobility for occupations, such as safe navigation in the kitchen during meal preparation tasks (AOTA, 2021).

Worksheet 5-6: Activities as Interventions—Using a Menu

Here are some suggestions although you may come up with others. While the methods listed here include the activity of role-playing, an occupational therapy practitioner should create opportunities to have clients perform real occupations, such as actually going to a restaurant or cafeteria.

Occupation	Client Factor/Performance Skill to Be Addressed	Specific Intervention Activity	Method (i.e., role play, menu choices, educate client)
IADL—Financial management	Improve calculation skills	Select an appetizer, entrée, and dessert that total less than $20.00 before tax and tip	Choose items from menu Teach math skills
Health management	Demonstrate healthy food choices Improve problem solving	Choose an entrée and side dish that are not deep fried	Choose items from menu Educate client regarding healthy versus unhealthy foods and emotional eating (e.g., comfort foods)
Health management	Demonstrate healthy beverage choices Improve coping skills	Choose a beverage that does not contain alcohol, or choose a beverage that will or will not add calories or specific nutrients, depending on the client's medical dietary needs	Choose items from menu Educate client regarding healthy versus unhealthy beverage choices and emotional eating Role-play and suggest coping strategies
Health management	Improve problem solving Improve safety awareness	Determine items that may contain allergens such as nuts, dairy products, or gluten	Choose items from menu Educate client regarding hidden ingredients
Leisure participation Social participation	Improve decision-making skills	Within a 5-minute period, choose a beverage, entrée, and dessert without changing mind, or choose a restaurant for the group to go to	Role-play and provide feedback
Health management	Demonstrate healthy eating habits Improve assertiveness skills	Ask server how an item is prepared, or ask for item to be specially prepared without butter, salt, and so forth.	Role-play and provide feedback
ADL—Feeding Social participation	Improve problem solving	Choose items that one can manage to eat without need for help or set-up	Choose items from menu (e.g., finger foods or fish fillet that does not need to be cut) Educate regarding compensatory strategies

Occupation	Client Factor/Performance Skill to Be Addressed	Specific Intervention Activity	Method (i.e., role play, menu choices, educate client)
Health management	Demonstrate healthy eating habits	Choose an appetizer, entrée, and beverage that total less or more than a specified amount of calories or sodium	Choose items from menu Educate client regarding healthy versus unhealthy foods and emotional response to food
IADL—Financial management	Improve calculation skills	Calculate tax and tip on specified items	Choose items from menu Teach math skills
IADL—Financial management	Improve calculation skills	Determine change back from a $50.00 bill after selecting several items	Choose items from menu Teach math skills
IADL—Financial management	Improve money management	Pay using exact change or perform credit card transaction properly	Role-play
Social participation	Improve interpersonal skills	Choose an appetizer or dessert that can be shared with the group Wait one's turn to order	Choose items from menu Role-play and provide feedback

Worksheet 5-7: Improving Basic and Instrumental Activities of Daily Living Occupations—More Practice

1. B. Plain apple juice and coffee are thin liquids that this client is not allowed to have. If thickeners were added to create the proper consistency, they might be acceptable. Scrambled eggs are soft, but semi-solid, and not considered to be puréed. It is essential to know what is acceptable or not acceptable for each client to eat. It is also important to ascertain if clients have other dietary requirements such as: dairy restrictions, food allergies, cultural considerations, or a special diet (e.g., low-sodium, low-calorie, or low-sugar) needed for other medical conditions.

2. B. As the client must use a wheelchair, an arm trough may be helpful to support and protect the involved arm. An airplane splint is a shoulder immobilization splint, which is not indicated for this condition. Pulleys may cause further damage to the shoulder if the arm is overstretched, and the client also does not have the requisite grasp to manage this device or to use therapy putty with the left hand.

3. C. The client does not have the requisite function of the involved arm to hold onto a rolling walker. The other devices may be used to teach the client compensatory techniques for ADL.

4. B. Macular degeneration is an eye disease. Only one of the choices relates to vision.

5. A. Vestibular problems may create vertigo or problems with balance. It is safer for the client to be seated while bathing. When going from sit to stand, the client should push up from the seated surface rather than pull up from a walker, which would be unsafe. Towel bars are not attached securely to the wall for use as a grab bar. There is no mention that this client has any hearing loss, so a personal sound amplifier is not indicated.

6. D. Presbycusis is age-related hearing loss. The only choice that relates to hearing is a telephone amplifier.

7.   C. Due to the client's diagnosis of COPD, the OTA should avoid activities that create dust (e.g., Fluidotherapy and sanding) or fumes (e.g., staining wood). While use of pulleys may involve grasp, this device is not the best choice to facilitate hand function. A functional fine-motor task, such as buttoning a shirt, is a more suitable choice.

8.   C. While A, B, and D are possible interventions that an occupational therapy practitioner might provide to clients receiving hospice care, these interventions are not needed for every client. An occupational therapy practitioner considers each client individually to determine appropriate interventions to help support the client's desired or needed occupational roles and quality of life (AOTA, 2020).

9.   C. An upper limb prosthesis classified as a passive terminal device does not have a battery. It also does not have sensory function. It is primarily used for cosmesis but can possibly be used as a gross assist (Papdapoulos & Deverix, 2013).

10.   A. A body-powered prosthesis can perform grasp but does not have sensory function, isolated motion of digits, or the ability to perform in-hand manipulation. Training includes working on ability to pick up various kinds of objects without damaging the objects (Papdapoulos & Deverix, 2013).

Worksheet 5-8: Fracture Interventions

Resources: Coppard & Padilla, 2019; Murphy & Lawson, 2018

1.   Y. Built-up pen

2.   Y. Pegboard

       However, it is better to work on functional activities and occupations involving fine-motor skills such as buttoning a shirt, writing, or self-feeding (using adaptive equipment as needed).

3.   Y. Built-up utensils

4.   N. Arm push-ups while sitting on mat

       Contraindicated at this time. May cause excessive pressure to healing fracture.

5.   Y. Universal cuff

6.   N. Paraffin to right hand

       Tremors would create a safety concern for splashing paraffin or touching sides of unit.

7.   N. Sock aid

       Client does not have the requisite motor function in hand and tremors would also create more difficulty with using this device.

8.   N. Retrograde massage

       No edema present.

9.   N. Vigorous stretching to increase wrist and finger ROM

       Fracture is likely not yet stable enough for vigorous stretching.

10.   Y. Elastic shoelaces

11.   N. MP extension resting orthosis

       Except for certain protocols (e.g., extensor tendon repair, MP joint replacement surgery) the hand generally should not be splinted in MP extension as this is not a functional position.

12.   Y. Wash mitt

13.   N. Practice transfers using a raised toilet seat

       Client is already independent in transfers, although the OTA may recommend this for future needs.

14.   N. Sensory retraining

       Sensation is intact.

15. Y. Towel scrunching with fingers
16. Y. Shoes with Velcro closures
17. Y. Hot pack to wrist and fingers
18. N. Hot pack to left hip

    Client was referred for an upper extremity diagnosis. A referral to physical therapy may be warranted to address the client's hip pain.

19. N. Pulleys

    Client's limited grip creates difficulty for holding the handle. Also, pulleys do not really address client's ROM deficits in hand and wrist sufficiently.

20. N. Walker

    Client is independent in ambulation. However, a referral to physical therapy may be warranted to determine if an ambulation device is appropriate for this client to minimize hip pain.

Worksheet 5-9: Chronic Obstructive Pulmonary Disease Interventions

Resource: Peralta et al., 2019

1. Y. Raised toilet seat.
2. N. One-arm-drive wheelchair

   Client has use of both arms and legs so does not require this specific type of wheelchair.
3. N. Instruction in joint protection

   Client does not have joint problems. Instruction on energy conservation would be more appropriate.
4. N. Buttonhook

   No fine-motor deficits noted.
5. N. Sanding and painting wood

   Creates dust and fumes.
6. Y. Commode
7. N. Hot pack to shoulders

   No shoulder problems are noted, and heat is contraindicated for severe cardiopulmonary conditions.
8. N. Disposable safety razor

   Client is on blood thinners so an electric razor would be safer.
9. Y. Exercise band

   May be useful to increase strength and endurance.
10. Y. Reacher
11. N. Ergonomics for yard work

    Resides in assisted living facility.
12. Y. Standing while playing a game

    Depending on the client's medical status and intervention plan, graded standing tasks could be useful to increase endurance for occupational performance.
13. N. Energy conservation for doing laundry

    Resides in an assisted living facility so laundry service is likely provided, eliminating the need for client to do own laundry. However, if laundry service is not provided, instruction in energy conservation techniques would be appropriate for any functional tasks the client must perform.
14. Y. Using ambulation device while getting clothes from dresser

Graded functional mobility tasks may be useful to increase endurance. However, a compensatory method, such as performing the task while seated in a wheelchair, may be needed to enable independent performance of this occupation.

15. N. Standing to cook at stove

To increase endurance, this could be used as a purposeful activity, but some or all meals are usually provided at an assisted living facility. Many facilities prohibit the use of cooking appliances due to safety concerns. However, depending on the specific facility, client might be allowed to use a microwave or coffeemaker so these tasks could be a possible choice to address. However, consider that a compensatory method, such as performing the task while seated, may be needed to enable independent performance of this occupation safely.

16. Y. Pursed lip breathing

17. Y. Long-handled shoehorn

18. N. Sawing and staining wood to make a picture frame

Creates dust and fumes, and client is also on blood thinners so caution should be used regarding use of sharp objects.

19. N. Teaching stair climbing

This is typically the role of physical therapy although occupational therapy can support functional mobility tasks (AOTA, 2021).

20. Y. Shampoo and soap dispenser in shower

Eliminates reaching for bottles or lifting them.

Worksheet 5-10: Meal Preparation Adaptations

Here are some suggestions for adaptive equipment and compensatory techniques for this client, although you may come up with others. Realize that the dominant hand is unable to perform grasp. Built-up handled objects would not be needed for the non-dominant hand.

Adaptive Equipment and Compensatory Methods	Scrambled Eggs	Bacon	Fresh Fruit Salad (e.g., apple, grapes, pear, strawberries)	Pancakes
Required tools/equipment (list adaptive equipment or compensatory methods)	Nonstick pan for easier clean-up Can use a microwave instead of stove Non-slip matting to secure bowl Use a bowl with a handle to pour	Can use a microwave instead of stove Nonstick pan for easier clean-up	Adapted cutting board with nails Non-slip matting Apple peeling device Can use an egg slicer to slice berries	Depending on method (e.g., frozen pancakes or using a mix), can use a toaster, toaster oven, microwave, electric griddle, or top of stove If making batter, use non-slip matting to secure bowl If making batter, use a bowl with a handle to pour or use a batter dispenser Nonstick pan for easier clean-up

Morreale, M. J. (2022). *Developing clinical competence: A workbook for the OTA* (2nd ed.). SLACK Incorporated.

Adaptive Equipment and Compensatory Methods	Scrambled Eggs	Bacon	Fresh Fruit Salad (e.g., apple, grapes, pear, strawberries)	Pancakes
Required supplies (food items)	Cooking spray to grease pan Liquid eggs in a carton Frozen prepared eggs	Pre-cooked bacon in grocery store refrigerated section Store-bought bacon bits	Pre-cut bags of fruit in frozen food or refrigerated section of supermarket Canned fruit Pre-cut fresh fruit from a grocery store/salad bar	Pancakes from a recipe versus a boxed mix; consider number of ingredients needed such as only water versus needing water, oil, and egg Premade store bought batter from a carton Frozen pancakes Cooking spray to grease pan
Required actions and timing	Sit, rather than stand, at stove Teach one-handed technique to break eggs Can use a carton holder with handle when pouring liquid eggs from a carton Keep items in higher shelves of refrigerator and accessible upper cabinets Rolling cart to move and carry items Apron with pockets to move and carry small objects	Use scissors to open package Sit, rather than stand, to prepare Keep items in higher shelves of refrigerator and accessible upper cabinets Rolling cart to move and carry items Apron with pockets to move and carry small objects	Can use a suction brush attached to sink to wash fruits Sit, rather than stand, to prepare Keep items in higher shelves of refrigerator and accessible upper cabinets Rolling cart to move and carry items Apron with pockets to move and carry small objects	If eggs are needed, teach one-handed technique to break eggs Sit, rather than stand, to prepare Keep items in higher shelves of refrigerator and accessible upper cabinets Rolling cart to move and carry items Can prepare batter ahead of time Teach compensatory method to open box of pancake mix Apron with pockets to move and carry small objects Can use a carton holder with handle when pouring milk or batter from a carton

Worksheet 5-11: Supported Employment

Resources for goal writing: Gateley & Borcherding, 2017; Morreale & Borcherding, 2017, Sames, 2015

Goals need to specify a time frame, measurable criteria, and delineate a desired client behavior relating to function. Goals should reflect what the client needs to achieve, not what the occupational therapy practitioner will do as interventions. Here are some suggested goals for this client. Realize that different settings or practice areas may use slightly different formats or terminology, as shown in the various examples following. Of course, the actual goals and time frames may be different for a "real" client.

1. Time management
   - *By the end of 1 month, Joe will demonstrate ability to pack 10 items in a grocery bag within a 2-minute period.*
   - *Joe will adhere to the allotted time for breaks with one verbal cue to set/use a timer, within 2 weeks.*
2. Activity transition
   - *After placing a grocery bag in customer's cart, Joe will continue packing remaining groceries without redirection to task, within 4 weeks.*
   - *At the end of his allotted break time, client will punch his timecard with two verbal cues, within 10 days.*
3. Social interaction
   - *With one verbal cue, client will ask customers if they prefer paper or plastic bags, 5 out of 5 opportunities, within 2 weeks.*
   - *Joe will greet customers with a smile and say "hello" 4/5 opportunities, by the end of the month.*
4. Packing groceries (specific aspect)
   - *Within 6 weeks, Joe will demonstrate ability to pack all cold items together and all produce items together with minimal verbal cues.*
5. Packing groceries (specific aspect)
   - *Client will demonstrate ability to place cans and heavier items on the bottom of grocery bag with stand-by assist, within 4 weeks.*
6. Packing groceries (specific aspect)
   - *Joe will place appropriate number of items to fill bag without risk of bag breaking when carried by handles, within 3 months.*

Worksheet 5-12: Creative Problem Solving

1. Here are several suggestions but you may come up with others.
   - *A piece of shelf liner*
   - *A flat rubber jar opener disc*
   - *A dampened dish towel or washcloth*
   - *Non-slip placemat*
2. Here are several suggestions but you may come up with others. The therapist must ensure that methods used are appropriate and safe for the particular client.
   - *Place commode in tub*
   - *Place a plastic lawn chair and rubber mat in tub*
3. Here are several suggestions but you may come up with others. Some alternate jewelry clasps/necklace extenders are readily available in craft stores and the items below can also be found by doing an internet search.
   - *Consider larger/bulkier jewelry which may be easier to manage*
   - *Adapt or purchase jewelry with alternate fastenings such as magnetic clasps, toggle, or "s" loop closures*
   - *Use larger length necklaces that can slip over the head (can extend existing necklaces with extra loops/necklace extender kits)*
   - *Elastic bracelets and watch bands (not too tight)*
   - *Watchband with a hook and loop closure*

- *Use a bracelet fastening tool*
- *A jeweler can adapt rings with adjustable/expandable ring shanks so that the rings can go over enlarged joints*
- *Use extra-large earring backs*
- *Use French wire earrings without backs*
- *If indicated, warm up hands and perform ROM exercises prior to task*

4. Here are several suggestions but you may come up with others.
   - *Color-code the straps and corresponding Velcro tabs*
   - *Number the straps and corresponding Velcro tabs*
   - *Take a picture of the correct placement of straps while client is wearing orthotic device*
   - *Use rivets to secure one end of each strap to the orthotic device*

5. When moving an attached catheter bag (such as threading it through garments) or hanging it when the client is resting, keep it below the level of the bladder to avoid backflow (Fairchild, 2018; George, 2018). Do not place the bag on the floor. Also, ensure that the catheter bag is moved accordingly during transfers, ambulation, and so forth, to avoid tension at the insertion site. Here are some suggestions for managing lower body clothing with a catheter in place (Malecare, Inc., 2020).
   - *Wear boxer shorts*
   - *Wear athletic type shorts or loose-fitting shorts*
   - *Wear looser pants such as sweatpants or pants with a drawstring closure*
   - *Wear basketball type pants with side snaps or zippers*
   - *Wear a dress or skirt*
   - *When resting at home, use a hospital gown, nightgown/nightshirt, short pajamas, or a bathrobe*

Reproduced with permission from Morreale, M. J., & Amini, D. (2016). *The occupational therapist's workbook for ensuring clinical competence.* SLACK Incorporated.

References

American Occupational Therapy Association. (2020). Occupational therapy practice framework: Domain and process (4th ed.). *American Journal of Occupational Therapy, 74*(Suppl. 2), 7412410010. https://doi.org/10.5014/ajot.2020.74S2001

American Occupational Therapy Association. (2021). *Scope of practice q & a: Gait assessment for falls risk.* Retrieved May 12, 2021, from https://www.aota.org/Practice/Manage/Scope-of-Practice-QA/gait.aspx

Bashar, J., & Hughes, C. A. (2018). Spinal cord injury. In H. M. Pendleton & W. Schultz-Krohn (Eds.), *Pedretti's occupational therapy practice skills for physical dysfunction* (8th ed., pp. 904-928). Elsevier Incorporated.

Coppard, B. M., & Padilla, R. (2019). Working with elders who have orthopedic conditions. In H. L. Lohman, S. Byers-Connon, & R. L. Padilla (Eds.), *Occupational therapy with elders: Strategies for the COTA* (4th ed., pp. 307-321). Elsevier Incorporated.

Fairchild, S. L., O'Shea, R. K., & Washington, R. D. (2018). *Pierson and Fairchild's principles & techniques of patient care* (6th ed.). Elsevier Incorporated.

Fike, M. L., Pendleton, K., & Hewitt, L. (2015). A telephone repairman with spinal cord injury. In K. Sladyk & S. E. Ryan (Eds.), *Ryan's occupational therapy assistant: Principles, practice issues, and techniques* (5th ed., pp. 269-288) SLACK Incorporated.

Gateley, C. A., & Borcherding, S. (2017). *Documentation manual for occupational therapy: Writing SOAP notes* (4th ed.). SLACK Incorporated.

George, A. H. (2018). Infection control and safety issues in the clinic. In H. M. Pendleton & W. Schultz-Krohn (Eds.), *Pedretti's occupational therapy practice skills for physical dysfunction* (8th ed., pp. 141-154). Elsevier Incorporated.

Gillen, G. (2011). *Stroke rehabilitation: A function-based approach* (3rd ed.). Elsevier Mosby.

Gillen, G. (2018). Cerebrovascular accident (stroke). In H. M. Pendleton & W. Schultz-Krohn (Eds.), *Pedretti's occupational therapy practice skills for physical dysfunction* (8th ed., pp. 809-840). Elsevier Incorporated.

Gower, D., & Bowker, M. (2015). A plumber and golfer with total hip arthroplasty. In K. Sladyk & S. E. Ryan (Eds.), *Ryan's occupational therapy assistant: Principles, practice issues, and techniques.* (5th ed., pp. 346-358). SLACK Incorporated.

Logigian, M. (2015). A businessman with a stroke. In K. Sladyk & S. E. Ryan (Eds.), *Ryan's occupational therapy assistant: Principles, practice issues, and techniques* (5th ed., pp. 374-389). SLACK Incorporated.

Malecare, Inc. (2020). *Clothing.* Retrieved May 12, 2021, from http://malecare.org/in-the-hospital/clothing

Morawski, D. L., Davis, T., & Padilla, R. (2019). Dysphagia and other eating and nutritional concerns with elders. In H. L. Lohman, S. Byers-Connon, & R. L. Padilla (Eds.), *Occupational therapy with elders: Strategies for the COTA* (4th ed., pp. 255-267). Elsevier Incorporated.

Morreale, M. J., & Amini, D. (2016). *The Occupational therapist's workbook for ensuring clinical competence.* SLACK Incorporated.

Morreale, M. J., & Borcherding, S. (2017). *The OTA's guide to documentation: Writing SOAP notes* (4th ed.). SLACK Incorporated.

Murphy, L. F. & Lawson, S. (2018). Orthopedic conditions: Hip fractures and hip, knee, and shoulder replacements. In H. M. Pendleton & W. Schultz-Krohn (Eds.), *Pedretti's occupational therapy practice skills for physical dysfunction* (8th ed., pp. 1004-1029). Elsevier Incorporated.

Papdapoulos, E., & Deverix, B. (2013). Amputation and prosthetics. In M. B. Early (Ed.), *Physical dysfunction practice skills for the occupational therapy assistant* (3rd ed., pp. 654-675). Mosby.

Peralta, A. M., Powell, S., & Byers-Connon, S. (2019). Working with elders who have pulmonary conditions. In H. L. Lohman, S. Byers-Connon, & R. L. Padilla (Eds.), *Occupational therapy with elders: Strategies for the COTA* (4th ed., pp. 331-336). Elsevier Incorporated.

Sames, K. M. (2015). *Documenting occupational therapy practice* (3rd ed.). Pearson Education.

Spinal Cord Injury Information Pages. (2020). *Spinal cord injury functional goals.* Retrieved March 15, 2020, from https://www.sci-info-pages.com/spinal-cord-injury-functional-goals/

Implementing Interventions to Support Occupations

Interventions to support occupations, such as physical agent modalities (PAMs), orthotic devices, therapeutic exercises, and sensorimotor techniques are used in occupational therapy to help develop, remediate, or manage specific client factors (e.g., range of motion [ROM], sensory processing, strength) and conditions (e.g., edema, pain, open wounds) with the goal of contributing to the client's occupational performance (American Occupational Therapy Association [AOTA], 2020). Although these methods and tasks supporting occupations can be an important part of a client's intervention plan, these interventions should supplement, but never replace, the use of activities and occupations (AOTA, 2020). The Accreditation Council for Occupational Therapy Education (ACOTE) sets forth standards for the attainment of knowledge and skills essential for entry-level occupational therapy assistant (OTA) practice (ACOTE, 2018). However, it is important to understand that state licensure laws delineate the specific kinds of PAMs and other types of interventions that may be used by an occupational therapist (OT) or OTA in that particular state plus any other continuing education requirements for their use (AOTA, 2018). OTs and OTAs must always adhere to regulatory guidelines and follow current clinical standards based on the evidence and other relevant factors, such as the client's health status and circumstances, precautions/contraindications, methods available, and safety. The worksheets and learning activities presented in this chapter address a variety of methods and tasks used in occupational therapy to support occupations for clients with physical conditions. Answers to worksheet exercises are provided at the end of the chapter.

Contents

Morreale, M. J. Developing Clinical Competence:
A Workbook for the OTA, Second Edition (pp. 245-292).
© 2022 SLACK Incorporated.

Worksheet 6-1

Therapeutic Exercises

1. An occupational therapy client who is an electrician is recovering from a shoulder fracture. To implement the intervention plan, an OTA is performing passive range of motion (PROM) to increase the ROM of the glenohumeral joint to enable client's return to work. When the client's arm is flexed to 140 degrees, the client states, "I feel a little stretch." What should the OTA do next?
    A. Discontinue PROM to the shoulder for this session
    B. Continue PROM, but only to 130 degrees flexion
    C. Keep joint positioned at 140 degrees flexion for a brief hold time
    D. Notify the referring physician

2. Teaching a client self-ROM is indicated for which of the following conditions?
    A. Flaccid extremity
    B. Adhesive capsulitis
    C. Extremity with fair minus muscle strength
    D. All of the above

3. To increase independence in self-care, an OTA is performing PROM on a shoulder of a client with Parkinson's disease who has been diagnosed with adhesive capsulitis. The client is positioned in supine with the client's shoulder in 90 degrees abduction. As the OTA moves the client's arm into 40 degrees of external rotation, the client reports sharp pain. Of the following choices, which is likely the OTA's better course of action?
    A. Document that the client has a low pain tolerance
    B. Do not attempt any passive external rotation beyond 40 degrees
    C. Attempt passive external rotation with shoulder adducted
    D. Move client to sitting position and attempt passive external rotation with shoulder positioned in 90 degrees abduction

4. An OTA is responsible for providing instruction to clients for home exercise programs using exercise bands for upper extremity strengthening. Which of the following instructions should the OTA give to each of the clients?
    A. Perform each exercise for two sets of 10 repetitions
    B. Perform exercises three times daily
    C. Inspect exercise bands for holes or tears
    D. Perform exercises only every other day

5. When using Thera-Band exercise bands, which of the following would indicate an upgrade of an exercise program or an increase in required effort?
    A. Use the same color exercise band in a shorter length than previously
    B. Use the same color exercise band in a longer length than previously
    C. Change from a red exercise band to a yellow exercise band
    D. Change from a blue exercise band to a green exercise band

Worksheet 6-1 (continued)

Therapeutic Exercises

6. A client recently diagnosed with rheumatoid arthritis (RA) has fair minus muscle strength for right shoulder flexion. Muscle strength of right elbow, wrist, and hand is within functional limits. Which of the following interventions would be more suitable to address this client's shoulder weakness in order to better manage household tasks?
   A. Codman's pendulum exercises
   B. Constraint-induced movement therapy
   C. Finger ladder
   D. Using a tabletop exercise skateboard

7. Which of the following one-handed activities is an example of an intervention to improve a child's finger to palm translation?
   A. Picking up beads from a table and moving them into palm
   B. Stacking 1-in. blocks with thumb, index, and middle fingers
   C. Holding a handful of coins and putting them in a piggy bank slot one at a time
   D. Pushing a miniature toy car along the floor

8. A client recovering from a Colles fracture is using a 1-lb weight to improve strength for wrist flexion and extension to enable self-care performance. The muscle contractions used for these exercises are:
   A. Isotonic
   B. Isometric
   C. Isothermal
   D. Isokinetic

9. A client is using an exercise band to improve the strength of the elbow flexors for lifting and carrying items at his job. The types of biceps contractions used to (1) pull the bands up and (2) slowly release them include all of the following except:
   A. Concentric
   B. Eccentric
   C. Isotonic
   D. Isometric

10. An OTA is working in a school setting with a child who has cerebral palsy. One of the goals in the child's Individualized Education Program (IEP) is to improve the child's voluntary grasp and release patterns to enable specific classroom tasks. During a tabletop activity of putting large pegs in a pegboard, the OTA should encourage the child to do which of the following?
    A. Maintain wrist flexion when placing pegs in holes
    B. Abduct shoulder to 90 degrees when placing pegs in holes
    C. Supinate forearm 45 degrees when placing pegs in holes
    D. Maintain wrist extension when placing pegs in holes

Worksheet 6-2

Open- and Closed-Kinetic-Chain Exercises

For each of the following *upper extremity* activities listed, indicate if it is an open-kinetic-chain exercise or closed-kinetic-chain exercise by putting an "O" or "C" next to each.

1. _____ Using exercise bands to improve shoulder strength

2. _____ Turning a heavy jump rope with another child holding the other end

3. _____ Weight bearing on forearm while writing with the contralateral hand

4. _____ Pushing a weighted toy shopping cart while walking around an obstacle course

5. _____ Putting cans in upper kitchen cabinets

6. _____ Using 1-lb weights to improve wrist strength

7. _____ Carrying a lunch tray in the cafeteria

8. _____ Sanding a wooden board using a sanding block

9. _____ Posing like a bear with hands and feet on floor

10. _____ Using a reacher to remove clothes from dryer

11. _____ Prone on elbows while watching a wind-up toy move

12. _____ Rolling dough into piecrust shape using a rolling pin

13. _____ Wringing out a washcloth

14. _____ Hanging clothes in closet while standing

15. _____ Pressing/flattening therapy putty with palm while standing at table

16. _____ Using cookie cutters to cut shapes out of a 1/2-in. thick clay circle on the table

Worksheet 6-2 (continued)
Open- and Closed-Kinetic-Chain Exercises

17. _____ Performing push-ups against the wall while standing

18. _____ Moving rings from one side of an exercise arc to the other side

19. _____ Applying lotion to extremities

20. _____ Arm push-ups while seated in preparation for transfers

21. _____ Cone stacking to improve grip

22. _____ Waving a ribbon wand to music

23. _____ Scrubbing a floor using a hand-held brush

24. _____ Painting on an easel while standing

25. _____ Sliding board transfer

Worksheet 6-3

Methods and Tasks to Support Occupations

1. An OTA is working with a client who had recent arthroscopic surgery to repair left rotator cuff. The client has been wearing a sling full-time since the surgery (except for showering and therapy) to protect the surgical site. Per the intervention plan, the OTA is instructing the client in Codman's pendulum exercises today. Which of the following choices better represents instructions the OTA might give to the client for these exercises?

   A. Stand with right side next to table or counter and remove sling carefully. Support self with right forearm on table/counter, lean over, and use a lower body rocking motion to gently swing the hanging left upper extremity (LUE) forward/backward and in circular motions passively.

   B. Stand with left side next to table and remove sling carefully. While standing upright, place LUE palm down on a towel on tabletop. Actively slide towel on table forward/back and in a side-to-side pendulum motion using LUE.

   C. Sit in a chair. Unfasten only distal part of sling so that left elbow can be removed carefully from it. Bend and straighten left elbow, wrist, and fingers passively using right upper extremity (RUE).

   D. Sit in a chair and remove sling carefully. Keeping both elbows flexed at 90 degrees, support LUE under forearm with RUE. Use RUE to flex both shoulders to 90 degrees then move bilateral upper extremity (BUE) side to side in a "rocking the baby" pendulum motion, keeping LUE passive.

2. An OTA is working with a client diagnosed with a closed crush injury to the dominant hand. The occupational therapy intervention plan includes methods to decrease hand edema and improve finger ROM to enable computer use and independent self-care. Which of the following interventions is a less suitable option to address these deficits?

   A. Hypertrophic scar massage

   B. Contrast baths

   C. Retrograde massage

   D. Overhead pumping

3. Rose is an 85-year-old female who sustained a Colles fracture and a T8 vertebral compression fracture due to a recent fall at home. She is presently in a skilled nursing facility for short-term rehabilitation and requires moderate assistance to ambulate and transfer. Which of the following is a possible choice for an OTA to recommend for pressure reduction to the client's ischial tuberosity area?

   A. Cushioned heel protectors

   B. Gel pad under wrist orthosis

   C. Foam seat cushion

   D. Gel back-support cushion

4. A left-handed 10-year-old child with a traumatic brain injury has increased muscle tone in RUE and fair sitting balance. While guarding the child for safety, how should the OTA position the child when working on graphomotor skills?

   A. Standing at desk, RUE in anatomical position with ipsilateral hand holding pencil

   B. Sitting at desk, feet supported, right forearm supinated on table with contralateral hand holding pencil

   C. Sitting at desk, feet supported, right forearm in midline position with ipsilateral hand holding pencil

   D. Sitting at desk, feet supported, right forearm pronated on table with contralateral hand holding pencil

Worksheet 6-3 (continued)

Methods and Tasks to Support Occupations

5. An OTA in a rehabilitation hospital is planning a lower body dressing session with a male client who has recently undergone surgery for a below-knee amputation. The OTA arrives at the client's room immediately following the client's shower. The client is dressed in a hospital gown but the long elastic bandage that has been used to shape his residual limb has not been reapplied. What action should the OTA take?
    A. Rewrap stump using a circular method to apply the bandage then work on lower body dressing
    B. Rewrap the stump using a figure-8 method to apply the bandage then work on lower body dressing
    C. Before performing dressing tasks, contact the physical therapist or physical therapist assistant and ask that person to rewrap the stump now
    D. Work on lower body dressing without reapplying the bandage

6. An OTA is working with a client diagnosed with right cerebrovascular accident (CVA) who has weakness in LUE and trunk. The client is seated at the edge of a mat with feet apart supported on the floor. To facilitate trunk flexion and anterior weight shift specifically (to enable self-care and transfers), which of the following interventions might the OTA have the client do (while client is guarded/assisted for safety)?
    A. Use LUE to reach up and forward for cones OTA is holding in front of client
    B. Use LUE to reach for cones placed on mat on client's left and right sides
    C. Use LUE to reach for cones placed on floor between client's feet
    D. Remain seated and perform alternating lower extremity stepping motions with hands resting on thighs

7. A client diagnosed with a CVA and left hemiparesis is beginning to exhibit some motor return in the affected upper extremity. An OTA using a Neurodevelopmental Treatment (NDT) approach is working with the client on LUE weight-bearing activities to improve proximal stability for dressing and bathing. The client is seated on a mat with affected arm extended at side and palm on the mat. Which of the following is not correct for the OTA to do?
    A. Flatten client's hand completely on the mat
    B. Support client's elbow in extension
    C. Have client shift weight gradually toward affected side
    D. Increase proprioceptive input to LUE

8. An OTA is working with a client using an exercise band to improve right shoulder external rotation strength needed for a fire fighter job. The OTA tied the exercise band to a doorknob. Which of the following instructions should the OTA give to the client for this task?
    A. Stand with right side of body nearer to doorknob. Use band in right hand and pull across front of body, keeping the weak shoulder adducted.
    B. Stand with right side of body nearer to doorknob. Use band in right hand and pull away from right side of body, keeping the weak shoulder adducted.
    C. Stand with left side of body nearer to doorknob. Use band in right hand and pull across front of body with right hand, keeping the weak shoulder adducted.
    D. Stand with left side of body nearer to doorknob. Use band in right hand and pull away from right side of body, keeping the weak shoulder adducted.

Worksheet 6-3 (continued)

Methods and Tasks to Support Occupations

9. A client is fully dressed and seated in a chair facing the OTA. The OTA is instructing the client in lightly resistive therapy putty exercises to improve overall hand function for activities of daily living (ADLs). Which of the following is less suitable for the OTA to instruct the client to do with the therapy putty at this time?
    A. Squeeze therapy putty into a ball
    B. Roll therapy putty into a log shape on client's thigh
    C. Pinch therapy putty with thumb, index, and long fingers
    D. Squeeze therapy putty between fingers

10. In occupational therapy, a musician recovering from carpal tunnel surgery is placing golf tees vertically in therapy putty to improve strength of muscles innervated by the affected nerve to resume playing musical instrument. This task was most likely chosen by the OTA to address which of the following?
    A. Interossei strength
    B. Tip pinch strength
    C. Lateral pinch strength
    D. Hypothenar muscle strength

Learning Activity 6-1: Client Factors and Motor Skills

For each of the client factors or performance skills in the table below, list two tasks supporting occupations plus two activities/occupations that may be used in occupational therapy to improve deficits in those areas. Examples are provided for each category. Also, determine three additional client factors or performance skills to add to this table. Considering each client factor/performance skill category, determine which of the interventions might be more meaningful or effective for a "real" client and the reasons why.

Client Factor/Performance Skill	*Tasks to Support Occupations*	*Activities and Occupations*
Shoulder ROM	*Pulleys* 1. 2.	*Put groceries in upper kitchen cabinet* 1. 2.
Upper extremity strength	*Exercise bands* 1. 2.	*Carry a laundry basket containing towels or clothes* 1. 2.
Cylindrical grasp	Stack cones 1. 2.	*Use large-handled utensils for feeding* 1. 2.
Hand strength	*Squeeze hand gripper* 1. 2.	*Knead bread dough* 1. 2.
Standing balance/tolerance	*Stand at table to use shoulder arc* 1. 2.	*Stand at kitchen counter to make a sandwich* 1. 2.
Sitting balance/tolerance	*Sit on mat to toss beanbags* 1. 2.	*Sit on tub bench when bathing* 1. 2.
3-point pinch/palmar pinch	*Stack small checkers* 1. 2.	*Put on lipstick* 1. 2.
Tip pinch	*Put small pegs in pegboard* 1. 2.	*Put pills in pill organizer (can use beans or small candies to simulate pills)* 1. 2.
Lateral pinch	*Pinch therapy putty* 1. 2.	*Hang towels on a clothesline using clothespins* 1. 2.
Dexterity/in-hand manipulation	*Pick up foam cubes one at a time and hold in palm* 1. 2.	*Sort a handful of coins into wrappers* 1. 2.
Other:	1. 2.	
Other:	1. 2.	
Other:	1. 2.	

Learning Activity 6-2: Process Skills

For each of the client factors or performance skills in the table below, list two tasks supporting occupations plus two activities/occupations that may be used in occupational therapy to improve deficits in those areas. Examples are provided for each category. Also, determine three additional client factors or performance skills to add to this table. Considering each client factor/performance skill category, determine which of the interventions might be more meaningful or effective for a "real" client and the reasons why.

Client Factor/Performance Skill	Tasks to Support Occupations	Activities and Occupations
Crossing midline	*Moving rings on a shoulder arc from one side to the other* 1. 2.	*Move kitchen utensils from dish drainer to drawer on opposite side* 1. 2.
Spatial relations	*Follow a pattern using blocks* 1. 2.	*Place cookie dough evenly spaced on a cookie sheet* 1. 2.
Bilateral integration	*Upper extremity pedal exerciser* 1. 2.	*Buttoning a shirt* 1. 2.
Short-term memory	*Memory matching game* 1. 2.	Use calendar to find/schedule appointments 1. 2.
Categorization	Sort shapes 1. 2.	*Sort utensils into a divided utensil tray* 1. 2.
Sequencing	*Sequencing cards* 1. 2.	*Follow a recipe* 1. 2.
Calculation skills	*Math worksheets* 1. 2.	*Use a restaurant menu and calculate cost of a meal including tax and tip* 1. 2.
Problem solving	Logic puzzles 1. 2.	Role play emergency situations 1. 2.
Body scheme	*Orient felt body pieces on a felt board* 1. 2.	*Dressing* 1. 2.
Awareness of left visual field	*Pick up beanbags on right side and place in bucket on left side* 1. 2.	*Locate grooming items on left side of counter when brushing teeth* 1. 2.
Other:	1. 2.	
Other:	1. 2.	
Other:	1. 2.	

Learning Activity 6-3: Physical Agent Modalities

ACOTE (2018, standard B.4.17., p. 49) delineates that entry-level OTAs demonstrate ability to "Define the safe and effective application of superficial thermal agents, deep thermal agents, electrotherapeutic agents, and mechanical devices as a preparatory measure to improve occupational performance. This must include indications, contraindications, and precautions." It is important to understand that state licensure laws delineate the specific kinds of PAMs that may be used by an OT or OTA in a particular state along with any continuing education or supervision requirements to demonstrate competency in their use (AOTA, 2018). OTs and OTAs must comply with regulatory requirements, demonstrate service competency and ethical use, and only implement PAMs as part of a comprehensive intervention plan designed to enhance occupational engagement (AOTA, 2018, 2020).

Instructions: Refer to AOTA's Position Statement *Physical Agents and Mechanical Modalities* (AOTA, 2018) to answer the following questions.

Define therapeutic modalities _____
_____
_____

List nine possible benefits that physical agents can provide:

1.

2.

3.

4.

5.

6.

7.

8.

9.

What three categories (not PAM properties) are delineated by AOTA as the beneficial therapeutic uses of PAMs as part of an occupational therapy intervention plan?

1.

2.

3.

Morreale, M. J. (2022). *Developing clinical competence: A workbook for the OTA* (2nd ed.). SLACK Incorporated.

Define the following terms:

Conduction:

Convection:

Conversion:

Briefly describe the basic difference between *electromagnetic* modalities and *electrotherapy*:

List four kinds of force various mechanical modalities can apply:

1.

2.

3.

4.

Identify two additional AOTA Official Documents that can help guide occupational therapy practice regarding the use of PAMs:

1.

2.

Worksheet 6-4

Physical Agent Modality Categories

Instructions: Indicate the pertinent category for each of the following PAMs or devices by their properties.

Physical Agent Modality	Superficial Thermal Agent	Deep Thermal Agent	Electrotherapeutic Agent	Electromagnetic Devices	Mechanical Device
Fluidotherapy					
Transcutaneous electrical nerve stimulation (TENS)					
Iontophoresis					
Hot pack					
Ultrasound					
Whirlpool					
Vasopneumatic device					
Cryotherapy					
Neuromuscular electrical stimulation (NMES)					
Functional electrical stimulation (FES)					
Continuous passive motion (CPM)					
Paraffin					
High-voltage pulsed current (HVPC)					
Cold pack					
Hydrotherapy					
Chemical heat packs					
Biofeedback					
Short-wave diathermy					
Vapocoolant spray					
Low-level laser (light) therapy					
Lymphedema pump					
Phonophoresis					
Microwaveable heat pack					
Contrast baths					
Controlled cold compression unit					

Worksheet 6-5

Selecting Physical Agent Modalities

For each of the following client conditions indicated, choose an appropriate modality or device from the list. Only use each modality or device once. Realize that these are merely examples of select conditions and potential uses of PAMs. Practitioners must always follow their state licensure laws and use professional reasoning in determining the specific PAMs suitable for a "real" client.

A. Whirlpool
B. CPM
C. Ultrasound
D. Fluidotherapy
E. Vasopneumatic pump
F. TENS
G. NMES
H. Cold pack
I. Hot pack
J. Paraffin
K. Iontophoresis
L. Biofeedback
M. Hydrotherapy
N. Contrast baths
O. Controlled cold compression unit

1. _____ Acute proximal interphalangeal (PIP) hyperextension injury with pain and edema

2. _____ Shoulder stiffness due to RA

3. _____ Muscle re-education to learn how to minimize involuntary upper trapezius muscle contraction

4. _____ Healed carpal tunnel release with stiffness, fair light touch sensation, intact protective sensation, and scar hypersensitivity

5. _____ Thumb carpometacarpal (CMC) arthritis with pain and stiffness

6. _____ Manage edema following soft tissue trauma

7. _____ Open wound requiring debridement

8. _____ Chronic biceps pain on discharge from occupational therapy

9. _____ Conditions requiring mechanical PROM

Worksheet 6-5 (continued)
Selecting Physical Agent Modalities

10. _____ Lateral epicondylitis requiring topical medication delivery through the skin

11. _____ CVA with hemiparesis and shoulder subluxation

12. _____ PIP joint contracture and scar adhesions following a healed laceration to volar index finger

13. _____ Used immediately following shoulder surgery to minimize postoperative pain and edema

14. _____ Client with complex regional pain syndrome needing home protocol to minimize hand stiffness, pain, and edema

15. _____ Client with fibromyalgia who may benefit from an aquatic exercise program to help relieve pain and stiffness

Morreale, M. J. (2022). *Developing clinical competence: A workbook for the OTA* (2nd ed.). SLACK Incorporated.

Worksheet 6-6
Using Physical Agent Modalities Safely

1. Which of the following conditions would be more of a fit for paraffin use?
    A. Crush injury resulting in pitting hand edema and finger stiffness
    B. Wrist fracture resulting in digital stiffness and insensate areas of thumb
    C. Healed Zone 2 flexor tendon repair of index and long fingers resulting in poor tendon gliding
    D. Laceration of thumb with sutures in place and decreased ROM of thumb and digits

2. The OT's intervention plan indicates that an outpatient client with a shoulder condition would benefit from superficial heat to help decrease shoulder stiffness for instrumental activities of daily living (IADL) performance. Before placing a hot pack on the client, the OTA should do which of the following?
    A. Ask client to remove watch and rings
    B. Use an anti-static mat under client to prevent electric shocks
    C. Wrap the hot pack with a terrycloth cover and place a plastic bag over it
    D. Check hydrocollator temperature

3. Of the following choices, which primary action should an OTA take when a client tells the OTA that a hot pack feels too hot?
    A. Lower temperature of hydrocollator
    B. Inform the client that the heat will gradually dissipate
    C. Remove hot pack
    D. Find the OT to inform them of the situation

4. Which of the following conditions would be more suitable for possible use of Fluidotherapy?
    A. RA flare-up causing painful hand and swollen finger joints
    B. Thumb CMC joint stiffness secondary to osteoarthritis
    C. Healed biceps tendon repair resulting in elbow pain and stiffness but no sensory loss
    D. Shoulder contracture secondary to complex regional pain syndrome

5. When using a cryotherapy gel pack on a client, the OTA should do which of the following?
    A. Apply it with continuous, slow circular motions over affected area
    B. When done, put gel pack immediately in a hydrocollator so it is ready for the next client
    C. Cover gel pack with a pillowcase before placing it over insensate area
    D. Explain that the client may experience a numb sensation

6. An inpatient client is morbidly obese and requires a mechanical lift to transfer him out of bed. He rolls side to side using bed rails but cannot roll onto his stomach. The client also has pain in his posterior deltoid, for which the doctor ordered occupational therapy, including hot packs. For the past 2 days the client has received hot packs on his shoulder while sitting in a chair. Today, when the OTA arrives with the hot pack, the mechanical lift is not available. What should the OTA do?
    A. Place the hot pack underneath the client's shoulder with client supine
    B. Place the hot pack on the client's shoulder with client side-lying
    C. Place the hot pack on the client's shoulder with client prone
    D. Defer use of hot pack

Worksheet 6-6 (continued)

Using Physical Agent Modalities Safely

7. When administering a paraffin treatment to a client who has stiffness in digits and intact skin, the OTA should do which of the following:
   A. Ask client to perform finger active range of motion (AROM) in paraffin bath
   B. Ask client to perform hand hygiene before using paraffin
   C. Place a plastic bag over client's hand then dip in paraffin and cover with a towel
   D. Ask client to immerse hand to the bottom of the unit to maximize coverage

8. An occupational therapy client with a wrist sprain has been receiving hot packs to involved wrist followed by ROM and functional activities per the intervention plan, to enable return to police officer job. When the client arrives today, the OTA notices the client has bad sunburn on both upper extremities which also extends over the injured wrist. What primary action should the OTA take?
   A. Administer a cold pack, then a hot pack followed by ROM and functional activities
   B. Defer treatment today and reschedule
   C. Defer hot pack and perform functional activities
   D. Call the client's physician

9. An occupational therapy client had recent surgery to remove basal cell carcinoma from right wrist and is presently receiving radiation to eliminate possible remaining malignant cells. The client reports right wrist pain 5/10 and has decreased ROM in right wrist and hand, which limit ADLs. Which of the following modalities would be indicated for this client?
   A. Hot pack
   B. Ultrasound
   C. Paraffin
   D. None of the above

10. Which of the following conditions would be more suitable for possible use of cryotherapy?
    A. Client with an acute wrist sprain and history of a carpal tunnel release 6 months ago with no loss of sensation
    B. Client with Raynaud's phenomenon and acute thumb tendinitis
    C. Client with upper extremity peripheral vascular disease and acute finger sprain
    D. Client with an elbow contracture secondary to biceps tendon tightness

Worksheet 6-7

Physical Agent Modality Basics

1. An OTA is working in a state that does not restrict occupational therapy practitioners from using PAMs. The OTA and the OT supervisor are competent in the use of superficial, deep thermal and electrotherapeutic agents. Which of the following intervention plans is not considered occupational therapy?
   A. Hot pack to shoulder, paraffin to hand, contrast baths
   B. PROM and NMES to hand, home management tasks
   C. Hot pack and TENS to shoulder, home management tasks
   D. Ultrasound and scar massage to wrist, ADLs

2. Which of the following PAMs transfer heat strictly by conduction?
   A. Fluidotherapy and hot packs
   B. Ultrasound and paraffin
   C. Paraffin and hot packs
   D. Fluidotherapy and hydrotherapy

3. Which of the following temperature ranges for paraffin are suitable for use with a client?
   A. 98 to 100 degrees
   B. 134 to 138 degrees
   C. 122 to 124 degrees
   D. 108 to 112 degrees

4. Which of the following is the technique of using ultrasound to deliver medication through the skin?
   A. NMES
   B. TENS
   C. Iontophoresis
   D. Phonophoresis

5. An OTA is working in a state that, regarding PAMs, allows OTAs to only use superficial thermal agents. The client has a diagnosis of carpal tunnel release and the occupational therapy intervention plan includes ultrasound, Fluidotherapy, and TENS to support occupations. Which of the following PAMs should the OTA use with the client to help decrease pain and improve ROM to enable client to resume hobbies of piano playing and knitting?
   A. Fluidotherapy
   B. Fluidotherapy and TENS
   C. Fluidotherapy, ultrasound, and TENS
   D. None of the above

6. A client was referred to occupational therapy following a laceration to the hand. The sutures were removed 1 week ago. The wound is healed, but the client is not yet able to return to flight attendant job due to scar hypersensitivity, decreased finger ROM, and moderate hand edema. Which of the following PAMs is a possible choice for an OTA to administer now, assuming it is delineated in the intervention plan?
   A. Fluidotherapy
   B. Paraffin
   C. Hot pack
   D. None of the above

Worksheet 6-7 (continued)
Physical Agent Modality Basics

7. An OTA who is competent in administering TENS has moved to a new state that prohibits OTAs from using electrotherapeutic agents. The sole OT at the rehabilitation facility is not competent in administering TENS. However, an occupational therapy client diagnosed with complex regional pain syndrome would likely benefit from TENS to help manage severe upper extremity pain. The prescription from the doctor says "PAMs PRN." What should the OTA do?
   A. The OTA should administer TENS only under the supervision of a physical therapist
   B. Ask the doctor to write an occupational therapy prescription specifically for TENS
   C. Have the OT administer TENS with the OTA supervising
   D. Do not use TENS

8. The OT intervention plan for a client with a PIP dislocation injury includes the following PAMs as needed (PRN) to support ADL performance: hot packs, Fluidotherapy, and cold packs. Today the client informs the OTA that she receives paraffin to her hands when getting manicures at the nail salon and enjoys it very much. The OTA feels that paraffin would indeed be beneficial to decrease the client's finger stiffness today. What should the OTA do during this session?
   A. Call the client's physician to obtain a prescription for paraffin
   B. Administer paraffin and notify the OT
   C. Document what the client said and administer paraffin
   D. Administer hot pack or Fluidotherapy

9. A client with thumb tendinitis is at the reconditioning phase in occupational therapy. During an intervention session, which of the following is most likely the proper sequence of interventions for this client, assuming they are all part of the intervention plan?
   A. Hot pack, activities/occupations, paraffin
   B. Hot pack, activities/occupations, cold pack
   C. Paraffin, activities/occupations, hot pack, cold pack
   D. Paraffin, activities/occupations, hot pack

10. Following a client's paraffin treatment, what should the OTA do with the used wax?
   A. Put it back in the paraffin unit
   B. Give it to the client to use at home for hand exercises
   C. Throw it away
   D. Save it in an individually labeled plastic bag for the client's next occupational therapy session

Worksheet 6-8

Deep Thermal and Electrical Modalities

Determine if the following statements are true (T) or false (F).

1. T ____   F ____   An ultrasound frequency of 1 MHz penetrates more deeply than a 3 MHz frequency.

2. T ____   F ____   Ultrasound coupling media can include gel pads, water immersion, and viscous aqueous gel.

3. T ____   F ____   An ultrasound duty cycle of 20% is suitable when a thermal effect is desired.

4. T ____   F ____   The anatomical area receiving the ultrasound treatment should be no larger than four times the size of the effective radiating area (ERA).

5. T ____   F ____   Contraindications for ultrasound include joint replacement with cement or plastic components in the affected area, pacemaker, and chronic tendinitis.

6. T ____   F ____   When documenting ultrasound intensity, the unit of measurement is W/cm^2.

7. T ____   F ____   Continuous ultrasound refers to continually moving the sound head during the treatment.

8. T ____   F ____   Three types of waveforms used in electrotherapy include pulsed current, direct current, and alternating current.

9. T ____   F ____   A monophasic pulsed current only flows in one direction for each pulse and pauses in-between pulses.

10. T ____   F ____   A drug commonly delivered transdermally with iontophoresis is dexamethasone.

11. T ____   F ____   Possible risks from electrotherapy include burns from electric currents and redness or skin irritation due to electrode adhesive or gel.

12. T ____   F ____   TENS with a short duration and pulse rate of 100 pps is considered low-rate or non-conventional TENS.

13. T ____   F ____   High-rate TENS elicits sensory effect and muscle contraction and, therefore, should not be used with acute conditions.

14. T ____   F ____   For chronic, stable conditions needing a longer duration of TENS to help manage pain, it is suitable to set pulse rate at less than 10 pps.

Worksheet 6-8 (continued)

Deep Thermal and Electrical Modalities

15. T ____   F ____   NMES uses electrical currents to produce contractions in muscles that are denervated.

16. T ____   F ____   When implementing NMES, an electrode is placed at the muscle's motor point which is typically at the musculotendinous junction.

17. T ____   F ____   In regard to NMES, on:off time refers to the timed intervals in-between therapy appointments.

18. T ____   F ____   Indications for NMES can include conditions such as weak upper/lower extremity muscles, dysphagia, spasticity, and urinary incontinence.

19. T ____   F ____   Clients that are debilitated, such as those with a cardiac pacemaker or implanted defibrillator, can benefit from NMES to help increase muscle strength and endurance.

20. T ____   F ____   When using NMES, ramp up/ramp down time refers to the amount of time that the force is gradually increased and decreased when producing and then relaxing the contraction.

Learning Activity 6-4: Generating Interventions

One of the unique aspects of occupational therapy is the occupational therapy practitioner's ability to use everyday objects for therapeutic purposes. In the following spaces, list specific ways that a deck of cards might be used to improve the various client factors or performance skills delineated in the *Occupational Therapy Practice Framework: Domain and Process, Fourth Edition* (OTPF—4; AOTA, 2020) to support occupations. Examples are provided for each category.

Joint, Bone, and Muscle Functions
Example: Improve ROM of the elbow—*Deal cards across the table to a partner*

1.

2.

3.

Motor Skills
Example: Improve standing tolerance—*Stand at table to play Solitaire for a designated length of time*

1.

2.

3.

Emotional Regulation/Social Interaction Skills
Example: Improve frustration tolerance—*Play a card game and wait patiently for one's turn*

1.

2.

3.

Mental Functions/Process Skills
Example: Improve counting and math skills—*Count a deck of cards accurately*

1.

2.

3.

Learning Activity 6-5: Generating More Interventions

This exercise will require you to think creatively. One of the unique aspects of occupational therapy is the occupational therapy practitioner's ability to use everyday objects for therapeutic purposes. In the following box, list specific ways that paper clips might be used to improve the various client factors and performance skills delineated in the *OTPF—4* (AOTA, 2020) to support occupations. Examples are provided for each category.

Joint, Bone, and Muscle Functions
Example: Improve tip pinch strength—*Use index finger and thumb to push paper clips vertically into therapy putty*

1.

2.

3.

Motor Skills
Example: Improve bilateral integration—*Stabilize paper on the table while attaching paper clips with the other hand*

1.

2.

3.

Emotional Regulation/Social Interaction Skills
Example: Improve interpersonal skills—*Ask a worker in office supply store where the paper clips are located*

1.

2.

3.

Mental Functions/Process Skills
Example: Safety awareness—*Avoid putting paper clips in mouth while working on a craft project*

1.

2.

3.

Learning Activity 6-6: Generating Creative Interventions

The media used in this exercise will require a bit more thinking "outside of the box." As previously noted, one of the unique aspects of occupational therapy is the occupational therapy practitioner's ability to use everyday objects for therapeutic purposes. In the following spaces, list specific ways that a container of uncooked rice might be used to improve various client factors, performance skills, and occupations delineated in the *OTPF—4* (AOTA, 2020) to support occupations. Examples are provided for each category.

Joint, Bone, and Muscle Functions
Example: Improve upper extremity strength—*Carry a 5-lb bag of rice*

1.

2.

3.

Motor Skills
Example: Improve coordination—*Move spoonfuls of rice from one container to another without spilling*

1.

2.

3.

Sensory Functions
Example: Reduce tactile hypersensitivity—*Locate objects embedded in rice*

1.

2.

3.

Emotional Regulation/Social Interaction Skills
Example: Express feelings—*Discuss significance of rice in one's own culture (e.g., rice and beans, fried rice, rice pudding)*

1.

2.

3.

Mental Functions/Process Skills
Example: Improve measuring skills—*Measure specified amounts of rice accurately*

1.

2.

3.

Occupations (ADLs/IADLs)
Example: Improve meal preparation skills—*Follow a recipe to make beans and rice for lunch*

1.

2.

3.

4.

5.

6.

Occupations (Play)
Example: Improve imaginary play skills—*Collaborate with another person and use rice to create a "beach" scene: decorating with shells, hidden "treasure," and dolls "suntanning"*

1.

2.

3.

4.

5.

6.

Worksheet 6-9

Orthotic Interventions

Match each of the orthoses or devices to one of the conditions that follow. Use each term only once.

    A. Resting hand orthosis
    B. Metacarpophalangeal (MP) extension blocking orthosis
    C. Airplane splint
    D. Palm protector
    E. Short opponens orthosis
    F. Dorsal blocking orthosis
    G. Forearm-based thumb immobilization orthosis
    H. Figure-8 finger orthosis
    I. Dynamic MP extension orthosis
    J. Ulnar deviation orthosis
    K. Volar wrist immobilization orthosis
    L. Anterior elbow orthosis
    M. PIP extension orthosis
    N. Forearm-based dorsal extension orthosis
    O. Distal interphalangeal (DIP) joint extension orthosis
    P. Ulnar gutter orthosis
    Q. Counterforce brace
    R. Body-powered prosthesis
    S. Composite flexion orthosis
    T. Tenodesis orthosis

1. _____ Carpal tunnel syndrome

2. _____ Boutonniere deformity ring finger

3. _____ Upper extremity amputation

4. _____ Small finger metacarpal fracture

5. _____ Dupuytren's release

6. _____ C6-C7 spinal cord injury

7. _____ Flexor tendon repair of digits

8. _____ Brachial plexus injury

9. _____ Swan neck deformity

Worksheet 6-9 (continued)
Orthotic Interventions

10. _____ Mallet finger

11. _____ Low level ulnar nerve injury

12. _____ Burns to hand/wrist

13. _____ Extrinsic extensor tightness of digits

14. _____ de Quervain's tenosynovitis

15. _____ Elbow flexion contracture

16. _____ MP joints requiring realignment secondary to RA

17. _____ Flexed digits of a client with end-stage dementia and skin breakdown in hand

18. _____ Low level median nerve injury

19. _____ Lateral epicondylitis

20. _____ Radial nerve palsy

Worksheet 6-10

Using Orthotic Devices

1. When fabricating a volar wrist immobilization orthosis for a client with a wrist sprain, an OTA must mold it carefully to avoid future skin breakdown at which of the following bony prominences:
   A. Radial head
   B. PIP joints
   C. Ulnar styloid
   D. Olecranon

2. A client with an unhealed fracture reports that he is perspiring under his thermoplastic orthosis. The OTA may take the following actions except:
   A. Punch air holes in the orthosis
   B. Provide washable stockinette liners
   C. Discontinue orthotic device
   D. Instruct client how to clean the orthotic device

3. When fabricating an orthotic device, the primary reason for making a paper pattern is:
   A. To avoid wasting expensive thermoplastic material
   B. To help ensure proper size and fit of orthosis
   C. To keep the pattern in the client's chart
   D. To avoid pen or pencil marks on thermoplastic material

4. After softening thermoplastic material in hot water for orthotic device fabrication, what should the OTA do next?
   A. Remove from water, blow on it for 10 to 15 seconds to cool it then place on client
   B. Trace the pattern on it
   C. Attach hook and loop fastener
   D. Dry off thermoplastic material and cool it until client can comfortably tolerate it

5. When fabricating a resting hand orthosis for a client with a flaccid extremity, the thumb should generally be positioned in:
   A. Palmar abduction
   B. Full adduction
   C. Full radial abduction
   D. 90 degrees MP flexion

6. When fabricating an orthotic device to address an index finger mallet injury, which of the following statements is not correct?
   A. Conform orthosis to transverse and longitudinal arches of palm
   B. Allow for full active MP flexion
   C. Position DIP joint in extension
   D. Leave thumb free

Worksheet 6-10 (continued)
Using Orthotic Devices

7. When fabricating a forearm-based thumb immobilization orthosis for a client with thumb CMC arthritis, which of the following principles does not apply?
   A. Orthosis should be half the length of the forearm
   B. Conform to transverse and longitudinal arches of hand
   C. Allow full thumb interphalangeal (IP) joint AROM
   D. Do not immobilize MP joints of other digits

8. A client diagnosed with a right CVA exhibits unilateral neglect and poor safety awareness regarding his non-functional left hand. The OT fabricated a volar resting hand orthosis to help keep the client's joints in a safe, functional position. The client's wrist spasticity keeps causing the Velcro wrist strap to detach. Besides possibly fabricating a different orthotic device for dorsum of hand, which of the following is likely a more suitable action for the OTA to remedy this problem?
   A. Remold the splint into a flexed wrist position
   B. Discontinue the splint
   C. Instruct the client to refasten the strap
   D. Use a D-ring and longer wrist strap

9. A primary purpose of an outrigger on a dynamic orthosis is:
   A. To ensure proper angle of pull
   B. To conform to the transverse and longitudinal arches
   C. To attach orthotic device to the forearm
   D. To make the orthosis more durable

10. A child with cerebral palsy was issued a hand-based thumb immobilization orthosis last week to promote prehension. Today the child arrives with his parent and tells the OTA that the orthosis is uncomfortable due to it rubbing at the thumb IP joint, and he does not want to wear it. The OTA notices that the edge of the orthosis is rough and observes slight redness at the thumb IP joint. The OT has already left for the day. Which of the following should the OTA do?
    A. Defer treatment and schedule an appointment with the OT tomorrow
    B. Fabricate a new orthosis
    C. Use a heat gun to smooth rough area of orthosis
    D. Document that the child is noncompliant with wearing the orthosis

Worksheet 6-11

Client Education

Imagine you have just fabricated and issued an orthotic device for a client who has osteoarthritis of her dominant thumb CMC joint. List at least eight things you need to educate the client about regarding the orthotic device.

1.

2.

3.

4.

5.

6.

7.

8.

Later that afternoon you receive a call from the referring physician. She tells you that this client phoned her office reporting that the orthosis was uncomfortable. It is 30 minutes from the end of the business day, and the OT has already left for home. What do you do?

Question adapted from Morreale, M. J., & Amini, D. (2016). *The occupational therapist's workbook for ensuring clinical competence.* SLACK Incorporated.

1.

2.

3.

4.

5.

Learning Activity 6-7: Custom Versus Prefabricated Orthotic Devices

Choose a specific type of orthotic device such as a resting hand orthosis, wrist extension orthosis, elbow extension orthosis, or dynamic MP extension orthosis. Make a list of all the materials and equipment needed to fabricate that specific orthotic device. Use a professional catalog to calculate the exact cost of materials for making the orthotic device, not including the practitioner's time or standard tools/equipment (e.g., heating unit, scissors). Also, determine if a similar prefabricated orthotic device is available for purchase. Compare the cost of materials for a custom orthosis versus the price of the prefabricated orthosis. Which option would you choose for a client? Explain your rationale.

Name of orthotic device:

List several conditions this orthotic device may be used for:

Materials Required	Package Cost and Quantity	Unit Cost for One Orthosis
Example: Loop fastener	$25 per 25-foot roll	24 in. = $2.00

Equipment Required	Tools Required	
Example: Electric heat pan	Example: Scissors	

Total cost of orthosis (excluding labor costs): $

Prefabricated orthosis cost: $

Rationale for Using a Custom Orthosis	Rationale for Using a Prefabricated Orthosis

Worksheet 6-12

Wound Care Basics

1. Although possibly a relevant term, which of the following is not considered one of the three primary phases of wound healing?
   A. Proliferative
   B. Pathological
   C. Inflammatory
   D. Remodeling

2. Which of the following is not a first-intention healing method?
   A. Skin graft
   B. Sutures
   C. Staples
   D. Surgical glue

3. When assessing a client's upper extremity wound, the OTA observes pale yellow, transparent exudate. This should be documented using which of the following terms?
   A. Serous
   B. Purulent
   C. Fibrinous
   D. Hemorrhagic

4. Which of the following is a main reason for wound debridement?
   A. To decrease granulation
   B. To increase eschar
   C. To increase shear force
   D. To expose healthy tissue

5. A client in occupational therapy has a stage 1 pressure injury on both heels. When working on dressing interventions, which of the following might an OTA expect to see on the heels when the client is donning and doffing socks?
   A. Pus
   B. Moist wound bed
   C. Necrotic tissue
   D. Erythema

6. Which of the following is correct regarding an unstageable pressure injury?
   A. The injury base is covered by slough or eschar
   B. There is partial-thickness skin loss
   C. Depth cannot be greater than 1.5 cm
   D. Depth cannot be greater than 20 mm

Worksheet 6-12 (continued)
Wound Care Basics

7. A client was referred to occupational therapy following recent surgery to remove a wrist ganglion cyst. Today the OTA sees that the client is exhibiting the four cardinal signs of inflammation at the surgical site. These four specific signs include all except which of the following (although that could also be present)?
   A. Erythema
   B. Pain
   C. Exudate
   D. Heat

8. An OTA in home care is working with an 88-year-old female client with dementia who is incontinent and non-ambulatory. The client lives with her daughter and son-in-law who are in relatively good health. The OTA is teaching them strategies to help prevent the client from developing pressure injuries. Which of the following recommendations is less suitable for the OTA to suggest for maintaining skin integrity?
   A. To protect heels, do not keep socks on the client when she is lying in bed
   B. Use a draw sheet when moving client in bed
   C. Have client maintain good hydration
   D. Use a topical moisture barrier

9. An OTA competent in basic wound care was delegated the task of changing an outpatient client's dressing and assessing the hand wound today. When attempting to remove the gauze pad on top of the wound, the OTA finds that it is sticking slightly to the wound. In general, which of the following choices is a more suitable option for the OTA to consider using?
   A. Pour some sterile saline over the adherent area to soften the exudate
   B. Pour some hydrogen peroxide over the adherent area to dissolve and soften the adherent exudate
   C. Pull the bandage off in a swift motion
   D. Do not remove the bandage today

10. An OTA is performing wound care with a client recovering from a finger laceration. In the initial evaluation performed 1 week ago, the OT described the wound as "yellow," and wound size as "9 mm long by 6 mm wide." Which of the following observations made by the OTA today would indicate that the wound is improving?
    A. Black color
    B. Red color
    C. 1 cm long by 0.6 cm wide
    D. 8 cm long by 5 cm wide

Worksheet 6-13

Upper Extremity Safety

Stella is an 82-year-old client with a diagnosis of right CVA, left hemiparesis. She is beginning to exhibit some limited motor return in her left shoulder and elbow, along with some active gross finger flexion. Stella also has poor LUE sensation, homonymous hemianopsia, and moderate unilateral neglect. When Stella sits in the wheelchair, she is unaware that her left arm tends to hang down over the side and get caught in the wheel. Imagine you are an OTA working with this client. List six different methods or tasks you might use to improve the safety of Stella's upper extremity while she is sitting in her wheelchair. Determine the pros and cons of each method or task.

Possible Intervention Options	Pros	Cons
1.		
2.		
3.		
4.		
5.		
6.		

Morreale, M. J. (2022). *Developing clinical competence: A workbook for the OTA* (2nd ed.). SLACK Incorporated.

Answers to Worksheets

Occupational therapy practitioners must always use professional reasoning and evidence-informed practice when planning and implementing interventions to support occupations (AOTA, 2020). OT practitioners must also consider multiple factors, such as the client's individual health status and circumstances, relevant precautions/contraindications, methods available, and safety. For clients with physical conditions, therapy programs often include a variety of interventions to support occupations (e.g., PAMs, orthotic devices, therapeutic exercises, manual techniques, sensory strategies). However, these methods and tasks should always work toward supporting occupational performance and include activities and occupations (AOTA, 2018, 2020). Although the worksheet answers in this chapter contain examples of best practices, it is important to realize they may not be suitable for all client situations.

Worksheet 6-1: Therapeutic Exercises

Resources: Avers & Brown, 2019; Fairchild et al., 2018; Rybski, 2019

1. C. It will depend on the specific circumstances but, in situations such as the one presented, a report of a minor complaint, such as "a little stretch" or "slight pull" is often not cause for major concern. Many clients in occupational therapy have painful conditions that rehabilitation must gradually work through, but professional reasoning is always needed to ascertain what level of pain is or is not acceptable, expected, safe, and the appropriate techniques to apply. Of course, if the client had a fragile wound, recent surgery such as a tendon or nerve repair, unstable joints, or reported a more severe complaint during ROM such as "severe pain" or "sharp pain," that would usually require more caution and different action taken by the OTA. Other considerations include joint end feel and if a client's pain is new, different, unexpected, or disproportionate to the task at hand.

    For the scenario depicted in this question, the OTA should not aggressively move or force the joint but might gently try to hold the joint at point of slight tension for a brief hold (per client tolerance without creating severe pain) to see if soft tissues relax and further ROM may be attained. Despite the old mantra of "no pain, no gain," always keep in mind that pain could indeed signify that something serious is happening, such as an infection, undiagnosed fracture, irritated nerve, or imminent risk of injury. When in doubt, always err on the side of caution and discuss with your OT supervisor.

2. D. The other answers all reflect inability to actively raise arm fully, which are indicators for self-ROM.

3. C. External rotation with the arm abducted is often a more challenging position to attain safely for clients with shoulder conditions. The OTA can first try an alternate position, (e.g., with shoulder adducted), to attempt gentle passive external rotation and determine if this will allow for safer, less painful gains in ROM. Review the general guidelines presented in the first answer regarding precautions/contraindications. When in doubt, err on the side of caution and collaborate with your OT supervisor. In instances such as a healing fracture, tendon or nerve repair, or other joint conditions, further communication with the referring physician may be warranted to determine client healing status and obtain guidance as to how aggressive therapy can be without risk of client injury.

4. C. A tear or hole in an exercise band may cause it to break when it is pulled taut, possibly harming the client. The frequency of exercises and number of repetitions must be individualized for each client (Performance Health, 2019a).

5. A. A shorter length will create more tension, thus needing more strength to pull band apart. Thera-Band resistance in order from weaker to stronger is yellow, red, green, blue, although additional colors (strengths) are available (Performance Health, 2019b).

6. C. A finger ladder is typically a narrow wood device attached to a wall. A client "walks" fingers up the ladder steps to increase shoulder ROM and strength. Codman's pendulum exercises are a specific kind of passive shoulder exercises in a dependent position. Constraint-induced movement therapy (CIMT) is not indicated for this client as it is a method used with neurological conditions (e.g., CVA). CIMT promotes active motion of affected limb through limiting movement of the non-affected limb. AROM on the table with a tabletop skateboard is in the gravity-minimized plane (needing only a muscle grade of poor) and would not really facilitate flexion of the shoulder. Functional activities should be incorporated and encouraged.

7.   A. Finger to palm translation means manipulating an object to move it from the fingers into the palm. Answers B, C, and D do not do that.

8.   A. Isotonic contractions include eccentric and concentric contractions, which are occurring in the wrist flexors and extensors.

9.   D. The biceps is actively shortening (as the elbow flexes) and lengthening (as the elbow extends) during the task.

10. D. Wrist extension during grasp and release is a typical mature pattern.

Worksheet 6-2: Open- and Closed-Kinetic-Chain Exercises

Closed-kinetic-chain exercises have a fixed end segment (such as in weight-bearing tasks), whereas open-kinetic-chain exercises have an end segment that is freely moveable (such as using dumbbells, exercise bands, reaching for objects, or holding items in space; Avers & Brown, 2019; Gillen, 2011; Rybski, 2019).

1.   O. Using exercise bands to improve shoulder strength
2.   O. Turning a heavy jump rope with another child holding the other end
3.   C. Weight bearing on forearm while writing with the contralateral hand
4.   C. Pushing a weighted toy shopping cart while walking around an obstacle course
5.   O. Putting cans in upper kitchen cabinets
6.   O. Using 1-lb weights to improve wrist strength
7.   O. Carrying a lunch tray in the cafeteria
8.   C. Sanding a wooden board using a sanding block
9.   C. Posing like a bear with hands and feet on floor
10. O. Using a reacher to remove clothes from dryer
11. C. Prone on elbows while watching a wind-up toy move
12. C. Rolling dough into piecrust shape using a rolling pin
13. O. Wringing out a washcloth
14. O. Hanging clothes in closet while standing
15. C. Pressing/flattening therapy putty with palm while standing at table
16. C. Using cookie cutters to cut shapes out of a 1/2-in. thick clay circle on the table
17. C. Performing push-ups against the wall while standing
18. O. Moving rings from one side of an exercise arc to the other side
19. C. Applying lotion to extremities
20. C. Arm push-ups while seated in preparation for transfers
21. O. Cone stacking to improve grip
22. O. Waving a ribbon wand to music
23. C. Scrubbing a floor using a hand-held brush
24. O. Painting on an easel while standing
25. C. Sliding board transfer

Worksheet 6-3: Methods and Tasks to Support Occupations

OTAs working in physical rehabilitation settings typically encounter clients who have impairment resulting from neurological conditions, such as CVA and traumatic brain injury. Traditional sensorimotor approaches to facilitate motor control have included Brunnstrom movement therapy, Rood, Proprioceptive Neuromuscular Facilitation (PNF) and Bobath/Neurodevelopmental Treatment (NDT; Schultz-Krohn & Mclaughlin-Gray, 2018). However, the evidence supports the use of newer approaches to motor learning, such as the task-oriented approach, which emphasizes functional interventions (Gillen, 2011, 2018; Phipps & Roberts, 2018). Additional methods, such as edema management or wound care, may be implemented as appropriate to address other factors and conditions.

It is important to incorporate the client's affected upper extremity into functional tasks so that it is not just a passive appendage. The OTA might use techniques for motor learning such as constraint-induced movement therapy, bilateral activities, mental imagery, and occupation-based activities that facilitate motor skills (Gillen, 2011, 2018; Phipps & Roberts, 2018). Practitioners should ensure any precautions/contraindications regarding the client's present situation are adhered to (such as fracture-healing status and post-operative protocols) and strive to use a function-based approach to promote awareness of the involved side, maintain mobility, and improve occupational performance (Gillen, 2011, 2018; Morawski et al., 2019; Phipps & Roberts, 2018).

1. A. Codman's pendulum exercises are a specific type of passive shoulder exercises as reflected in answer A. Realize that the instructions to an actual client would be more thorough than the minimal instructions presented in choice A. The surgeon will determine when the client can begin ROM of the distal extremity and progression to passive and active shoulder exercises according to healing status (Murphy & Lawson, 2018).

2. A. This scenario indicates that the client did not sustain any open wounds so external scarring should not be present.

3. C. Ischial tuberosity are the "sit bones" so a foam seat cushion will help to relieve pressure when seated in wheelchair.

4. D. The child's feet need to be supported for trunk stability. It is not productive for the child to write with the non-dominant hand. The affected hand should be positioned to stabilize the paper with forearm in pronation for weight bearing to help inhibit tone and provide postural stability (Schultz-Krohn & Mclaughlin-Gray, 2018).

5. B. The OTA should have the clinical skill to perform stump wrapping. The appropriate method is a figure-8 diagonal application (Fairchild et al., 2018).

6. C. Answer A promotes trunk extension and anterior weight shift, B promotes weight shifting to the side and trunk rotation, and D promotes hip flexion (Gillen, 2018).

7. A. To protect the client's hand, the OTA should ensure the hand is not completely flattened and the hand arches are maintained (Morawski, Padilla, & Jewell, 2019). A weak upper extremity may cause the elbow to buckle, which is unsafe. Gradual weight shifting/leaning toward the affected side will help to promote weight bearing through that affected extremity so that it can provide stability during functional tasks. Weight shift toward the unaffected side will help elongate muscles of the weak arm and trunk. A function-based approach should be used to incorporate the involved extremity in weight-bearing activities for daily occupations, such as stabilizing objects, wiping a table, using extremity as a postural support while dressing, and so forth (Gillen, 2011, 2018; Morawski et al., 2019; Phipps & Roberts, 2018).

8. D. The arm must move away from the body to have tension in the exercise band for external rotation. Standing with the right side closest to doorknob would not allow for tension in the band.

9. B. Although all the exercises indicated are suitable, it is best to not use exercise putty directly over clothing, as putty may stick to it and possibly ruin clothing.

10. B. Median nerve compression involved in carpal tunnel syndrome may affect strength of the intrinsic muscles in the thenar eminence which control thumb MP flexion, palmar abduction, and opposition, thus affecting tip pinch (American Academy of Orthopaedic Surgeons, 2020). Thumb adduction (used in lateral pinch) is ulnar nerve innervated, so that is not the best answer; although it is possible diminished thumb sensation could hinder lateral pinch. Hypothenar muscles on ulnar side of hand (opponens digiti minimi, flexor digit minimi, and abductor digiti minimi) and interossei are intrinsic muscles innervated by ulnar nerve and involve motions of the small finger and abduction/adduction of digits.

Worksheet 6-4: Physical Agent Modality Categories

Indicate the pertinent category for each of the following PAM listed by their properties (AOTA, 2018; Bracciano, 2017; Cameron, 2018).

Physical Agent Modality	Superficial Thermal Agent	Deep Thermal Agent	Electrotherapeutic Agent	Electromagnetic Devices	Mechanical Device
Fluidotherapy	*				
Transcutaneous electrical nerve stimulation (TENS)			*		
Iontophoresis			*		
Hot pack	*				
Ultrasound		*			
Whirlpool	*				
Vasopneumatic device					*
Cryotherapy	*				
Neuromuscular electrical stimulation (NMES)			*		
Functional electrical stimulation (FES)			*		
Continuous passive motion (CPM)					*
Paraffin	*				
High-voltage pulsed current (HVPC)			*		
Cold pack	*				
Hydrotherapy	*				
Chemical heat packs	*				
Biofeedback			*		
Short-wave diathermy				*	
Vapocoolant spray	*				
Low-level laser (light) therapy				*	
Lymphedema pump					*
Phonophoresis		*			
Microwaveable heat pack	*				
Contrast baths	*				
Controlled cold compression unit	*				

Worksheet 6-5: Selecting Physical Agent Modalities

Resources: Bellew et al., 2016; Bracciano, 2008, 2017; Cameron, 2018

1. H. Acute PIP hyperextension injury with pain and edema (*cold pack*)
2. I. Shoulder stiffness due to RA (*hot pack*)
3. L. Muscle reeducation to learn how to minimize involuntary upper trapezius muscle contraction (*biofeedback*)
4. D. Healed carpal tunnel release with stiffness, fair light touch sensation, intact protective sensation, and scar hypersensitivity (*Fluidotherapy*)

    The moving particles can be used to reduce hypersensitivity and the modality temperature can be lowered to avoid harm due to client's slightly decreased sensation.
5. J. Thumb CMC arthritis with pain and stiffness (*paraffin*)
6. E. Manage edema following soft tissue trauma (*vasopneumatic pump*)
7. A. Open wound requiring debridement (*whirlpool*)
8. F. Chronic biceps pain upon discharge from occupational therapy (*TENS*)
9. B. Conditions requiring mechanical PROM (*CPM*)
10. K. Lateral epicondylitis requiring topical medication delivery through the skin (*iontophoresis*)
11. G. CVA with hemiparesis and shoulder subluxation (*NMES*)
12. C. PIP joint contracture and scar adhesions following a healed laceration to volar index finger (*ultrasound*)

    Ultrasound can provide thermal and nonthermal effects to promote tissue changes and healing.
13. O. Used immediately following shoulder surgery to minimize post-operative pain and edema (*controlled cold compression unit*)
14. N. Client with complex regional pain syndrome needing home protocol to minimize hand stiffness, pain, and edema (*contrast baths*)
15. M. Client with fibromyalgia who may benefit from an aquatic exercise program to help relieve pain and stiffness (*hydrotherapy*)

Worksheet 6-6: Using Physical Agent Modalities Safely

Resources: Bellew et al., 2016; Bracciano, 2008, 2017; Cameron, 2018

1. C. Paraffin is contraindicated for areas containing open wounds, severe edema, or poor sensation. Superficial heat is used to help minimize joint stiffness and promote tendon gliding.
2. D. In this scenario, the hot pack is used on the client's shoulder so there is no need to remove jewelry from wrist and hand. An anti-static mat or plastic bag is not indicated for this modality.
3. C. The client is at risk for a burn, so the hot pack should be removed and client's skin checked before the OTA spends time looking for the OT. The hydrocollator temperature should be checked before a hot pack is placed on a client. The OTA might determine that extra towels are needed to minimize heat transfer from hot pack.
4. B. Due to how an extremity must be placed in the Fluidotherapy unit, this modality is not appropriate for shoulder or elbow use. Heat should not be applied to a rheumatic joint that is acutely inflamed.
5. D. Cryotherapy is use of a cold thermal agent which when applied, causes the client to experience a progression of effects in that area such as cold intensity, then burning sensation, aching, and eventually numbness (Cameron, 2018; Fruth & Michlovitz, 2016). Answer A indicates ice massage (i.e., cryotherapy probe or water frozen in paper cup) and not gel pack procedure. In preparation for cryotherapy, gel packs are placed in a freezer or chiller unit rather than a hydrocollator (which heats water for hot packs). A cover is used over the gel pack before placing it on the skin where it typically remains stationary for the allotted time. It is important to monitor

what the client is feeling from a gel or ice pack and understand the client is at risk for tissue damage if cold is administered for an extended time period or applied on areas with absent sensation (insensate).

6. B. Care should be taken to protect the client's neck from the hot pack possibly touching it. Clients should not lie directly on a hot pack as a burn could result from excessive pressure against the pack or the pack's gel or excess water oozing out of it onto the skin.

7. B. Clients should wash and dry hands before a paraffin treatment. A plastic bag is placed over the client's hand after the hand has been dipped in the paraffin. The client's affected hand should typically remain still during paraffin dips to avoid breaking the paraffin "glove," which would allow hot wax to seep underneath and possibly burn the skin. The client should avoid touching the bottom or sides of the unit as these areas could be especially hot, possibly causing a burn.

8. C. It is contraindicated to apply heat to a burn. There is probably no need to contact the client's physician for simple sunburn unless the client is exhibiting other adverse effects such as dehydration, sunstroke, infection, skin rash, or hives. The client should be able to work on other aspects of the intervention plan, such as functional activities.

9. D. Application of superficial heat modalities or ultrasound is contraindicated over areas with tumors and malignancy. Phonophoresis involves use of an ultrasound device with a topical agent.

10. A. Cold is beneficial to help reduce acute inflammation and spasticity but is contraindicated for clients with cold intolerance and poor circulation (Cameron, 2018). Heat modalities, rather than cold, are typically used when soft tissue extensibility is desired. In this scenario, the carpal tunnel release should be well healed at this time and there is no indication of resulting sensory deficits in this scenario.

Worksheet 6-7: Physical Agent Modality Basics

Resources: Bellew et al., 2016; Bracciano, 2008, 2017; Cameron, 2018

1. A. The use of PAMs alone is not considered occupational therapy (AOTA, 2018).

2. C.

3. C.

4. D.

5. A. Ultrasound and TENS are not superficial thermal agents, so the OTA cannot legally administer them in that specific state.

6. A. Fluidotherapy can be used for both desensitization and AROM and the unit temperature can be lowered to minimize heating effect as necessary (Rennie & Michlovitz, 2016).

7. D. Service competency for a modality is needed for an OT to include it in an intervention plan and properly supervise an OTA administering it to ensure safe and effective use (AOTA, 2015, 2018). If the client needs a modality that the OT is not competent to supervise, the client should be referred to another practitioner. (PRN stands for "as needed.")

8. D. The OTA should only implement the modalities delineated in the OT's intervention plan. However, the OTA may document what the client said and speak to the OT to determine if the intervention plan should be modified to include paraffin.

9. B. Superficial heat is often used in therapy to decrease pain, relax muscles, and improve tissue extensibility in preparation for therapeutic exercises/tasks to support occupations. Cold can be used following exercises/activities to help prevent further pain, inflammation, or flare up of the condition. Normally it is not indicated to implement both hot packs and paraffin to the same area during a single session.

10. C. The used wax removed from the client's hand should always be discarded to help keep the paraffin unit clean. Paraffin hardens completely so it will not be useful for exercises at home.

Worksheet 6-8: Deep Thermal and Electrical Modalities

Resources: Bellew et al., 2016; Bracciano, 2008, 2017; Cameron, 2018

1. T. An ultrasound frequency of 1 MHz penetrates more deeply than a 3 MHz frequency.
   (Cameron, 2018; Lake, 2016).

2. T. Ultrasound coupling media can include gel pads, water immersion, and viscous aqueous gel.
   (Lake, 2016).

3. F. An ultrasound duty cycle of 20% is suitable when a thermal effect is desired.
   This duty cycle produces a mechanical, nonthermal effect (Cameron, 2018; Lake, 2016).

4. T. The anatomical area receiving the ultrasound treatment should be no larger than four times the size of the effective radiating area (ERA).
   (Lake, 2016).

5. F. Contraindications for ultrasound include joint replacement with cement or plastic components in the affected area, pacemaker, and chronic tendinitis.
   Although presence of a pacemaker or joint replacement with plastic or cement components (in the treatment area) are contraindications for ultrasound, a condition of chronic tendinitis could be appropriate for ultrasound use (Cameron, 2018).

6. T. When documenting ultrasound intensity, the unit of measurement is W/cm^2.

7. F. Continuous ultrasound refers to continually moving the sound head during the treatment.
   Continuous ultrasound refers to a duty cycle of 100%.

8. T. Three types of waveforms used in electrotherapy include pulsed current, direct current, and alternating current.
   (Bellew, 2016b; Cameron et al., 2018b).

9. T. A monophasic pulsed current only flows in one direction for each pulse and pauses in-between pulses.
   (Bellew, 2016b; Cameron et al., 2018b).

10. T. A drug commonly delivered transdermally with iontophoresis is dexamethasone.
    (Bellew, 2016a).

11. T. Possible risks from electrotherapy include burns from electric currents and redness or skin irritation due to electrode adhesive or gel.
    (Bellew, 2016a).

12. F. TENS with a short duration and pulse rate of 100 pps is considered low-rate or non-conventional TENS.
    This is considered high-rate or conventional TENS (Cameron et al., 2018a).

13. F. High-rate TENS elicits sensory effect and muscle contraction and, therefore, should not be used with acute conditions.
    High-rate or conventional TENS is sensory-level electrical stimulation which does not produce muscle contraction and, therefore, can be appropriate for acute conditions (Cameron et al., 2018a).

14. T. For chronic, stable conditions needing a longer duration of TENS to help manage pain, it is suitable to set pulse rate at less than 10 pps.
    These parameters reflect low-rate TENS that produces muscle contraction (Cameron et al., 2018a).

15. F. NMES uses electrical currents to produce contractions in muscles that are denervated.
    NMES produces contractions in innervated muscles (Bellew, 2016a; Cameron et al., 2018b).

16. F. When implementing NMES, an electrode is placed at the muscle's motor point which is typically at the musculotendinous junction.

    A muscle's motor point is typically located at the muscle belly (Bellew, 2016a; Cameron et al., 2018a).

17. F. In regard to NMES, on:off time refers to the timed intervals in-between therapy appointments.

    On:off time refers to the amount of time set for the muscles to contract and relax for each cycle (Cameron et al., 2018a).

18. T. Indications for NMES can include conditions such as weak upper/lower extremity muscles, dysphagia, spasticity, and urinary incontinence.

    (Johnston, 2016).

19. F. Clients that are debilitated, such as those with a cardiac pacemaker or implanted defibrillator, can benefit from NMES to help increase muscle strength and endurance.

    Cardiac conditions such as a pacemaker or implanted defibrillator are contraindications for NMES (Cameron et al., 2018b).

20. T. When using NMES, ramp up/ramp down time refers to the amount of time that the force is gradually increased and decreased when producing and then relaxing the contraction.

    (Cameron et al., 2018a).

Worksheet 6-9: Orthotic Interventions

Resources: Coppard & Lohman, 2015; Lashgari et al., 2018; West-Frasier & Vennix, 2015

1. K. Carpal tunnel syndrome (*volar wrist immobilization orthosis*)
2. M. Boutonniere deformity ring finger (*PIP extension orthosis*)
3. R. Upper extremity amputation (*body-powered prosthesis*)
4. P. Small finger metacarpal fracture (*ulnar gutter orthosis*)
5. N. Dupuytren's release (*forearm-based dorsal extension orthosis*)
6. T. C6-C7 spinal cord injury (*tenodesis orthosis*)
7. F. Flexor tendon repair of digits (*dorsal blocking orthosis*)
8. C. Brachial plexus injury (*airplane splint [shoulder abduction orthosis]*)
9. H. Swan neck deformity (*figure-8 finger orthosis [PIP hyperextension block orthosis]*)
10. O. Mallet finger (*DIP joint extension orthosis*)
11. B. Low level ulnar nerve injury (*MP extension blocking orthosis*)
12. A. Burns to hand/wrist (*resting hand orthosis*)
13. S. Extrinsic extensor tightness of digits (*composite flexion orthosis*)
14. G. de Quervain's tenosynovitis (*forearm-based thumb immobilization orthosis [long opponens orthosis, radial gutter orthosis]*)
15. L. Elbow flexion contracture (*anterior elbow orthosis*)
16. J. MP joints requiring realignment secondary to RA (*ulnar deviation orthosis*)
17. D. Flexed digits of a client with end-stage dementia and skin breakdown in hand (*palm protector, can also use a soft hand cone*)
18. E. Low level median nerve injury (*short opponens orthosis*)
19. Q. Lateral epicondylitis (*counterforce brace [tennis elbow strap]*)
20. I. Radial nerve palsy (*dynamic MP extension orthosis*)

Worksheet 6-10: Using Orthotic Devices

Resources: Coppard & Lohman, 2015; Lashgari et al., 2018; West-Frasier & Vennix, 2015

1. C. A volar wrist extension orthosis begins proximal to the MPs and continues two-thirds the length of the forearm. A potential pressure area is the ulnar styloid.

2. C. The OTA should not discontinue the orthosis without physician approval and the OT's collaboration, particularly for an unhealed fracture.

3. B. While a pattern may be placed in the client's chart for future reference, it is not necessary to do so. As patterns are usually traced onto the thermoplastic material, that will not avoid marks. Making a pattern does help prevent costly mistakes by not using a trial and error approach. However, the primary purpose of a pattern is to help ensure proper orthosis size and fit, determine best design, and fabricate the orthosis more efficiently.

4. D. Never place thermoplastic material directly from the heating source onto the client, as the high heat could cause a skin burn. Cooling times vary by type and thickness of thermoplastic material and it is not sanitary to blow on it. The pattern should be traced onto the thermoplastic before the material is heated. Hook and loop fasteners are added after the thermoplastic material is molded and fitted.

5. A. The orthotic device should position the thumb in a functional position.

6. A. A mallet finger orthosis typically only immobilizes the DIP joint.

7. A. The orthosis should generally be two-thirds the length of the forearm.

8. D. Looping the strap through a D-ring and creating more hook and loop fastener contact will increase stability. However, it is essential to ensure that this new strap configuration does not cause any harmful pressure on the client's wrist or cut off circulation. This strap option should be considered before fabricating a completely new orthosis or remolding the orthosis into a sub-optimal flexed position. While answer C would work, it is only a temporary solution and not the best option.

9. A. Dynamic orthoses require outriggers carefully placed to allow a proper angle of pull (normally 90 degrees), to avoid traction or compression of a joint.

10. C. The OTA should be able to easily modify the orthosis with a heat gun (to smooth the rough edge) so the orthosis is better tolerated by the child. The OTA's observation of redness indicates the child is not simply making up an excuse. Education should be provided to the parent and child regarding precautions and monitoring of skin integrity. A follow-up orthotic check should be scheduled and the OT also notified.

Worksheet 6-11: Client Education

Resources: Coppard & Lohman, 2015; Lashgari et al., 2018; West-Frasier & Vennix, 2015

1. Purpose of orthosis
2. Wearing schedule
3. How to don and doff orthotic device
4. Home exercise program to prevent stiffness of immobilized joints
5. Care and cleaning of orthotic device
6. Skin integrity (e.g., keeping skin dry, check for pressure areas)
7. Possible problems that may arise (e.g., pressure areas, pain, edema)
8. Orthosis protection (e.g., keep orthosis away from heat sources, do not leave in car on hot day)
9. Contact information if problems should arise
10. Follow-up appointment (bring orthosis)

Steps must be taken to ensure that the client is not at risk for skin break down or injury because the orthosis is ill-fitting. Consider the following options (Morreale & Amini, 2016):

- Contact the supervising OT to notify of the situation and discuss an action plan.
- Phone the client and explain that you heard from the physician. Ask the client for more details about concerns.
- Suggest that the client come back to the OT department today to have the orthosis assessed and adjusted. Plan to stay at the office until the client can return.
- If the client is unable to return today, you might ask if placing a soft material such as cotton, gauze, or a band-aid under the problem area will resolve the problem. Because the orthosis is not being used for a condition that would greatly create risk without the device (such as recent surgery for a flexor tendon repair), you might tell the client to discontinue wearing the orthosis until her next appointment.
- Schedule the client for a visit as soon as possible.

Adapted from Morreale, M. J., & Amini, D. (2016). *The occupational therapist's workbook for ensuring clinical competence.* SLACK Incorporated.

Worksheet 6-12: Wound Care Basics

1. B. (Fairchild et al., 2018).
2. A *A skin graft is an example of second-intention healing* (Fairchild et al., 2018).
3. A. (Fairchild et al., 2018).
4. D. *To promote wound healing, debridement removes unhealthy/necrotic tissue (eschar) to expose healthy tissue.* (Fairchild et al., 2018).
5. D. *The other choices represent more advanced stages of a pressure injury.* (Fairchild et al., 2018)
6. A. *Although an unstageable pressure injury does not have a specific depth limitation, it involves full-thickness loss of skin/tissue and eschar/slough at the base which limits depth assessment* (Fairchild et al., 2018).
7. C. *The fourth sign is edema.* (Fairchild et al., 2018)
8. A. *The client could benefit from pressure reduction for heels using a cushioned covering such as soft double socks or commercial heel protectors* (Fairchild et al., 2018). *Ensure the foot coverings are not too tight. Moisture barrier ointments/creams are used to protect skin from excessive moisture such as from incontinence or sweating.*
9. A. *In this case, the OTA should continue to attempt the delegated task. A small amount of sterile saline poured over the area is a common remedy that can help loosen the exudate so the bandage can more easily be removed. Pulling on the bandage could reopen the wound which is not desirable.* (Fairchild et al., 2018; Walsh & Chee, 2018).
10. B. *Answers C and D indicate an increase/worsening of wound size. Wounds are classified as red (healing granulation tissue), yellow (has exudate such as pus), or black (necrotic tissue)* (Fairchild et al., 2018; Von der Heyde & Evans, 2011; Walsh & Chee, 2018).

Worksheet 6-13: Upper Extremity Safety

While proper body alignment is essential, it is also important to incorporate the client's involved upper extremity into functional tasks as much as possible so that it is not just a passive appendage. For clients with hemiparesis, the OTA might use various techniques such as weight bearing, guiding, bilateral activities, constraint-induced movement therapy, task-oriented reaching, and so forth, incorporated into occupations to facilitate functional motor skills at appropriate stages of recovery (Gillen, 2011, 2018; Phipps & Roberts, 2018). The inclusion of the client's affected extremity in everyday tasks helps to promote awareness of that side, maintain mobility, and improve its function (Gillen, 2011, 2018; Morawski et al., 2019; Phipps & Roberts, 2018). The existing evidence and the pros and cons of possible intervention options for each client must be considered carefully in determining which method (or combination of methods) is more appropriate, safe, and effective to use.

Possible Intervention Options	Pros	Cons
1. Support LUE on a lap tray	Safer position for LUE than dangling Decreased potential for injury LUE in visual field May improve trunk upright posture	May be considered a restraint Arm may slide off lap tray Potential for skin breakdown Passive position
2. Support LUE on an arm trough/side arm support	Safer position for LUE than dangling Decreased potential for injury LUE may be in visual field May improve trunk upright posture	Upper limb may slide off the arm trough/support May not be a naturally comfortable position for client's upper extremity Potential for skin breakdown Passive position
3. Educate client on proper position of LUE and risk of injury. Provide verbal and written reminders. Encourage client to self-correct arm position with unaffected hand.	Increases client awareness of problem and self-correction of problem	Unilateral neglect or cognitive deficits may interfere with carryover. Client may not be able to reach and position extremity with unaffected hand
4. Provide sling for LUE	Keeps arm from getting caught in wheel	Places arm in a nonfunctional, passive position May lead to contracture for shoulder adduction and internal rotation Arm may slide out of sling May cause pressure around neck Impedes emerging voluntary motion
5. Have client look in mirror and determine what is problematic with her wheelchair posture	Increases client awareness of problem and self-correction of problem	Unilateral neglect or cognitive deficits may interfere with carryover
6. Use bilateral techniques and active involvement of involved arm to incorporate the extremity in functional task performance	Increases client awareness of extremity Promotes functional movement patterns and motor learning for occupations Assists in joint mobility Helps prevent disuse	Client may overstretch joints or may drop the arm and cause injury if too aggressive, inattentive, or not careful Unilateral neglect or cognitive deficits may interfere with carryover

References

Accreditation Council for Occupational Therapy Education. (2018). 2018 Accreditation Council for Occupational Therapy Education (ACOTE) standards and interpretive guide (effective July 31, 2020). *American Journal of Occupational Therapy, 72*(Suppl. 2), 7212410005. https://doi.org/10.5014/ajot.2018.72S217

American Academy of Orthopaedic Surgeons. (2020). *Carpal tunnel syndrome.* https://orthoinfo.aaos.org/en/diseases--conditions/carpal-tunnel-syndrome/

American Occupational Therapy Association. (2015). Standards of practice for occupational therapy. *American Journal of Occupational Therapy, 69*(Suppl. 3), 6913410057. http://dx.doi.org/10.5014/ajot.2015.696S06

American Occupational Therapy Association. (2018). Physical agent and mechanical modalities. *American Journal of Occupational Therapy, 72*(Suppl. 2), 7212410055. https://. doi.org/ 10.5014/ajot.2018.72S220

American Occupational Therapy Association. (2020). Occupational therapy practice framework: Domain and process (4th ed.). *American Journal of Occupational Therapy, 74*(Suppl. 2), 7412410010. https://doi.org/10.5014/ajot.2020.74S2001

Avers, D., & Brown, M. (2019). *Daniels and Worthingham's muscle testing: Techniques of manual examination and performance testing* (10th ed.). Elsevier Incorporated.

Bellew, J. W. (2016a). Clinical electrical stimulation: Application and techniques. In J. W. Bellew, S. L. Michlovitz, & T. P. Nolan (Eds.), *Michlovitz's modalities for therapeutic intervention* (6th ed., pp. 287-327). F. A. Davis Company.

Bellew, J. W. (2016b). Foundations of clinical electrotherapy. In J. W. Bellew, S. L. Michlovitz, & T. P. Nolan (Eds.), *Michlovitz's modalities for therapeutic intervention* (6th ed., pp. 253-285). F. A. Davis Company.

Bellew, J. W., Michlovitz, S. L., & Nolan, T. P. (2016). *Michlovitz's modalities for therapeutic intervention* (6th ed.). F. A. Davis Company.

Bracciano, A. G. (2008). *Physical agent modalities: Theory and application for the occupational therapist* (2nd ed.). SLACK Incorporated.

Bracciano, A. G. (2017). Physical agent modalities. In K. Jacobs & N. MacRae (Eds.), *Occupational therapy essentials for clinical competence.* (3rd ed., pp. 501-519). SLACK Incorporated.

Cameron, M. H. (2018). *Physical agents in rehabilitation: An evidence-based approach to practice.* (5th ed.). Elsevier Incorporated.

Cameron, M. H., Shapiro, S., & Ocelnik, M. (2018a). Electrical currents for pain control. In M. H. Cameron (Ed.), *Physical agents in rehabilitation: An evidence-based approach to practice.* (5th ed., pp. 258-270). Elsevier Incorporated.

Cameron, M.H., Shapiro, S., & Ocelnik, M. (2018b). Introduction to electrotherapy. In M. H. Cameron (Ed.), *Physical agents in rehabilitation: An evidence-based approach to practice.* (5th ed., pp. 219-237). Elsevier Incorporated.

Coppard, B. M., & Lohman, H. (2015). *Introduction to orthotics: A clinical-reasoning & problem-solving approach* (4th ed.). Elsevier Incorporated.

Fairchild, S. L., O'Shea, R. K., & Washington, R. D. (2018). *Pierson and Fairchild's principles & techniques of patient care* (6th ed.). Elsevier Incorporated.

Fruth, S. J., & Michlovitz, S. L. (2016). Cold therapy modalities. In J. W. Bellew, S. L. Michlovitz, & T. P. Nolan (Eds.), *Michlovitz's modalities for therapeutic intervention* (6th ed., pp. 21-60). F. A. Davis Company.

Gillen, G. (2011). *Stroke rehabilitation: A function-based approach* (3rd ed.). Elsevier Mosby.

Gillen, G. (2018). Cerebrovascular accident (stroke). In H. M. Pendleton & W. Schultz-Krohn (Eds.), *Pedretti's occupational therapy practice skills for physical dysfunction* (8th ed., pp. 809-840). Elsevier Incorporated.

Johnston, T. E. (2016). NMES and FES in patients with neurological diagnoses. In J. W. Bellew, S. L. Michlovitz, & T. P. Nolan (Eds.), *Michlovitz's modalities for therapeutic intervention* (6th ed., pp. 399-433). F. A. Davis Company.

Lake, D. (2016). Therapeutic ultrasound. In J. W. Bellew, S. L. Michlovitz, & T. P. Nolan (Eds.), *Michlovitz's modalities for therapeutic intervention* (6th ed., pp. 89-134). F. A. Davis Company.

Lashgari, D., Atkins, M., & Baumgarten, J. (2018). Orthotics. In H. M. Pendleton & W. Schultz-Krohn (Eds.), *Pedretti's occupational therapy practice skills for physical dysfunction* (8th ed., pp. 728-765). Elsevier Incorporated.

Morawski, D. L., Padilla, R., & Jewell, V. (2019). Working with elders who have had cerebrovascular accidents. In H. L. Lohman, S. Byers-Connon, & R. L. Padilla (Eds.), *Occupational therapy with elders: Strategies for the COTA* (4th ed., pp. 268-281). Elsevier Incorporated.

Morreale, M. J., & Amini, D. (2016). *The Occupational therapist's workbook for ensuring clinical competence.* SLACK Incorporated.

Murphy, L. F. & Lawson, S. (2018). Orthopedic conditions: Hip fractures and hip, knee, and shoulder replacements. In H. M. Pendleton & W. Schultz-Krohn (Eds.), *Pedretti's occupational therapy practice skills for physical dysfunction* (8th ed., pp. 1004-1029). Elsevier Incorporated.

Performance Health. (2019a). *Theraband care and safety.* Retrieved June 22, 2021, from https://www.theraband.com/care-and-safety

Performance Health. (2019b). *Theraband products color progression.* Retrieved June 22, 2021, https://www.theraband.com/products/rehab-therapy/resistance-bands-tubes/theraband-professional-latex-resistance-bands-6-yard-roll.html

Phipps, S., & Roberts, P. (2018). Motor learning. In H. M. Pendleton & W. Schultz-Krohn (Eds.), *Pedretti's occupational therapy practice skills for physical dysfunction* (8th ed., pp. 798-808). Elsevier Incorporated.

Rennie, S., & Michlovitz, S. L. (2016). Therapeutic heat. In J. W. Bellew, S. L. Michlovitz, & T. P. Nolan (Eds.), *Michlovitz's modalities for therapeutic intervention* (6th ed., pp. 61-88). F. A. Davis Company.

Rybski, M. F. (2019). *Kinesiology for occupational therapy* (3rd ed.). SLACK Incorporated.

Schultz-Krohn, W., & Mclaughlin-Gray, J. (2018). Traditional sensorimotor approaches to intervention. In H. M. Pendleton & W. Schultz-Krohn (Eds.), *Pedretti's occupational therapy practice skills for physical dysfunction* (8th ed., pp. 766-797). Elsevier Incorporated.

Walsh, J. M., & Chee, N. (2018) Hand and upper extremity injuries. In H. M. Pendleton & W. Schultz-Krohn (Eds.), *Pedretti's occupational therapy practice skills for physical dysfunction* (8th ed., pp. 972-1003). Elsevier Incorporated.

West-Frasier, J. M., & Vennix, C. L. (2015). Basic splinting. In K. Sladyk & S. E. Ryan (Eds.), *Ryan's occupational therapy assistant: Principles, practice issues, and techniques* (5th ed., pp. 484-495). SLACK Incorporated.

Von der Heyde, R. I., & Evans, R. B. (2011). Wound classification and management. In T. M. Skirven, A.L. Osterman, J. M. Fedorczyk, & P. C. Amadio (Eds.), *Rehabilitation of the hand and upper extremity* (6th ed., pp. 219-232). Elsevier/Mosby.

CHAPTER 7

Assessing and Documenting Client Function

Occupational therapy practitioners use professional reasoning in determining a client's level of function through various means, such as skilled observation, formal and informal assessments, and interviews with client or family/significant others. The occupational therapist (OT) is responsible for directing and documenting the initial evaluation and establishing the occupational therapy intervention plan (American Occupational Therapy Association [AOTA], 2015, 2020). An occupational therapy assistant (OTA) collaborates with the OT to perform select, delegated tasks to help assess and document client function and implement skilled interventions—all in accordance with regulatory guidelines and payer requirements (AOTA, 2015, 2020). Pertinent underlying client factors and performance skills are assessed by occupational therapy practitioners to determine which of these hinder or support an individual client's occupational performance (AOTA, 2020). During an intervention session, occupational therapy practitioners use their professional reasoning skills to assess safety and ascertain changes in the client's situation, areas of progress, and specific factors impeding progress. This chapter provides worksheets and learning activities to help you determine and document levels of function accurately and implement various kinds of assessments correctly. Answers to worksheet exercises are provided at the end of the chapter.

Contents

Morreale, M. J. Developing Clinical Competence:
A Workbook for the OTA, Second Edition (pp. 293-327).
© 2022 SLACK Incorporated.

Worksheet 7-1

Determining Assist Levels

Indicate the specific type of cues or level of assistance (e.g., contact guard, moderate, maximum) you would document for each of the following client scenarios.

1. The client donned socks by herself using a sock aid.

2. After assessing the resident's transfer skills, the OTA determined the resident needs someone next to her for safety in case the resident forgets to lock the wheelchair brakes or moves too quickly.

3. At lunchtime, the client needed three reminders to look to the left in order to find all the food on the plate.

4. The client required a mechanical lift to transfer from bed to wheelchair.

5. The resident needed both the OTA and physical therapist assistant to help him transfer from the wheelchair to the mat, but he was able to bear some weight on his weak leg.

6. During a toothbrushing task, the client could not put the paste on the brush, manipulate or hold the brush; but she did open her mouth, rinse, and spit on command.

7. The OTA noted that after the containers are opened and food is cut, the resident can feed herself.

8. The student zippered her jacket by herself, and the OTA told her she did a good job.

Worksheet 7-1 (continued)

Determining Assist Levels

9. The OTA put the crayon in the child's weak hand, helped him hold it, and guided the child's arm so the child could draw a circle.

10. The OTA let the client know that the lunch tray was in her room, so the client returned to her room and fed herself.

11. When donning his shirt, the client needed a little help to bring the shirt around his back and line up the first button.

12. During craft group, because sharp objects were present, the OTA sat next to the client who is suicidal.

13. During recess, the OTA looked out the window periodically to monitor and help ensure the child was playing cooperatively with the other children on the playground.

14. While the client was cooking at the stove, the OTA put an arm lightly around the client's back in case the client became unsteady.

15. The client who has end-stage renal disease (ESRD) unloaded the dishwasher, but needed several rest breaks in order to complete the task.

16. The client with left neglect could read the newspaper article only after the OTA put a red line at the left margin.

Worksheet 7-1 (continued)

Determining Assist Levels

17. During mealtime, the OTA had to touch the client's arm a few times to prompt the client to bring food to mouth.

18. The child needed help for about half of the shoe-tying task.

19. The client would only remember to take her medicine when her cell phone timer buzzed.

20. The student demonstrated ability to use her power wheelchair well, so the OTA put a smiley face sticker on the wheelchair.

Morreale, M. J. (2022). *Developing clinical competence: A workbook for the OTA* (2nd ed.). SLACK Incorporated.

Worksheet 7-2

Assessing Feeding

Chen, a 75-year-old male from China, sustained a myocardial infarction 4 days ago while on vacation visiting his adult children in New York. He remains hospitalized since that time. Yesterday the physician ordered occupational therapy and the OT evaluated Chen. The intervention plan includes goals for increasing Chen's activity tolerance for feeding and grooming while seated in a chair. Today the OTA is working with Chen at breakfast and observes that Chen does not make eye contact, is not picking up the utensils, and is shaking his head "no." What do you think might be a reason for Chen's behavior and refusal to eat? List at least 10 possibilities.

Examples: *Chen could be showing signs of depression following his recent heart attack.*
Chen may not feel hungry at this time or might have just eaten something else.

1.

2.

3.

4.

5.

6.

7.

8.

9.

10.

Morreale, M. J. (2022). Developing clinical competence: A workbook for the OTA (2nd ed.). SLACK Incorporated.

Learning Activity 7-1: Client Interview

Occupational therapy practitioners gather important information by interviewing clients and family/significant others. The focus of an interview and specific questions asked will vary depending on the client's diagnosis and circumstances, the type of practice area, specific services provided, and priorities for care. In addition to carefully considering the client's responses, occupational therapy practitioners employ skilled observations to assess the client's mood, demeanor, social interaction skills, cognitive abilities, motor skills, and so forth, using professional reasoning. For example, is the client able to maintain attention for the duration of the interview? Does the client make sustained eye contact? Can the client maintain an upright, symmetrical sitting posture? Are tremors or spasticity exhibited? Does the client demonstrate difficulty recalling or understanding information?

To practice your interview skills, use the form in Figures 7-1A and 7-1B to interview a family member, classmate, or friend. While this form may help to determine a client's social history, develop an occupational profile, or screen for problem areas, it may need to be adapted for different populations or situations. Additionally, this form does not include all of a client's demographic data or insurance information that might be present on a "real" form. Be sure to explain the purpose of the interview and let the person you are interviewing know they can choose not to answer any of the questions. It is also important to keep the information confidential, so do not use the person's real name or date of birth on the form. Of course, for an actual client, identifying information would always be included and the occupational therapy practitioner would use therapeutic communication techniques to probe further if the client was not forthcoming or particular concerns were noted. Review Chapter 1 for tips regarding active listening and asking open versus closed questions.

Following the interview, elicit feedback about your performance from the person you interviewed. For example, did you speak too quickly or use too much technical jargon? Did you ask questions clearly, confidently, and concisely? Did the interview "flow"? Did the person interviewed feel that you appeared interested in their responses? Did you spend too much time looking at the form and writing rather than focusing directly on that person? Reflect on any difficulties you may have encountered during this experience. Determine what you might have done better or how you could have worded your questions differently. It is also useful to practice interviewing people from different age groups (e.g., a pre-teen and an older adult) to compare and contrast your interview experiences, such as amount of time needed, style of questioning, demeanor of the individuals being interviewed, their life views, and types of responses.

Feedback elicited:

Difficulties encountered:

Changes needed:

Client Interview Form

Client name: _____   Date: _____
Date of birth:_____   Age: _____
Gender: _____

Diagnosis/health concerns: _____
_____

Marital status: ☐ Married   ☐ Widowed   ☐ Divorced   ☐ Single   ☐ Domestic partnership
    ☐ Other_____

Emergency contact: _____
Contact phone number: _____
Relationship to client:_____

Personal Factors/Cultural Considerations: _____

Communication: ☐ Intact   ☐ Impaired   ☐ Hard of hearing   ☐ Hearing aid   ☐ Aphasia
    ☐ Other_____

*Level of Education Completed:*_____
Special training/skills:_____
Desired skills or education: _____

Work: Type of occupation _____
    ☐ Presently working   ☐ Works full-time   ☐ Works part-time   ☐ Works from home
    ☐ Works occasionally   ☐ Retired   ☐ Never worked   ☐ Volunteers _____
What does client like/dislike about present work?_____

Living Situation:
    ☐ Owns home   ☐ Condo/co-op   ☐ Apartment   ☐ Relative's home   ☐ Assisted living facility
    ☐ Institution   ☐ Rents a room   ☐ Other _____
Children: ☐ Yes   ☐ No _____
Lives with others: ☐ Yes   ☐ No _____
Stairs/architectural barriers:_____
Pets: ☐ Yes   ☐ No _____

Emergency Preparedness:
    ☐ Smoke alarm   ☐ CO_2 detector   ☐ Flashlight/batteries   ☐ Fire extinguisher
    ☐ Personal emergency response system/panic button   ☐ Portable/cell phone   ☐ Bottled water
    ☐ Nonperishable food and manual can opener

Pertinent Environmental Factors: _____

ADLs/IADLs:
Daily living skills that client needs help with:_____
_____
Dietary considerations: _____

Figure 7-1A. Client interview form (page 1).

Client Interview Form (continued)

Functional Mobility: Assistance needed ☐ Yes   ☐ No
   ☐ No devices used   ☐ Cane   ☐ Quad cane   ☐ Walker   ☐ Rollator   ☐ Crutches
   ☐ Manual wheelchair   ☐ Power wheelchair   ☐ Power mobility scooter   ☐ Other _____

Community Mobility: Transportation adequate for needs: ☐ Yes   ☐ No
   ☐ Drives own car   ☐ Relative drives   ☐ Friend drives   ☐ Walks   ☐ Uses a taxi   ☐ Bus   ☐ Train
   ☐ County/town transit for elderly/disabled   ☐ Uses a ride sharing service

Rest and Sleep:
Reported stress level (0 to 10 scale): _____
Hours of sleep per night?_____   Takes naps?_____
Sleep interrupted by: ☐ Pain   ☐ Bathroom needs   ☐ Caregiver responsibilities   ☐ Anxiety   ☐ Noise
   ☐ Other_____

Play/Leisure:
List three favorite activities and frequency:
1. _____
2. _____
3. _____
Hobbies/special interests or talents:_____
Hours per day watching television:_____
Does client read: ☐ Books   ☐ Newspapers   ☐ Magazines
Amount and type of daily/weekly exercise: _____

Habits Impacting Health:
Tobacco use: _____   Alcohol use: _____
Other: _____

Computer Skills:
   ☐ Excellent   ☐ Good   ☐ Fair   ☐ Poor   ☐ Do not use
Hours per day using computer: ☐ Work_____   ☐ Leisure _____
Computer or leisure skills desired: _____

Social Participation:
Clubs, groups, religious organizations: _____
_____
Easily engages in activities: ☐ Yes   ☐ No
Satisfied with amount of friends: ☐ Yes   ☐ No
Prefers: ☐ Individual activities   ☐ Group activities   ☐ Activities at home   ☐ Activities in community
Barriers to leisure or social participation: _____

Personal Goal: _____
_____
_____

OTA/OT signature: _____

Figure 7-1B. Client interview form (page 2).

Learning Activity 7-2: Administering a Standardized Test

Imagine you are completing your Level II fieldwork and are expected to administer a specific standardized test to meet objectives for fieldwork. You have not learned about this assessment in school and have not yet seen it used in fieldwork. You would like to implement the standardized test properly so that you will receive a passing grade for fieldwork. Consider how you might approach this dilemma.

For this exercise, choose a standardized assessment with which you are not familiar. You might ask one of your academic instructors or your fieldwork educator for access to a standardized test (that is appropriate for an OTA to administer in collaboration with the OT), such as one that assesses particular development in children, visual-motor skills, or coordination. Complete the following questions regarding the assessment you selected:

Name of assessment:

1. What steps can you take to become more knowledgeable about this test?
   a.

   b.

   c.

   d.

   e.

2. What kinds of information does this test provide?
   a.

   b.

   c.

   d.

   e.

3. List three possible conditions this test might be used for:
   a.

   b.

   c.

4. Indicate the age range appropriate for use with this test:

5. Is this test valid and reliable?　　　☐ Yes　　　☐ No

6. Indicate the type of setting where this test may be administered (e.g., quiet room with privacy, rehab gym, playground, classroom):

7. Indicate the general format for the assessment (i.e., interview, gross or fine-motor activities, activities of daily living, visual, constructional, written responses):

8. How much time is needed to administer this test?

9. What is the format for providing instructions to the client?

☐ Written instructions   ☐ Word-for-word verbal instructions   ☐ Paraphrase verbal instructions   ☐ Other

10. Indicate all the equipment or supplies you will need to gather in order to administer this test (i.e., table, paper, pencil, timer, blocks, leather lacing project, occlusion board):

11. What possible factors may interfere with test administration?

12. Find three evidence-based articles that support or discourage the use of this assessment and cite them below:
    a.

    b.

    c.

13. Indicate how the results of this assessment may relate to a client's occupational performance:

14. List several alternate assessments to the one you chose that measure similar client factors, performance skills, or occupations.

Worksheet 7-3

Assessing Client Factors

1. The OT asked an OTA to use a visual analog scale with a specific client. This type of scale is used to measure which of the following?
   A. Weight
   B. Oxygen level
   C. Visual acuity
   D. Pain

2. The handle of a hydraulic hand dynamometer (e.g., Lafayette or Jamar) can be adjusted to how many different grip positions?
   A. 3
   B. 4
   C. 5
   D. 6

3. When using a hydraulic hand dynamometer (e.g., Lafayette or Jamar) the OTA should place the client's upper extremity in which of the following positions?
   A. 90 degrees shoulder flexion, adduction, 90 degrees elbow flexion, forearm in neutral position
   B. 0 degrees shoulder flexion, adduction, 90 degrees elbow flexion, forearm in neutral position
   C. 90 degrees shoulder flexion, adduction, 90 degrees elbow flexion, supination
   D. 0 degrees shoulder flexion, 90 degrees abduction, 90 degrees elbow extension, forearm in neutral position

4. When using a manual sphygmomanometer with a client, an OTA notices it is not inflating at all when the device is initially squeezed. Which of the following actions should the OTA try doing next with this device?
   A. Plug it into a different electrical outlet
   B. Turn the valve in the opposite direction
   C. Change the handle position
   D. Reset the device to zero

5. When using a hand-held pinch meter to test lateral pinch, the OTA should place the client's upper extremity in which of the following positions?
   A. 90 degrees shoulder flexion, adduction, 90 degrees elbow flexion, full pronation
   B. 90 degrees shoulder flexion, adduction, 90 degrees elbow flexion, forearm in neutral position
   C. 0 degrees shoulder flexion, adduction, 90 degrees elbow flexion, forearm in neutral position
   D. 0 degrees shoulder flexion, adduction, 90 degrees elbow flexion, full supination

6. To test a client's pinch strength, an OTA is using a hand-held pinch meter with a manual reset knob. The OTA determines that the pinch meter needle is already set at zero. When the client squeezes the device, the OTA observes that the needle does not move from the zero position to register pinch strength like the device did earlier in that day. This is the only pinch meter in the clinic. Which of the following actions is more suitable for the OTA to do first?
   A. Turn the pinch meter over and have the client squeeze the device again
   B. Turn the pinch meter knob the opposite way and have the client squeeze the device again
   C. Notify the OT that the device is broken
   D. Contact the facility maintenance/engineering department to ascertain if the device can be fixed

Worksheet 7-3 (continued)

Assessing Client Factors

7. When using a volumeter to assess edema, the client should immerse the upper extremity until the plastic stop is between which two digits?
   A. Thumb and index
   B. Ring and small
   C. Index and long
   D. Long and ring

8. During the initial evaluation, an OT assessed a client's right-hand edema using a volumeter containing tap water. The OT documented the results as 560 mL. One week later, the OTA retested the client's same hand and documented the results as 520 mL. However, as there was a problem with the clinic's water supply at that time, the OTA used bottled water to fill the volumeter for this reassessment. The change from 560 to 520 mL is most likely due to:
   A. Decreased edema
   B. Increased edema
   C. OTA tester error
   D. Different chemicals in the two water sources

9. A client sustained a dislocation injury to his right index finger proximal interphalangeal (PIP) joint. An OTA is taking circumferential measurements of this joint and documents the joint measurement as 6.2 cm. A week earlier the same joint measured 5.7 cm. The client's left index finger PIP joint has a measurement of 5.4 cm. As a result, the OTA should document that the client's right PIP joint demonstrates:
   A. Decreased range of motion (ROM)
   B. Decreased edema
   C. Increased edema
   D. An infection

10. An OTA is working with a client diagnosed with COPD who receives oxygen through a nasal cannula. As the client has been exhibiting dyspnea upon exertion, the OT asked the OTA to assess and document vital signs during the client's self-care routine today. Of the following choices, which is less of a fit for the OTA to assess during this session?
    A. Blood oxygen saturation levels
    B. Heart rate
    C. Systolic pressure
    D. Body temperature

Morreale, M. J. (2022). *Developing clinical competence: A workbook for the OTA* (2nd ed.). SLACK Incorporated.

Learning Activity 7-3: Evidence-Informed Practice—Grip Strength

With a partner, use a hydraulic hand dynamometer that has adjustable grip positions. Lafayette and Jamar are common brands of these devices, but various others are also available for use in rehabilitation settings. The person being tested should squeeze the dynamometer with the device set at each of the adjustable handle positions. Note grip scores in order, beginning from the narrowest grip position and progressing to the widest handle position. The device should be reset to zero after each squeeze and the person being tested should exert maximum effort for each trial. Plot the measurements on a graph and connect the dots.

1. _____ lb

2. _____ lb

3. _____ lb

4. _____ lb

5. _____ lb

Measure grip strength again with the dynamometer set at each of the handle positions, resetting to zero after each squeeze. However, this time the person being tested should give less than maximal effort to misrepresent actual strength (as a malingering client might do to avoid showing progress). Note grip scores in order, beginning from the narrowest grip position and progressing to the widest handle position. Plot the measurements on a graph and connect the dots.

1. _____ lb

2. _____ lb

3. _____ lb

4. _____ lb

5. _____ lb

Now compare the two graphs. Are they similar or different in terms of shapes or slopes? Find five evidence-based articles to determine if graphing the five grip positions is clinically valid when attempting to determine if a client is exerting the maximum effort or not. List the five citations below. Discuss the information presented in the articles and compare it to your partner's test results.

1.

2.

3.

4.

5.

Worksheet 7-4

Assessing Additional Client Factors

1. An OTA is assessing static two-point discrimination for a client who has undergone surgery for a digital nerve repair to his right index finger. When using a Disc-Criminator or aesthesiometer on the fingertip, which of the following measurements would be considered in the normal range?
   A. 1 cm
   B. 5 cm
   C. 5 mm
   D. 8 mm

2. How much pressure should the OTA apply when administering a static two-point discrimination test?
   A. Until the filament begins to bend
   B. 5 mm of pressure
   C. Until the client reports ability to feel the stimulus
   D. Until the skin blanches

3. An OTA is using Semmes-Weinstein monofilaments to assess a client's sensation. In mapping out these results, the progression of colors indicating sensation level in order from better to worse is:
   A. Green, blue, purple, red
   B. Green, yellow, red, blue
   C. Blue, green, purple, red
   D. Blue, purple, red, black

4. The primary use of a pulse oximeter is to assess which of the following?
   A. Blood glucose levels
   B. Blood pressure
   C. Body mass index
   D. Blood oxygen saturation levels

5. An OTA is assessing a client's right upper extremity passive range of motion (PROM). Which of the following observations noted by the OTA would indicate an abnormal end feel?
   A. Shoulder external rotation: Capsular stretch
   B. Wrist flexion: Hard
   C. Elbow flexion: Soft
   D. Elbow extension: Hard

6. An OTA is assessing a client's right upper extremity PROM. Which of the following observations noted by the OTA would indicate a normal end feel?
   A. Shoulder flexion: Springy block
   B. Shoulder abduction: Capsular stretch
   C. Thumb metacarpophalangeal (MP) flexion: Hard
   D. Elbow extension: Soft

Worksheet 7-4 (continued)

Assessing Additional Client Factors

7. An outpatient client has a diagnosis of adhesive capsulitis. An OTA is assessing the client's active range of motion (AROM) for shoulder flexion. The OTA observes that when the client raises her affected arm, the client elevates her right scapula excessively. In general, which of the following is less suitable for the OTA do?
   A. Ask client to perform active shoulder flexion again but tell her to "relax the shoulder"
   B. Document that the client has poor motor planning
   C. Have client perform AROM in front of a mirror
   D. Provide a tactile cue

8. An OT asked the OTA to assess AROM for a client who has cognitive deficits. When the OTA verbally asks the client to follow various upper extremity commands (e.g., "Lift your arm up over your head"), the OTA observes that the client is attending but is not performing the motions correctly. What primary action is more suitable for the OTA to do?
   A. Write down simple instructions for these motions
   B. Document that the client is noncompliant
   C. Speak in a louder voice
   D. Demonstrate the active motions

9. An OTA plans to assess sitting balance for an adult client who sustained a cerebrovascular accident. The client needs moderate assistance to perform bed mobility and transfers. Of the following activities, which would generally provide the OTA with a more accurate picture of the client's dynamic sitting balance? Assume the OTA is implementing appropriate guarding/assist for client safety.
   A. Client sitting on edge of bed and remaining stationary with arms folded in lap
   B. Client positioned in Fowler's position in bed while self-feeding
   C. Client sitting on the mat and reaching with both arms for items on either side
   D. Client sitting in wheelchair in front of sink while shaving

10. An OTA is assessing a client's muscle tone for the biceps muscle. Which of the following is a typical technique for the OTA to use to determine muscle tone?
    A. PROM with a quick stretch
    B. PROM with a slow stretch
    C. Active resisted flexion
    D. Active resisted extension

Assessing Muscle Strength

The questions in Worksheets 7-5 and 7-6 assume that the occupational therapy practitioner is performing a conventional manual muscle test (MMT) rather than a functional screening to assess the strength of a muscle or muscle groups for specific joint motions. When administering an MMT, the examiner considers the effects of gravity and places the client in test-specific positions (e.g., supine, prone, side-lying, sitting, standing) according to the motions being tested. Depending on a particular client's situation (e.g., diagnosis, precautions/contraindications, available time, treatment priorities, client mobility), an occupational therapy practitioner might use professional reasoning to modify standard techniques or positions and perform a functional strength test instead. A functional strength test, rather than a standard MMT, could entail having a client remain lying supine in bed or sitting in a wheelchair for all muscle groups being tested. For example, it may be contraindicated or not feasible for a client with a recent total hip replacement or a frail, older client to assume a prone position. The methods used should be clearly documented in the client's chart. Use Figure 7-2 to help you with the clinical decision-making process for performing an MMT.

It is important to realize that, although most sources are generally consistent in defining the muscle grades of Normal (N), Good (G), Fair (F), Poor (P), Trace (T), and Zero (0), differences in scoring are evident in the definitions of plus (+) and minus (-) muscle grades and whether plus and minus grades should even be used at all (Avers & Brown, 2019; Clarkson, 2013; Jacobs & Simon, 2020; Kaskutas, 2018; Liska & Gonzalez, 2013; Reese, 2012; Rybski, 2019). Note that for purposes of the worksheets and learning activities in this chapter, the muscle grades of Fair- (F-) will be delineated as incomplete ROM against gravity (greater than 50%) and Poor+ (P+) as incomplete ROM against gravity (less than 50%; Clarkson, 2013; Liska & Gonzalez, 2013; Reese, 2012). In conventional muscle grading, numbers also correspond to the words. Table 7-1 shows different ways in which muscle grades can be documented. Always use the specific grading system and methods standard for your facility. It is also important to be consistent when testing and retesting a client's muscle strength and recording the results.

Table 7-1 Documenting Muscle Grades			
Normal	N	5	5/5
Good	G	4	4/5
Fair	F	3	3/5
Poor	P	2	2/5
Trace	T	1	1/5
Zero	0	0	0/5

Some Clinical Tips When Performing a Manual Muscle Test

- **Always adhere to any precautions and contraindications based on the individual client's condition and situation**. Not all clients will require an MMT. Not all clients will be able to assume standard test positions safely. Application of resistance (or even AROM only) may be contraindicated for certain conditions or situations, such as an unhealed tendon repair or fracture.

- Use easy-to-understand instructions instead of technical jargon when asking a client to perform a particular active motion. For example, for shoulder flexion, rather than saying, *"Flex your shoulder,"* you might say, *"Lift your arm up over your head"* or *"Reach up to the ceiling."* It is helpful to demonstrate the desired motions.

- An easier way to remember and visualize proper client position is to consider that motions against gravity move upward toward the ceiling (e.g., flexion and abduction while seated or standing, horizontal adduction in supine) and the positions minimizing the effects of gravity allow for motions to be performed parallel to the floor (e.g., scapula elevation while prone, horizontal abduction while seated, shoulder flexion while side-lying).

- If you observe that the client does not exhibit full AROM, do not automatically assume that weakness or joint problems exist. If you simply provide an additional verbal cue, such as, *"Can you lift your arm up any higher than that?"* or *"Can you turn your hand over any further?"* the client will often exhibit more complete motion.

- A main defining factor in MMT decision making, a baseline, is determining if the client can perform full available AROM against gravity (at least a muscle grade of Fair). If the client is able to do this, resistance is applied and the resulting muscle grade can then only be: Fair, Fair+, Good, or Normal. (Some facilities also use G+ and G-). If the client does not meet that baseline, there are two options: (1) the client has already demonstrated the criteria for F- or P+ (depending on amount of motion exhibited) and the test is complete, or (2) based on the criteria, the client must be positioned in a gravity reduced position to determine a muscle grade of Poor, Trace, or Zero.

- As means to help with remembering, the author's students have dubbed the muscle grade of F+ as "shake and break," meaning that the muscle can sustain a minimal amount of resistance but struggles (shakes) with any greater resistance and lowers downward (breaks).

- A joint limitation or contracture does not necessarily indicate decreased strength. When performing an MMT, if AROM and PROM of a particular joint are equal (client moves through available joint range), then resistance should be applied to determine strength (Reese, 2012). For example, a bodybuilder with pectoralis muscle bulk may demonstrate limited ROM for the antagonist of horizontal abduction. However, this is would not necessarily signify that the bodybuilder has decreased muscle strength for horizontal abduction.

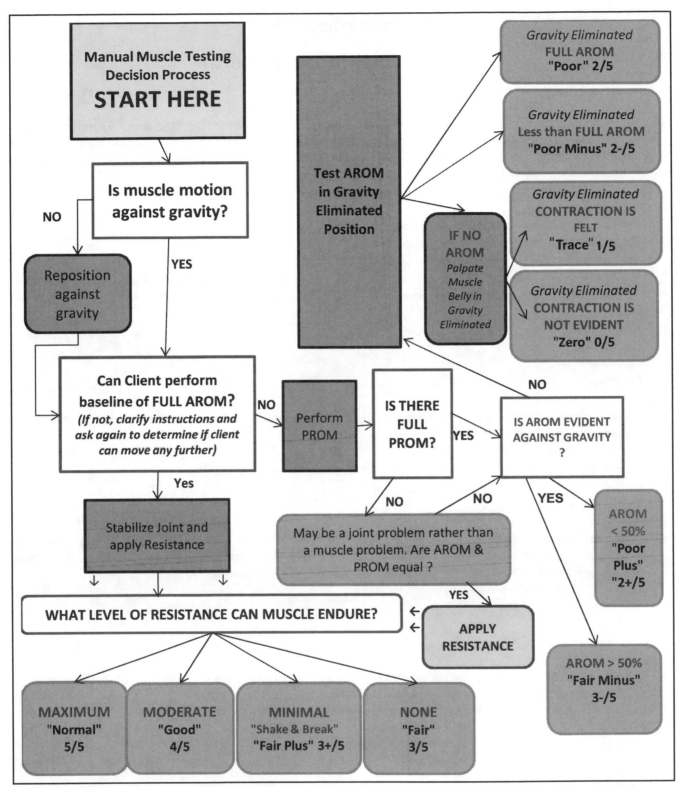

Figure 7-2. MMT flow chart. (Adapted from Marie J. Morreale course lecture notes and developed by Elaine Trainor, COTA.)

Worksheet 7-5

Assessing Muscle Strength

Instructions: For the scenarios in this worksheet, assume the client can safely undergo standard MMT procedures.

1. An OTA is performing a standard MMT bedside to determine a client's muscle strength for right shoulder flexion. The client, who is seated at the edge of the bed, is unable to initiate lifting his arm into shoulder flexion but exhibits full PROM. To complete the MMT for shoulder flexion, the OTA should place the client in which of the following positions?
   A. Side-lying in bed
   B. Supine
   C. Prone with arm hanging off side of bed
   D. Not applicable as the test is now complete

2. An athlete with a shoulder condition is receiving outpatient occupational therapy. When performing a standard MMT for shoulder external rotation, the OTA should initially position the client in which of the following positions?
   A. Sitting in a chair
   B. Side-lying in bed
   C. Supine
   D. Prone

3. When performing a standard MMT for wrist flexion, on what aspect of the client's upper extremity should the OTA apply resistance?
   A. Volar forearm
   B. Volar palm
   C. Volar digits
   D. Dorsal hand

4. While performing a standard MMT on a 35-year-old client who has good balance and mobility, the OTA observes that a client cannot shrug his shoulders while sitting in a chair. To complete the test for this motion, the next position for the OTA to place the client in is which of the following?
   A. Kneeling on a mat
   B. Sitting on edge of bed
   C. Standing
   D. Prone

5. When assessing muscle strength for wrist extension, a client can perform full AROM with his hand resting sideways on the ulnar side (on a tabletop). However, the client is unable to initiate wrist extension with the palm resting face down on the table. The muscle grade is most likely which of the following?
   A. Fair
   B. Fair-
   C. Poor
   D. Trace

Worksheet 7-5 (continued)

Assessing Muscle Strength

6. When performing a standard MMT, the OTA observes a client can perform full active supination against gravity. To complete the MMT for this motion, what should the OTA do next to determine the client's muscle grade for this motion?
   A. Nothing, as the test is completed and muscle grade is Fair
   B. Nothing, as the test is completed and muscle grade is 5/5
   C. Perform PROM to forearm
   D. Apply resistance

7. A patient with COPD exhibits both AROM and PROM for shoulder flexion as 0 to 100 degrees. The client is unable to sustain any resistance applied to the shoulder flexor muscles. What muscle grade should this be documented as?
   A. Poor
   B. Fair
   C. Poor+
   D. Fair+

8. A client exhibits full passive elbow ROM but can only actively flex his elbow ¾ of the range when seated. What muscle grade should this be documented as?
   A. Fair
   B. Fair+
   C. Fair-
   D. Poor

9. When performing a standard MMT to test muscle strength for horizontal adduction, the OTA should place the client in which start position?
   A. Supine
   B. Sitting
   C. Side-lying
   D. Prone

10. An OTA is performing a standard MMT to test a client's muscle strength for shoulder extension (hyperextension). After completing the initial step, the OTA determines the client must be placed in a gravity-reduced position to complete the test which, for that motion, is which of the following positions?
    A. Sitting
    B. Standing
    C. Side-lying
    D. Prone

Morreale, M. J. (2022). *Developing clinical competence: A workbook for the OTA* (2nd ed.). SLACK Incorporated.

Worksheet 7-6

Assessing Muscle Strength—More Practice

1. When assessing strength for internal rotation, which of the following clients is a more suitable candidate to be positioned in the standard MMT initial test position?
   A. A 40-year-old carpenter presently in the reconditioning phase of therapy following rotator cuff surgery
   B. A 35-year-old athlete with adhesive capsulitis who is also 3 weeks status post open-heart surgery
   C. A 70-year-old homemaker 3 days status post total hip replacement who requires upper body strengthening for walker use
   D. A 45-year-old female status post mastectomy 1 week ago with resultant upper limb weakness

2. When performing a standard MMT to test muscle strength for shoulder abduction, the OTA observes that the client exhibits 100 degrees AROM and 160 degrees PROM. The OTA should determine that the muscle grade is which of the following?
   A. Fair
   B. Fair+
   C. Fair-
   D. Undetermined, need to further test in a gravity-eliminated position

3. A client can fully flex his biceps muscle against gravity. To complete the MMT for the biceps, the OTA should do which of the following?
   A. Nothing, as the test is now complete and muscle grade is 3/5
   B. Nothing, as the test is now complete and muscle grade is 5/5
   C. Place client in gravity-minimized position
   D. Apply resistance

4. When performing a standard MMT to test muscle strength for shoulder internal rotation, the OTA should apply resistance to what aspect of the client's upper extremity?
   A. Distal forearm with client prone
   B. Distal forearm with client supine
   C. Distal forearm with client sitting
   D. Distal humerus with client prone

5. An OTA is performing a standard MMT to test a client's muscle strength for MP extension. The OTA should place the client's upper extremity in which start position?
   A. Palm supported facing down
   B. Hand sideways with ulnar side of hand resting on table
   C. Hand sideways with thumb side of hand resting on table
   D. Palm supported on table facing up

Worksheet 7-6 (continued)
Assessing Muscle Strength—More Practice

6. A male client can actively touch his thumb to index and long fingers but not the others. The OTA determines the client has full PROM and muscle weakness. Of the following muscles, which is more likely affected in this scenario?
   A. Flexor digitorum profundus
   B. Opponens pollicis
   C. Abductor digiti minimi
   D. Flexor pollicis longus

7. A client is unable to actively flex his MPs to 70 degrees while simultaneously extending his PIPs and distal interphalangeals (DIPs). PROM is within normal limits (WNL). Which of the following muscles is more likely affected?
   A. Lumbricals
   B. Extensor carpi radialis
   C. Flexor digitorum superficialis
   D. Flexor digitorum profundus

8. A client is demonstrating difficulty with tendon gliding following a Zone 2 flexor tendon repair. Today an OTA has been delegated the task of teaching this client tendon gliding exercises to improve hand function for ADLs. To implement this intervention, the OTA should primarily work toward facilitating movement of which of the following muscles?
   A. Opponens pollicis and opponens digiti minimi
   B. Extensor pollicis longus and extensor pollicis brevis
   C. Flexor carpi radialis and flexor carpi ulnaris
   D. Flexor digitorum profundus and flexor digitorum superficialis

9. An OTA is working with a client diagnosed with carpal tunnel syndrome. The occupational therapy evaluation performed several days ago indicates the client is exhibiting weakness of median innervated intrinsic muscles only. Thus, the OTA might expect to see deficits in which of the following muscle groups?
   A. Adductor pollicis, flexor pollicis brevis, opponens pollicis
   B. Flexor pollicis brevis, opponens pollicis, abductor pollicis longus
   C. Opponens pollicis, adductor pollicis, abductor pollicis brevis
   D. Flexor pollicis brevis, opponens pollicis, abductor pollicis brevis

10. A client has a diagnosis of low-level ulnar nerve lesion. Which of the following observations by an OTA would be a fit with that condition?
    A. Inability to perform palmar abduction
    B. Inability to flex thumb MP
    C. Inability to flex small finger MP
    D. Inability to flex index finger MP

Learning Activity 7-4: Assessing Pain

As part of a group exercise, participants should create a combined list of situations for which they have experienced (or are currently experiencing) physical pain. Some suggestions are listed as follows, but the group may come up with others. According to each member's comfort level for voluntary disclosure of any personal information, members should describe their personal pain experiences. Consider the particular words needed to specifically describe pain patterns, and to quantify and qualify pain. For example, was the pain throbbing, burning, knife-like, prickly, or achy? Where exactly did the pain occur? Did the pain travel? Was pain constant, intermittent, or perhaps only aggravated by specific motions or activities? What methods, if any, helped to reduce the pain? Compare and contrast the description of pain by several members who have experienced the same conditions. Participants might also discuss the personal effects of pain regarding their occupational performance. Determine what formal or informal pain scales could be used to assess pain for each participant's condition or situation. Try not to use the same pain scale more than once for this exercise.

Broken bone	Infection (sinus, ear, wound, urinary tract)
Sprained ankle	Headache/migraine
Childbirth	Pneumonia/pleurisy
Kidney stone	Surgery
Exercising/working out at the gym	Toothache
Back injury/sciatica	Compressed nerve

Specific Condition	Pain Description	Effect on Occupational Performance	Formal Pain Scales That Could Be Used	Informal Pain Scales That Could Be Used

Now list five pain assessments that may be used with children or clients that are unable to communicate:

1.

2.

3.

4.

5.

Worksheet 7-7

Improving Observation Skills—Appearance and Hygiene

Clients with conditions such as brain injuries, intellectual and developmental disabilities, or mental health conditions require assessment of various factors and skills that reflect mental function, process skills, and ability to interact within social norms. What might you observe and document regarding your client that would indicate a well-groomed appearance versus poor hygiene, health factors, or an unkempt/untidy appearance? In the boxes below, list *objective* factors pertaining to clothing, skin, face, hair, and so forth.

Good Hygiene/Well-Groomed Appearance	Poor Hygiene or Health Factors, Unkempt/Untidy Appearance

Morreale, M. J. (2022). *Developing clinical competence: A workbook for the OTA* (2nd ed.). SLACK Incorporated.

Worksheet 7-8

Improving Observation Skills—Mood and Behavior

Clients with conditions such as brain injuries, intellectual and developmental disabilities, or mental health conditions require assessment of various factors and skills that reflect mental function, process skills, and ability to interact within social norms. Consider *observable* client actions and communications that an OTA might note as indicators of a client's present demeanor, mood, or level of cognition. In the boxes below, create a list of possible objective factors an OTA might look for while observing a client, such as specific kinds of client behaviors and verbal expressions.

Behavioral Observations (give specific examples of what the client actually did)	Client's Verbalizations (give specific examples of what the client actually said)
Example: Arms crossed in front of chest or not	*Example: Client uses courteous words (Please, Thank You, May I…) or profane words/curses at family, staff, and peers on unit*
Example: Attentive or easily distracted (due to what specific internal or external factors)	*Example: Verbalizes understanding of one's own deficits or not*

Learning Activity 7-5: Practicing Observation Skills

With a partner or group, choose an episode of a television show (a drama or situation comedy) to watch. One character in that show should be agreed upon for all to observe. Each group member should separately jot down objective "clinical observations" to assess demeanor, hygiene, mood, behavior, health, and mental functions that the character is exhibiting. Next to each item, indicate if that is an asset/positive trait (+) or a limiting factor/negative trait (-). You can refer to the lists created in Worksheets 7-7 and 7-8 to help determine the kinds of things to look for. When all observations of the designated character have been completed, partners/group members should compare lists and discuss similarities and differences.

Realize that with a real client, occupational therapy practitioners use professional reasoning to determine what specific observations have clinical importance and are relevant to record in that client's chart. For example, an OTA might observe that an outpatient orthopedic client has a new haircut and is wearing full make-up today. Normally, this would not be considered of major importance or necessary to document in the medical record. However, if this same client has been diagnosed with depression and neglecting personal appearance, these observations might then be very relevant to record.

Observations of Television Character

Examples:

- *Character expressed her anger by cursing and throwing a book at spouse (-)*
- *When cooking at barbeque grill, character demonstrated good safety awareness by using long-handle cooking utensils and silicone mitt, maintaining proper distancing from heat/flames, and turning off gas when done (+)*
- *Character is missing two front teeth, has a left black eye and swollen upper lip (-)*

Indicators of health/hygiene/demeanor:

Behaviors as indicators of the character's mood and mental functions (give specific examples of what the character did):

Verbalizations as indicators of the character's mood and mental functions (give specific examples of what the character said):

Answers to Worksheets

Worksheet 7-1: Determining Assist Levels

Resources: Centers for Medicare & Medicaid Services (CMS), 2019; Jacobs & Simon, 2020; Morreale & Borcherding, 2017

Settings may vary in the specific terminology and criteria used to describe levels of function. Always use the methods that are standard for your facility, practice setting, and payer requirements. Examples of commonly used terms and definitions are listed below in Table 7-2.

Table 7-2	
Levels of Assistance	
Total assistance (TOT)	Individual requires 100% assistance to safely complete task. Individual does not assist at all.
Maximum assistance (MAX)	Individual requires 75% of physical/cognitive assistance to safely complete task. Individual assists 25%.
Moderate assistance (MOD)	Individual requires 50% of physical/cognitive assistance to safely complete task. Individual assists 50%.
Minimal assistance (MIN)	Individual needs no more than 25% physical/cognitive assistance. Individual assists 75%.
Stand-by assistance (SBA)	Supervision or stand-by assistance for safe, effective task performance.
Set-up assistance	Individual requires set-up of necessary items to perform tasks.
Independent (IND)	No assistance or supervision is required. Able to perform independently. Safety is demonstrated during tasks.

Reproduced with permission from Jacobs, K., & Simon, L. (Eds.). (2020). *Quick reference dictionary for occupational therapy* (7th ed.). SLACK Incorporated.

1. *Modified independence.* The client donned socks by herself using a sock aid.

2. *Stand-by assist.* After assessing the resident's transfer skills, the OTA determined the resident needs someone next to her for safety in case the resident forgets to lock the wheelchair brakes or moves too quickly.

3. *Three verbal cues or minimal verbal cues.* At lunch time, the client needed three reminders to look to the left in order to find all the food on the plate.

4. *Dependent or total assistance.* The client required a mechanical lift to transfer from bed to wheelchair.

5. *Maximum assistance of two persons (max assist X 2).* The resident needed both the OTA and physical therapist assistant to help him transfer from the wheelchair to the mat, but he was able to bear some weight on his weak leg.

6. *Maximum assistance.* During a toothbrushing task, the client could not put the paste on the brush, manipulate or hold the brush; but she did open her mouth, rinse, and spit on command.

7. *Independent with set-up.* The OTA noted that after the containers are opened and food is cut, the resident can feed herself.

8. *Independent.* The student zippered her jacket by herself, and the OTA told her she did a good job.

9. *Hand-over-hand assistance.* The OTA put the crayon in the child's weak hand, helped him hold it, and guided the child's arm so the child could draw a circle.

10. *Independent.* The OTA let the client know that the lunch tray was in her room, so the client returned to her room and fed herself.

11. *Minimal assistance.* When donning his shirt, the client needed a little help to bring the shirt around his back and line up the first button.

12. *Supervision within arm's length or close supervision.* During craft group, because sharp objects were present, the OTA sat next to the client who is suicidal.

13. *Distant supervision or supervision within line-of-sight.* During recess, the OTA looked out the window periodically to monitor and help ensure the child was playing cooperatively with the other children on the playground.

14. *Contact guard assistance.* While the client was cooking at the stove, the OTA put an arm lightly around the client's back in case the client became unsteady.

15. *Modified independence.* The client who has ESRD unloaded the dishwasher but needed several rest breaks in order to complete the task.

16. *Visual cue.* The client with left neglect could read the newspaper article only after the OTA put a red line at the left margin.

17. *Several tactile cues or minimal physical prompting.* During mealtime, the OTA had to touch the client's arm a few times to prompt the client to bring food to mouth.

18. *Moderate assistance.* The child needed help for about half of the shoe-tying task.

19. *Auditory cue.* The client would only remember to take her medicine when her cell phone timer buzzed.

20. *Independent.* The student demonstrated ability to use her power wheelchair well, so the OTA put a smiley face sticker on the wheelchair.

Worksheet 7-2: Assessing Feeding

It is important to look at the client holistically, consider all the possibilities, and use professional reasoning to help determine which of these factors are applicable to Chen's situation.

1. Chen may be awaiting medical tests for which he is not allowed to eat prior to the test.

2. Chen may not like the food choices, as they may be quite different than the typical food he is used to eating in China.

3. If ethnic food is available, it may be bland or not appealing due to a possible low-salt or low-fat diet.

4. Chen may normally use chopsticks and may not be comfortable using silverware (Asher, 2006).

5. Food may not conform to the client's values or beliefs, such as specific religious tenets or if Chen is a vegetarian and meat was served.

6. Chen may be embarrassed to have someone helping him or watching him eat, particularly if the person is a different gender.

7. Chen may have difficulty chewing due to missing teeth or a painful jaw.

8. Chen may have dentures that are not currently in place or are ill-fitting and painful.

9. Chen may be experiencing discomfort from reflux, nausea, indigestion, constipation, or stomachache due to medication side effects or an underlying physical or mental condition.

10. Chen may be very tired or experiencing pain.

11. Chen may have a poor body image or may have an eating disorder.

12. Chen may have underlying cognitive impairment or perceptual problems.

13. Chen may be waiting for his family to arrive before he eats.

Worksheet 7-3: Assessing Client Factors

It is important to look at the client holistically, consider all the possibilities, and use professional reasoning to help determine which of these factors are applicable to Chen's situation.

1. D. This is a basic, commonly used pain scale (Engel, 2018).
2. C. (Lafayette Instrument, 2020; Walsh & Chee, 2018).
3. B. (Clarkson, 2013; Lafayette Instrument, 2020).
4. B. A sphygmomanometer is a blood pressure device. When using a manual blood pressure device, if the bulb's air valve (knob) is not turned in the proper direction to close it, the cuff will not inflate. This device does not use electricity and automatically starts at zero when the cuff is deflated.
5. C. (Clarkson, 2013; Walsh & Chee, 2018).
6. B. In this instance, the knob was probably turned the wrong way so that the peak-hold needle (which indicates the measurement) is behind, rather than in front of, the gauge needle that is supposed to push it.
7. D. (Walsh & Chee, 2018).
8. A. Bottled versus tap water should not have any effect on test results. Less water was displaced, indicating decreased edema.
9. C. When taking circumferential measurements, an increased number usually indicates increased edema (although girth can also increase due to other factors, such as a nodule, ganglion, cyst, etc.). While it is possible the client could be getting an infection, there are no clinical signs indicated for that, such as increased pain, redness, or increased warmth of digit. ROM measurements are not noted in this example.
10. D. The OTA should measure the client's blood pressure, blood oxygen saturation levels (with a pulse oximeter), pulse rate, and note respiration rate and any shortness of breath. While it may be appropriate to assess temperature in certain situations, such as for a suspected fever or joint infection, it is not indicated in this situation.

Worksheet 7-4: Assessing Additional Client Factors

1. C. (Abrams & Ivy, 2018).
2. D. (Abrams & Ivy, 2018).
3. A. (Abrams & Ivy, 2018).
4. D.
5. B. (Clarkson, 2013; Shurtleff & Kaskutas, 2018).
6. B. (Clarkson, 2013; Shurtleff & Kaskutas, 2018).
7. B. With this condition, the client is likely compensating for muscle weakness in shoulder flexors and/or exhibiting joint limitations/stiffness rather than poor motor planning. The OTA should try methods to minimize muscle substitution and compensatory motions.
8. D. Demonstration would help the client to better process the desired motions. Written instructions could be more confusing and, unless the client has hearing impairment or is exhibiting poor attention, a louder voice would not really help the situation.
9. C. Of the choices provided, sitting unsupported on a mat and weight shifting to either side would better challenge dynamic sitting balance. However, it would be even more challenging if the client were reaching for objects and weight shifting while seated on edge of bed (which is an unstable surface) with feet unsupported rather than a stable mat surface. Use appropriate guarding/assist for safety.
10. A. A quick stretch to a muscle is the usual method to determine if resistance (i.e., spasticity) occurs as a response to the movement (Gillen, 2011; Preston, 2018).

Worksheet 7-5: Assessing Muscle Strength

Resources: Avers & Brown, 2019; Clarkson, 2013; Reese, 2012

Professional reasoning is needed to determine if modifications are needed for a specific client. These answers are based on standard MMT procedure. As previously noted, motions against gravity move upward toward the ceiling (e.g., flexion and abduction while seated/standing, horizontal adduction in supine) and the positions minimizing the effects of gravity allow for motions to be performed parallel to the floor (scapula elevation while prone, horizontal abduction while seated, shoulder flexion while side-lying). Again, it is important to realize that it may not be safe or feasible for some clients to assume a standard test position or even undergo an MMT.

1. A. The OTA needs to position the client in a gravity-reduced position, which, in this situation, is side-lying. The OTA should support the client's arm or use a powder board.
2. D. The against-gravity start position for external rotation is a prone position. However, this position may be too difficult for elderly clients or contraindicated for some conditions.
3. B. The test begins with client's arm resting on the table with palm facing up. The client flexes the wrist and the OTA applies pressure on the palm in a downward direction.
4. D. A prone position minimizes effects of gravity for scapula elevation. Assuming a prone position may be difficult for elderly clients or contraindicated for some conditions.
5. C. The muscle grade is poor as the client is able to perform the motion in a gravity-reduced plane but cannot move against gravity.
6. D. The test is not yet complete. The OTA has determined the client demonstrates at least a Fair (F) muscle grade but needs to apply resistance to complete the MMT.
7. B. The client's present maximum joint range is 100 degrees. While the ROM deficit is documented as a joint contracture, active and passive ranges are equal, so the client has at least Fair muscle strength. Resistance is then applied to complete the test, which, in this case, the client cannot sustain so the muscle grade is Fair.
8. C. The client is unable to perform full AROM against gravity but performs more than 50% of the motion.
9. A. A supine position allows for horizontal adduction to be performed against gravity.
10. C. The gravity-reduced position for shoulder extension is side-lying. The OTA should support the client's arm or use a powder board.

Worksheet 7-6: Assessing Muscle Strength—More Practice

Resources: Avers & Brown, 2019; Clarkson, 2013; Reese, 2012

Professional reasoning is needed to determine if modifications are needed for a particular client. These answers are based on standard MMT procedure.

1. A. Resistance is applied to distal forearm with client prone. The other clients have medical conditions that entail contraindications for application of resistance and/or a prone position.
2. C. The client demonstrates incomplete AROM against gravity but more than 50% of available joint range.
3. D. The client demonstrates full AROM against gravity, so the next step is to apply resistance.
4. A. The against-gravity start position for internal rotation is a prone position. The position may not be feasible for frail, elderly patients or may be contraindicated for certain conditions (e.g., recent total hip replacement).
5. A. The against-gravity start position for MP extension is with the palm facing down.
6. B. The opponens pollicis allows for thumb opposition.
7. A. This motion is performed using the lumbricals.

8. D. A flexor tendon injury in Zone 2 affects differential tendon gliding of the flexor digitorum profundus and flexor digitorum superficialis. Of course, other muscles and joints may also be affected due to complications from the injury and/or surgery with possible additional intervention needed.

9. D. The adductor pollicis is ulnar nerve innervated. The abductor pollicis longus is an extrinsic muscle and is not innervated by the median nerve.

10. C. Inability to perform palmar abduction or MP flexion of thumb could indicate median nerve impairment. Inability to flex finger MPs may indicate weakness of the lumbricals, which are innervated by both the median nerve (index and long fingers) and ulnar nerve (ring and small fingers).

Worksheet 7-7: Improving Observation Skills—Appearance and Hygiene

Resources: Morreale & Borcherding, 2017

A client's personal appearance and hygiene could be an indicator of the client's self-image, mood, health, or cognitive status. However, the mere presence of any unkempt/untidy factors listed in the answer table does not necessarily correlate to deficits in mental functions or social skills and does not necessarily need to be documented. For example, a client coming to therapy directly from a landscaping or construction job may be wearing garments with large dirt stains or tears. You might even have once had a piece of spinach inadvertently stuck in your teeth! It is also important not to make value judgments based on one's personal fashion preferences, moral standards, or religious beliefs (Morreale & Borcherding, 2017). The occupational therapy practitioner must distinguish between factors, such as a client who may have a long beard to meet religious requirements versus a client who has suddenly stopped shaving due to depression, defiance against his parents' wishes, or not understanding a job's dress code. If a client arrives with make-up applied only to one side of face or with lipstick circling the nose, clinical reasoning will ascertain if these behaviors are influenced by specific deficits, such as unilateral neglect or perhaps a psychotic episode. As another example, a teenager wearing flannel pajama pants at a coffee shop may consider as fitting in with peers, whereas an 80-year-old adult might consider the teen's fashion choice as inappropriate for outside of the home. However, other observations, such as a client with disordered clothing, needle track marks, or a skeletal appearance, may be quite noteworthy. Professional reasoning is used to assess patterns of behavior and determine if clinical observations are pertinent or significant to the client's present circumstances for documenting in the client's chart. Although the boxes below contain many examples, it should not be considered an all-inclusive list.

Good Hygiene/Well-Groomed Appearance	Poor Hygiene or Health Factors, Unkempt/Untidy Appearance
Clean face and skin, no visible dirt or food particles present	Visible dirt or food on face/skin, presence of soap or make-up residue, strong body odor
Hair clean, combed, styled neatly	Hair greasy, dirty, uncombed, matted, presence of lice
Clean teeth, no food particles noted in mouth	Food particles stuck in teeth; gum disease; missing, discolored, or loose teeth
Clothing without wrinkles, neatly pressed, intact	Clothing wrinkled, torn, number/size of holes, presence of multiple lint balls, or large hanging threads/missing buttons
Clothing clean, without stains	Clothing unclean (e.g., has food, grass, or dirt stains; bugs crawling)
Clothing fits properly	Clothing ill-fitting: described as inability to fasten buttons or zipper due to clothing not fitting, clothing several sizes too big, undergarments visible, skirt dragging on floor, and so forth.
Buttons lined up properly, fastenings closed, shoelaces tied	Fastenings open or misaligned, shoelaces untied or missing
Clothing right side out	Clothing disordered, inside out, or backward
Hat centered on head, socks pulled up	Hat worn backward or falling off, socks down to ankle

Good Hygiene/Well-Groomed Appearance	Poor Hygiene or Health Factors, Unkempt/Untidy Appearance
Clothing matches and is complete and appropriate for occasion and weather; attention to detail with accessories	Missing an item, such as a sock or shoe, clothing does not match or is not appropriate for weather or occasion.
Clean shaven, facial hair neatly trimmed	Stubble (e.g., several days facial hair growth), length of beard/mustache, blood present from shaving cuts
Make-up applied neatly	Make-up streaked; lipstick, eye liner, or shadow grossly uneven or beyond typical boundaries
Nails clean, neatly shaped, and polished	Visible dirt beneath nails, length or unevenness of nails, brittleness or fungus present
Smooth, intact skin	Flaky skin, rough/scaly patches, thick callous, open sores, acne, rash, presence of needle track marks, scars from self-mutilation/cutting, nicotine stains
Weight in proportion to height	Weight not in proportion to height (e.g., skeletal, morbidly obese), note specific weight and height or body mass index (BMI)

Adapted from Morreale, M. J., & Borcherding, S. (2017). *The OTA's guide to documentation: Writing SOAP notes* (4th ed.). SLACK Incorporated.

Worksheet 7-8: Improving Observation Skills—Mood and Behavior

Avoid "judgmental" words when describing relevant client actions objectively and use professional reasoning to determine how those observations are pertinent to the client's condition/situation and what is noteworthy to document (Morreale & Borcherding, 2017). For example, instead of documenting, "Client is paranoid," a more suitable choice of words based on behavior could be, "Client is exhibiting suspicious behavior such as disassembling his phone and alarm clock several times daily to check if those items are bugged." The boxes below contain many examples but should not be considered an all-inclusive list.

Behavioral Observations (give specific examples of what the client actually did)	Client's Verbalizations (give specific examples of what the client actually said)
Facial expression (e.g., flat affect or smiling, laughing, frowning, tearful/crying)	Identifies own mood, such as feelings/thoughts of persecution, depression, happiness, anger, grief, anxiety, guilt, and so forth.
Eyes open or closed, level of eye contact, looks away	Positive or negative statements about one's own appearance, abilities, or how others perceive client
Attentiveness, ability to concentrate, easily startled or distracted	Flight of ideas, confusion, lucidity, logical or illogical statements
Posture sitting/standing, head and trunk upright or shoulders hunched, client stooped over or leaning to side	Changes answers/opinions, vacillates, repetitiveness of answers, or replies without thinking
Personal space boundaries	Specific statements that reflect various defense mechanisms (identify with examples)
Arms/legs crossed or open, leans forward or away	Stated opinion regarding future /outlook, past/present rehabilitation, or potential to change
Affectionate behaviors (hugs, kisses) within social norms or not, readily shakes hands, avoids personal contact	Expresses obsessive thoughts, hallucinations, or delusions

Behavioral Observations (Give Specific Examples of What the Client Actually Did)	Client's Verbalizations (Give Specific Examples of What the Client Actually Said)
Repetitive behavior/rituals or motor activity (e.g., hand wringing, shaking/trembling, tics, nail-biting, thumb-sucking, rocking, spinning, and so forth.)	Tone and quality of speech, fluency
Client exhibits behaviors such as hitting, kicking, spitting, or hurting others	Client exhibits profane language, yells, screams, or makes other sounds
Threatening approach (points, jabs, is "in one's face")	Client acknowledges or denies problems or deficits
Pacing, timing, and level of energy exhibited (give examples of sedentary, active, manic, impulsive, cautious, reckless, suspicious behavior, and so forth.)	Client expresses specific realistic or unrealistic fears/anxieties or abilities
Alert, awake, energetic versus groggy, sleepy, listless	Client expresses willingness or unwillingness to change thoughts or behavior
Goal-directed behaviors or agitation, restlessness, wandering aimlessly	Client's stated attitude toward completion of task
Sits alone or engages easily with others	Verbalizes understanding of deficits or not
Tantrums or other types of acting-out behaviors noted	Length of responses, uncommunicative, rambles, or guarded responses
Handling of objects (rough, destroys or throws items, handles carefully, and so forth.)	Uses tactful, courteous, respectful words or expresses frustration, is argumentative/tries to pick a fight
Avoids or seeks specific sensory stimulation	Stated sleep patterns or changes
Shares items willingly or not (e.g., sitting space, food, cigarettes, craft materials, books/magazines, tools)	Stated changes in weight (in what time period)
Other:	Asks staff, family, or peers for help when needed
Other:	

Adapted from Morreale, M. J., & Borcherding, S. (2017). *The OTA's guide to documentation: Writing SOAP notes* (4th ed.). SLACK Incorporated.

References

Abrams, M. R., & Ivy, C. C. (2018). Evaluation of sensation and intervention for sensory dysfunction. In H. M. Pendleton & W. Schultz-Krohn (Eds.), *Pedretti's occupational therapy practice skills for physical dysfunction* (8th ed., pp. 580-593). Elsevier Incorporated.

American Occupational Therapy Association. (2015). Standards of practice for occupational therapy. *American Journal of Occupational Therapy, 69*(Suppl. 3), 6913410057. http://dx.doi.org/10.5014/ajot.2015.696S06

American Occupational Therapy Association. (2020). Guidelines for supervision, roles, and responsibilities during the delivery of occupational therapy services. *American Journal of Occupational Therapy, 74*(Suppl. 3), 7413410020. https://doi.org/10.5014/ajot.2020.74S3004

Asher, A. (2006). Asian Americans. In M. Royeen & J. L. Crabtree (Eds.), *Culture in rehabilitation: From competency to proficiency* (pp. 151-180). Pearson Education.

Avers, D., & Brown, M. (2019). *Daniels and Worthingham's muscle testing: Techniques of manual examination and performance testing* (10th ed.). Elsevier Incorporated.

Centers for Medicare & Medicaid Services. (2019). *IRF-PAI manual version 3.0 (chapter 2: section GG)*. https://www.cms.gov/Medicare/Medicare-Fee-for-Service-Payment/InpatientRehabFacPPS/IRFPAI

Clarkson, H. M. (2013). *Musculoskeletal assessment: Joint motion and muscle testing* (3rd ed.). Lippincott Williams & Wilkins.

Engel, J. M. (2018). Pain management. In H. M. Pendleton & W. Schultz-Krohn (Eds.), *Pedretti's occupational therapy practice skills for physical dysfunction* (8th ed., pp. 701-709). Elsevier Incorporated.

Gillen, G. (2011). Upper extremity function and management. In G. Gillen (Ed.), *Stroke rehabilitation: A function-based approach* (3rd ed., pp. 218-279). Elsevier Mosby.

Jacobs, K., & Simon, L. (Eds.). (2020). *Quick reference dictionary for occupational therapy* (7th ed.). SLACK Incorporated.

Kaskutas, V. (2018). Evaluation of muscle strength. In H. M. Pendleton & W. Schultz-Krohn (Eds.), *Pedretti's occupational therapy practice skills for physical dysfunction* (8th ed., pp. 512-579). Elsevier Incorporated.

Lafayette Instrument. (2020). *Lafayette hydraulic hand dynamometer user instructions.* Retrieved June 22, 2021, from http://www.limef.com/Downloads/MAN32261-j00105-forpdf-rev2.pdf

Liska, C., & Gonzelez, T. R. (2013). Assessment of muscle strength. In M. B. Early (Ed.), *Physical dysfunction practice skills for the occupational therapy assistant* (3rd ed., pp. 132-155). Mosby.

Morreale, M. J., & Borcherding, S. (2017). *The OTA's guide to documentation: Writing SOAP notes* (4th ed.). SLACK Incorporated.

Preston, L. A. (2018). Evaluation of motor control. In H. M. Pendleton & W. Schultz-Krohn (Eds.), *Pedretti's occupational therapy practice skills for physical dysfunction* (8th ed., pp. 444-469). Elsevier Incorporated.

Reese, N. B. (2012). *Muscle and sensory testing* (3rd ed.). Elsevier Saunders.

Rybski, M. F. (2019). *Kinesiology for occupational therapy* (3rd ed.). SLACK Incorporated.

Shurtleff, T., & Kaskutas, V. (2018). Joint range of motion. In H. M. Pendleton & W. Schultz-Krohn (Eds.), *Pedretti's occupational therapy practice skills for physical dysfunction* (8th ed., pp. 477-511). Elsevier Incorporated.

Walsh, J. M., & Chee, N. (2018). Hand and upper extremity injuries. In H. M. Pendleton & W. Schultz-Krohn (Eds.)., *Pedretti's occupational therapy practice skills for physical dysfunction* (8th ed., pp. 972-1003). Elsevier Incorporated.

Applying Knowledge and Skills in Group Leadership and Mental Health Practice

Implementing effective interventions and programs to support a client or population's occupational performance entails that occupational therapists (OTs) and occupational therapy assistants (OTAs) in all service delivery areas use professional reasoning along with incorporating therapeutic use of self and empathy (AOTA, 2020; Taylor, 2019; 2020). Occupational therapy practitioners must also demonstrate other essential traits and skills such as creative problem-solving ability, safety awareness, good behavioral observation skills, and professionalism. In the areas of mental health (behavioral health) and other activity programs (such as adult day care or assisted living), OTs and OTAs must also be able to lead groups effectively and implement suitable activities and occupations that work toward attaining clients' therapeutic goals for occupational participation. The worksheets and learning activities in this chapter are designed to help you learn and practice various approaches and methods used in mental health practice. Answers to worksheet exercises are provided at the end of the chapter.

Contents

Morreale, M. J. *Developing Clinical Competence:*
A Workbook for the OTA, Second Edition (pp. 329-357).
© 2022 SLACK Incorporated.

Worksheet 8-1

Mental Health Situations

1. A client with severe violent tendencies needs a one-on-one session to review a leisure checklist. When delegated this task, which is more suitable for an OTA to do?
    A. Keep the door closed for privacy
    B. Refuse to treat the client
    C. Ask a staff member to remain in the vicinity
    D. Review the leisure checklist during an occupational therapy leisure group

2. An OTA is working with a client who exhibits hostility and is attending an anger management program. When planning an occupational therapy group that this client will attend, which of the following activities is generally less suitable as a possible choice to help reduce this client's tension?
    A. Sweeping the floor
    B. Wiping tables
    C. A 15-minute walk
    D. Sanding a small wood project

3. An OTA brings a client with an eating disorder over to the craft supply closet. The OTA asks the client to choose a craft project from among the items on the shelves. The client exhibits passivity, insecurity, and says repeatedly, "I don't know what I should do" and "I can't decide." What primary action should the OTA take?
    A. Use a timer to facilitate decision making
    B. Give the client a choice of two craft projects
    C. Have another client choose a project for this client
    D. Have the OTA choose a project for this client

4. An OTA in a mental health setting is leading a sensorimotor group for clients with chronic schizophrenia. Which of the following activities is a more suitable choice as a possible primary activity for this group?
    A. Writing down feelings with lively music playing in background
    B. Discussing bright colors of flowers and rainbows
    C. Tossing and hitting a beach ball
    D. Lying on yoga mats while listening to calming music

5. A client in a group the OTA is leading is becoming aggressive, out of control, and appears ready to hit someone. Of the following choices, the last course of action the OTA should consider taking is?
    A. Try to physically restrain the client
    B. Ask another client to go get help
    C. Talk to the client in a calm voice
    D. Remove other clients from the area

6. An OT and OTA are working on an acute behavioral health unit. They are collaborating to develop a policy and procedure manual for all the occupational therapy groups to ensure safety and meet therapeutic goals. Of the following craft group procedures, which is less suitable for the OT and OTA to include in the manual?
    A. Hand out sharps individually to clients needing them for the activity
    B. Count the number of scissors before and after the group
    C. Avoid using permanent markers and oil-based stains
    D. Give clients the autonomy to retrieve craft supplies, scissors, yarn, and so forth from the occupational therapy supply closet

Worksheet 8-1 (continued)
Mental Health Situations

7. A client with schizophrenia has been attending a community mental health program but has not shown up for the past week. Today the client arrives and begins talking about how her neighbors are watching her through the television. She also states they come in her apartment at night and move her belongings, even though her doors have a deadbolt lock. In collaboration with the OT, which of the following activities is generally more suitable as a possible choice for the OTA to use with client?
   A. Writing in a journal
   B. Peeling potatoes in an instrumental activities of daily living (IADL) group
   C. Painting a picture to represent feelings in a crafts group
   D. Discussing feelings in an expressive group

8. During an occupational therapy activity group, a client is focused on picking lint off his clothing. He also keeps trying to pick lint off the other clients' clothing, despite the OTA asking him repeatedly to stop this behavior. The other clients are becoming irritated at being touched. The OTA should document the lint-picking behavior in the client's chart and describe it using which of the following terms?
   A. Obsessive behavior
   B. IADL retraining
   C. Compulsive behavior
   D. Attention to detail

9. A client attending a partial hospitalization program has a diagnosis of anxiety disorder. The client is exhibiting a panic attack, is trembling, crying, and stating she is going to die. What primary action should the OTA take?
   A. Encourage the client to take slow, deep breaths
   B. Call an ambulance
   C. Call the client's doctor
   D. Go get the OT

10. An OTA is leading a group for clients on an acute behavioral health unit who are diagnosed with depression. The group members are making items to decorate their individual hospital rooms. Of the following choices, which would likely be more suitable as a possible intervention?
    A. A painted ceramic piggy bank
    B. A decorative wreath made with artificial flowers glued to a wire hanger
    C. A painted picture made with the use of stencils
    D. A colorful macramé wall hanging

The Occupational Therapy Group Process

Groups in occupational therapy work toward desired outcomes, such as interaction within social norms, expression of feelings, insight into one's actions, improved coping skills and behavior, a positive self-image, and acquisition of skills needed to support occupational roles. Various leaders in psychology (e.g., Freud, Skinner, Piaget, Erikson) and occupational therapy (e.g., Fidler, Mosey, Allen) have contributed important theories concerning mental functions and group process that are beyond the scope of this book. The reader is encouraged to review the primary frames of reference and models that have guided occupational therapy mental health practice. Many of these have been clearly summarized by Cole (2018) who describes the following approaches: psychodynamic, developmental, sensorimotor, cognitive-behavioral continuum, Allen's Cognitive Disabilities, and various approaches that use the Model of Human Occupation. Following the development of Gail Fidler's task-oriented group model, which uses a psychodynamic approach, Anne Cronin Mosey applied a developmental perspective and identified five stages for group functioning: parallel groups, project groups, egocentric-cooperative groups, cooperative groups, and mature groups (Cole, 2018; Tufano, 2015). Each of these stages addresses acquisition of specific skills. Taylor's Intentional Relationship Model (2008, 2019, 2020) defines the interpersonal dynamic between the OT and client and describes six interpersonal communication modes that occupational therapy practitioners use frequently in therapeutic relationships. These six ways of relating to clients individually and in groups are described by Taylor as advocating, collaborating, empathizing, encouraging, instructing, and problem-solving (Taylor, 2008, 2019, 2020).

As a group leader, the occupational therapy practitioner needs to determine how much direction and structure the specific group requires, depending on the activity demands of the specific task, member abilities, limitations, and therapeutic goals (Cole, 2018; Scaffa, 2019). To lead occupational therapy groups effectively, an OTA, in partnership with the OT, must demonstrate the ability to choose the methods and activities to meet therapeutic goals, encourage and motivate group members, set limits, recognize defense mechanisms, handle problem behaviors, use therapeutic qualities and communication skills (e.g., sensitivity, genuineness, attending, empathy, limited self-disclosure, modeling of appropriate behavior), understand individual and group member roles, and determine capacities and limitations of members (Cole, 2018; Tufano, 2015: Scaffa, 2019). Cole (2018) describes, at length, seven steps for effective group leadership in occupational therapy, which she adapted from Pfeiffer and Jones' *Reference Guide to Handbooks and Annuals* (1977). Cole's Seven-Step Format for Groups method, briefly summarized below, is a very useful process for highest level groups and can also be modified to meet other groups' needs (Cole, 2018).

Cole's Seven-Step Groups (2018)

1. Introduction—The start of a group should include an introduction of the occupational therapy practitioner and participants, along with a warm-up to set the mood and encourage attention. The leader explains the group's purpose, outlines the session, and delineates the time frame and expectations.

2. Activity—The leader chooses an activity designed to meet therapeutic goals. The activity is based on multiple factors, such as time constraints, the members' mental and physical abilities, and the leader's skill/knowledge. Other considerations for the activity include adaptations needed; amount of intended structure, creativity, or social interaction; and the specific method of instruction to implement the task.

3. Sharing—Group members show their work or explain their feelings. The group leader encourages participation and acknowledges each person verbally or nonverbally.

4. Processing—Group members express their feelings about the group experience and interactions with peers and leader. The underlying group dynamics may be explored.

5. Generalizing—The leader summarizes the learning aspects and general cognitive principles ascertained through the group process.

6. Application—The identified principles are applied to life situations. Practical methods are discussed, and the leader may provide limited self-disclosure to model solutions.

7. Summary—Important aspects of the group are emphasized briefly, such as goals and knowledge achieved. The leader notes any changes of behavior, and acknowledges and thanks members for their participation.

Learning Activity 8-1: Using Cole's Seven-Step Format— Eating Disorders

Imagine the facility you are working at is starting a new program for young adults with eating disorders. You are collaborating with the OT to develop an activities of daily living (ADL) group that will be implemented in this program. Consider occupational therapy discussion topics or activities relating to areas such as dressing, eating, shopping for food or clothing, health maintenance, and so forth. Choose a specific ADL or IADL and use Cole's Seven-Step Format for Group Leadership (2018) to help plan an entire group session for six clients. Determine how much time you will allocate for each stage of this group. Realize that actual activities used in an intervention program will depend upon the specific approach or frame of reference that the OT (and team) determines is appropriate for that setting and particular group of clients.

Frame of reference for activity: _____

Occupation to be addressed: _____

Activity: _____

Length of group: _____

1. *Introduction*: Time allocated: _____ minutes

    What specific words or actions will you use to greet the members and warm-up the group? How will you outline the group's purpose and expectations?

2. *Activity*: Time allocated: _____ minutes

    What specific activity will the group do? How and where will you set up the activity and position the clients? List the activity demands, such as equipment or supplies needed, specific content of any worksheets/written materials used, method of instruction, sequence of steps, and so forth.

3. *Sharing*: Time allocated: _____ minutes

    What would you like the members to share? What will you ask and do to encourage member participation?

4. *Processing*: Time allocated: _____ minutes

    What will you ask or say to encourage member participation? What aspects of the group process will you focus on?

5. *Generalizing*: Time allocated: _____ minutes

    What concepts do you want the clients to learn?

6. *Application*: Time allocated: _____ minutes

    How can this experience be applied to other life situations? What limited self-disclosure might you offer?

7. *Summary*: Time allocated: _____ minutes

    What will you say to summarize and provide a closing for the group?

Adapted from Cole, M. B. (2018). *Group dynamics in occupational therapy: The theoretical basis and practice application of group intervention* (5th ed.). SLACK Incorporated.

Worksheet 8-2

Social Skills Group—Picnic

Imagine you are leading an occupational therapy social skills group for clients with high cognitive abilities who have been allowed to go on a supervised community outing. The varied diagnoses of the group members include anxiety disorder, mood disorder, obsessive-compulsive disorder, and borderline personality disorder. After collaboration with the OT, you have determined that the group should plan and prepare a picnic lunch over the course of several sessions. Food items may be obtained from the facility's food service department (with 24 hours notice), and the facility has a transportation service. Consider some ways in which you can facilitate interaction among the group members to plan out this occupation. For each conversation starter idea you list for this egocentric-cooperative group, indicate a practical method (an activity) for implementing that discussion. Here is an example:

1. Topic:

    Encourage group members to determine a common menu, considering likes, dislikes, food allergies, dietary restrictions, and availability of items.

    Possible activity/method:

    Group leader provides each client with a worksheet listing 10 food choices. Clients number them in order of priority from 1 to 10.

    or

    Each client is provided with a list of all available food items to check off or circle one desired item in each category (e.g., beverage, dessert).

    Worksheet answers can be listed on a white board or flip chart. Group members discuss answers and decide on menu. Consider factors such as decision-making skills, cooperation, assertiveness, conflict resolution, and so forth.

2. Topic:

    Activity/Method:

3. Topic:

    Activity/Method:

4. Topic:

    Activity/Method:

Worksheet 8-2 (continued)
Social Skills Group—Picnic

5. Topic:

    Activity/Method:

6. Topic:

    Activity/Method:

7. Topic:

    Activity/Method:

8. Topic:

    Activity/Method:

9. Topic:

    Activity/Method:

10. Topic:

    Activity/Method:

Learning Activity 8-2: Four Current Events Groups

Imagine you are leading four separate occupational therapy current events groups (and collaborating with an OT when required by law for that setting). For each of the groups, choose a recent, interesting article from a newspaper to discuss with the group members. Pick a different article for each group, considering the therapeutic needs of the specific group. For each article, develop eight open-ended questions you might use as conversation starters to facilitate interaction among the group members. Determine the therapeutic purpose for each of the groups and incorporate occupational therapy group process skills. Indicate the lessons that members can learn from discussing the article and application to life situations.

For example, you might ask the group questions such as:

- *What is your opinion about that?*
- *What do you think will happen next?*
- *Why do you agree or disagree with that proposed law?*
- *Why is that important?*
- *What are the pros and cons of that?*
- *Can you describe a similar experience you had?*
- *What would you have done in the same situation?*
- *Why do you think he committed that crime?*
- *Do you think the punishment fits the crime? Why or why not?*

1. **Inpatient Behavioral Health Unit: Substance Use Disorder**

   You are an OTA working on an acute inpatient behavioral health unit. The group participants have high cognitive abilities and are diagnosed with substance use disorder.

   Topic of article:_____

   Purpose of group:_____

   General principles to be discussed/applied:_____

   Conversation starter questions:

   A.

   B.

   C.

   D.

   E.

   F.

   G.

   H.

2. **Senior Citizen Program**

You are an activity leader for a local senior citizen day program.

Topic of article:_____

Purpose of group:_____

General principles to be discussed/applied:_____

Conversation starter questions:

A.

B.

C.

D.

E.

F.

G.

H.

3. **Social Day Program: Intellectual and Developmental Disability**

You are an activity leader working in a social day program for young adults who live with their families. Each participant has a developmental disability with mild to moderate intellectual impairment. However, each participant has functional verbal skills.

Topic of article:_____

Purpose of group:_____

General principles to be discussed/applied:_____

Conversation starter questions:

A.

B.

C.

D.

E.

F.

G.

H.

4. **School Program: Bullying**

You are an OTA working in a school program designed to prevent bullying and are leading a small group of middle-school students.

Topic of article:_____

Purpose of group:_____

General principles to be discussed/applied:_____

Conversation starter questions:

A.

B.

C.

D.

E.

F.

G.

H.

Worksheet 8-3

Social Skills Group—Collage Craft

Imagine you are leading an occupational therapy social skills group for clients who have high cognitive abilities and varied mental health conditions, including mood disorders, anxiety, and substance use disorder. After collaboration with the OT, you have determined that the group members should work together to make one big collage. List 10 possible ways to facilitate interaction among group members as they are making the collage.

Here is an example: *Group participants must decide on a common theme such as "Happiness" or "Family."*

1.

2.

3.

4.

5.

6.

7.

8.

9.

10.

Morreale, M. J. (2022). *Developing clinical competence: A workbook for the OTA* (2nd ed.). SLACK Incorporated.

Learning Activity 8-3: Interventions in Mental Health— Frames of Reference

For each of the following occupational therapy groups, list the frame of reference you will utilize plus three activities appropriate for adult clients with *depression*. For these exercises, assume that you have collaborated with the OT.

Activity Group

Frame of reference:_____

List three craft projects that the client can choose from and explain why you chose each craft. For example, is the craft a quick-success project, or does it allow the client to express emotions? You will also need to decide if tasks will be performed individually or as a collaborative effort.

1.

2.

3.

According to the frame of reference, this particular activity was chosen because_____

_____

_____

Expressive Group

Frame of reference:_____

List three discussion topics or activities for this group and explain why you chose each one. For example, does the activity facilitate interpersonal skills or exploration of feelings?

1.

2.

3.

According to the frame of reference, this particular activity was chosen because_____

_____

ADL/IADL Group

Frame of reference:_____

List three possible ADL/IADL activities for this group and explain why you chose each one. For example, does the activity facilitate role performance or promote healthy habits?

1.

2.

3.

According to the frame of reference, this particular activity was chosen because_____

_____

_____

Learning Activity 8-4: More Interventions in Mental Health

For each of the following occupational therapy groups, list three activities appropriate for young adults diagnosed with *substance use disorder*. For this exercise, assume that you have collaborated with the OT.

Activity Group

Frame of reference:_____

List three craft projects that the client can choose from and explain why you chose each craft. For example, is the craft a quick-success project, or does it allow the client to express emotions? You will also need to decide if tasks will be performed individually or as a collaborative effort.

1.

2.

3.

According to the frame of reference, this particular activity was chosen because_____

_____

_____

Expressive Group

Frame of reference:_____

List three discussion topics or activities for this group and explain why you chose each one. For example, does the activity encourage client to express emotions or teach coping strategies?

1.

2.

3.

According to the frame of reference, this particular activity was chosen because_____

_____

_____

Leisure Group

Frame of reference:_____

List three possible activities for this group and explain why you chose each one. For example, does the activity develop leisure skills or help alleviate stress?

1.

2.

3.

According to the frame of reference, this particular activity was chosen because_____

_____

_____

Five-Stage Group Format Designed by Ross

Ross (1997) designed a Five-Stage Group format based on neurophysiological principles for clients who have low cognitive or social abilities, developmental disability, nonverbal/limited communication, or behavioral problems (e.g., hostility, acting out). Ross advocates a structured progression of sensory stimulation as a means to motivate the group, improve behavior and social skills, and help members process and organize information. Desired responses are elicited through sensory activities (e.g., vestibular, tactile, proprioceptive, visual) and these activities' effect on the central nervous system (Ross, 1997). Ross's Five-Stage Group format is briefly summarized below (Ross, 1997):

- Stage 1: Orientation—Introductions and a simple 1-minute activity (i.e., handle simple instruments, pass around items, use scents, noisemakers) to increase alertness, facilitate calmness and relaxation, and provide sensory stimulation.

- Stage 2: Movement—This stage consists of motor activities, such as reaching, walking, hopping, dance, or activities using props such as a parachute, ball, ribbon wand, scarves, hoops, and so forth.

- Stage 3: Visual-motor perceptual activities—Consists of more challenging tasks, such as puzzles, activities addressing body parts (e.g., Simon Says), and eye-hand coordination (e.g., golf putting, plastic bowling).

- Stage 4: Cognitive stimulation and function—Activities such as stories, short poems, discussions, memory and guessing games, and so forth are used to increase communication and help organize thoughts and behavior.

- Stage 5: Closing the session—A brief, familiar routine is used to signal the end of the session and provide positivity (e.g., a song, snack, hold hands).

Learning Activity 8-5: Assisted Living Facility— Using Ross's Five-Stage Group Format

Imagine you are an activity leader for the Alzheimer's unit in an assisted living facility. You would like to provide the residents with meaningful opportunities to reminisce, handle objects, engage in familiar activities, and socialize. Use Ross's Five-Stage Group format (1997) to design a group session. Create an activity box relating to a familiar occupation and plan the group around this theme. Keep in mind any safety concerns or dietary restrictions. An example of an activity box and relevant group activities for a session are provided.

Occupation	*IADL: Baking*	
Activity box contents	Egg beater, wooden spoon, spatula, small muffin tin, sifter, plastic measuring cups, measuring spoons, small rolling pin, cookie cutters	
Stage 1	Greeting and introduction Smell spices used in baking (e.g., vanilla, cinnamon, ginger)	
Stage 2	Roll out prepared sugar cookie dough with a rolling pin	
Stage 3	Cut out cookies with a cookie cutter and place on a cookie sheet	
Stage 4	Each group member selects a kitchen item to handle and name Reminisce about baking, favorite desserts	
Stage 5	Closing remarks, provide a snack that clients are medically allowed to eat (the baked cookies or an alternate snack)	

Worksheet 8-4

Therapeutic Responses

Provide the therapeutic response indicated to the client comments that follow.

1. "I am so confused by all of the rules and regulations surrounding Medicare reimbursement, I may just scream"

   Reflective listening response

   _____

   _____

2. "I just completed a 5K marathon in 6 hours"

   Affirmation

   _____

   _____

3. "I am looking forward to graduation"

   Open-ended question to gain specific information

   _____

   _____

4. "I had a couple of drinks last night, but I deserve it since I had not had one for 2 weeks"

   Therapeutic paradox

   _____

   _____

5. "I am sure you have never seen anyone with a stroke as bad as the one I have had; I will never do anything again"

   Normalizing statement

   _____

   _____

Worksheet 8-5

Behavioral Observation Skills in Mental Health

For each category, list specific behaviors that an occupational therapy practitioner might expect to see in a client who is depressed. Describe briefly how those behaviors might interfere with occupational performance.

Social Participation (include the following areas):

Intrapersonal factors:

Interpersonal behaviors:

Task behaviors:

Occupations:

ADL:

Rest and sleep:

Leisure:

Work/education:

After completing your list of behaviors, review the following case study carefully. Based on the client information provided, consider each of the behaviors you listed. Identify and circle any items on your list that are *actually observed* for Laurie while she is on the unit.

Case Study

Laurie, a 38-year-old bank teller, was admitted to an acute behavioral health unit with a diagnosis of depression. Following her spouse's death from cancer 3 months ago, Laurie states she has stopped attending her weekly college business class and her daily routine of going to the gym. She reports having frequent headaches and muscle tension in her upper back for the past 4 weeks. For the 2 weeks prior to admission, Laurie stayed in bed all day in her pajamas; missed work; lost weight due to decreased appetite; and did not answer phone calls, text messages, or email. She states that she is *"not good enough"* to return to work. When asked if she has contacted her college or job to discuss a medical leave, Laurie replied, *"Why bother?"* She denies suicidal ideation at this time. Laurie does not have any children. She has one sister who lives in the next town, and her parents live in a retirement community 1000 miles away.

Learning Activity 8-6: Schizophrenia— Using Allen's Cognitive Disabilities Model

Occupational therapy practitioners work with clients who have various mental health or physical conditions impacting functional cognition. One model used in occupational therapy practice is Claudia Allen's Cognitive Disabilities Model (1985), which can aid therapists in evaluation and intervention planning. Allen (1985) describes global characteristics for six distinct levels of cognitive function. Current information about this model and specific assessments used can be found at www.allen-cognitive-network.org.

For this exercise, imagine you are collaborating with your occupational therapy supervisor regarding three adults diagnosed with schizophrenia, each presently at one of the three levels designated in the boxes. The clients do not have any physical limitations but have been referred to occupational therapy to assess existing functional abilities, improve safety and occupational performance, and provide education to primary caregivers. From the following list, select 1 of the 14 activities/occupations that you will address with all three of these clients. Compare and contrast the kinds of occupational therapy interventions needed to meet the varied abilities of each client. Consider if each client is expected to achieve independence in this occupation or if the assistance of another person is likely needed to complete this activity safely. Use activity analysis to determine how the individuals will perform sequence of steps involved in this activity and consider any safety concerns. Assume you are partnering with the OT and describe the compensatory methods, equipment or occupational adaptations that are indicated for each client; specific types of cues needed (e.g., verbal, tactile, visual); and any family/caregiver education required (Morreale & Amini, 2016).

Activity/Occupation List:

1. Bowel and bladder management
2. Grooming (e.g., shaving, applying make-up, brushing teeth, nail care)
3. Dressing
4. Bathing
5. Using a cell phone or landline (include situations such as social calls, contacting service providers, dealing with telemarketers)
6. Feeding (e.g., managing finger foods, utensils, knife, cup)
7. Hair care (e.g., wash, get a haircut, self-style)
8. Health management (e.g., managing symptoms, obtaining medication, physical activity, nutrition)
9. Banking and paying bills
10. Care of a pet
11. Grocery shopping
12. Preparing breakfast (e.g., tea and toast)
13. Preparing lunch (e.g., soup and sandwich)
14. Community mobility

Occupation Selected That Requires Intervention	Client with Schizophrenia: Allen Level 2	Client with Schizophrenia: Allen Level 4	Client with Schizophrenia: Allen Level 5
Attainable assist level/ desired outcome (e.g. modified independence, mod, max assist)			
Probable setting where the client resides and where intervention will take place			
Safety concerns for task			
Aspects of task likely requiring set-up/assistance			
Compensatory methods, adaptive equipment and/ or durable medical equipment indicated			
Sequence of steps and instructional methods			
Family/caregiver education needed for this task			

Adapted from Morreale, M. J., & Amini, D. (2016). *The occupational therapist's workbook for ensuring clinical competence.* SLACK Incorporated.

Answers to Worksheets

Worksheet 8-1: Mental Health Situations

1. C. For safety reasons, the OTA should keep the door open and ensure that a staff member is in the vicinity in case the client becomes aggressive. Information provided indicates client needs an individual session.

2. A. A client can use a mop or broom as a weapon (Early, 2009).

3. B. While a timer could possibly work, it is not the best option as it could create more stress for the client and lessen feelings of self-control. A full closet of craft options may be too overwhelming for this client, so minimizing the choices to two options would be more suitable to facilitate decision making. Having others choose the project would not allow for the client to experience any self-control or decision making.

4. C. The only choice consisting of a gross-motor activity is the beach ball activity.

5. A. If a client is becoming out of control, it is best for the OTA to call for help, talk in a calm voice, and remove other clients from the area. Physically restraining a client should be avoided and used only as a last resort (Early, 2009).

6. D. To help ensure safety, an occupational therapy practitioner must carefully keep track of sharps and other hazardous objects, such as string and yarn. Items with fumes (e.g., stains, dyes) can also be dangerous (Early, 2009).

7. B. A client experiencing hallucinations would benefit from activities that are structured (i.e., familiar tasks to help the client to maintain appropriate focus [Early, 2009]).

8. C. The client is acting on his obsessive thoughts and demonstrating compulsive behavior.

9. A. An OTA should always use professional reasoning to distinguish between a true medical emergency versus the client's pattern of panic attacks and act accordingly. For a panic attack, generally the first course of action is to encourage the client to take slow, deep breaths to help the anxiety to pass.

10. C. A wire hanger, glass, and cords can be used by a client to harm self or others (Early, 2009).

Worksheet 8-2: Social Skills Group—Picnic

In general, the OTA should facilitate positive interaction among group members; provide necessary feedback regarding appropriate and inappropriate language/behavior exhibited; and provide opportunities for socialization, leisure, and learning, such as application of the group experience to life and strategies (Cole, 2018). Here are some practical suggestions to facilitate interaction among group members for this picnic task but you may come up with other ideas that could also be appropriate. Realize these are only examples of best practice and may not be suitable for each group of clients. Actual implementation and choice of a specific method or activity will depend upon the particular approach or frame of reference that the OT (and team) determines is appropriate for a particular group of clients.

1. Topic:

    Encourage group members to determine a common menu, considering likes, dislikes, food allergies, dietary restrictions, and availability of items.

    Possible activity/method:

    Group leader provides each client with a worksheet listing 10 food choices. Clients number them in order of priority from 1 to 10.

    or

    Each client is provided with a list of all available food items to check off or circle one desired item in each category (e.g., beverage, dessert).

Worksheet answers can be listed on a white board or flip chart. Group members discuss answers and decide on menu. Consider factors such as decision-making skills, cooperation, assertiveness, conflict resolution, and so forth.

2. Topic:

    Group members can discuss feelings/attitudes toward picnics or going outdoors, considering past experiences, and anticipation of task.

    Activity/Method:

    Have client anonymously write a word or phrase on an index card describing personal feelings toward the upcoming picnic activity, such as fun, anxious, relaxing, boring, and so forth, and place it in a basket for discussion.

    or

    Worksheet: Each client circles or checks off from a list of emotions to describe how the client is feeling regarding the upcoming picnic, then discusses.

3. Topic:

    Once menu has been decided, group members must determine a list of all items needed for the picnic.

    Activity/Method:

    Group leader (or member) writes down member suggestions on a large flip chart or white board. Can list by categories (specific food items/condiments, eating and serving equipment, recreational items, etc.).

4. Topic:

    Group members must determine time frames for preparatory tasks (e.g., order food 2 days prior, bake cupcakes 1 day prior, make sandwiches morning of the picnic).

    Activity/Method:

    Group leader (or member) writes down list of steps and member suggestions on a large flip chart or white board. Discuss factors such as organization and time management.

5. Topic:

    Group members must decide on a picnic location within a certain radius.

    Activity/Method:

    Group leader provides each client with a worksheet listing five choices of locations. Clients are asked to number them in order of priority from 1 to 5 and then discuss and decide on location. The pros and cons can be written on a flip chart or white board.

6. Topic:

    Group members should discuss alternatives if it rains.

    Activity/Method:

    Worksheet: Clients write down two alternative solutions or choose from a list of possible alternatives. Member suggestions can be written on a flip chart or white board for discussion.

7. Topic:

Group members can plan for other recreational activities at picnic site, such as sedentary or active leisure tasks.

Activity/Method:

Each member fills out leisure inventory/checklist. Clients choose two items to suggest to the rest of group or write them on index cards and place in a basket for discussion. Consider factors of cooperation and compromise.

8. Topic:

Group members must plan how food items will be prepared (e.g., Will the food service department provide premade sandwiches? Will each person prepare their own sandwich? Will each member prepare a component of the meal for everyone? Will the group bake a batch of cookies together?)

Activity/Method:

List options on flip chart or white board, discuss, and decide. Consider factors such as food safety, decision making, cooperation.

9. Topic:

Cooperation/compromise/conflict resolution.

Activity/Method:

Perform a meal preparation task, such as baking cookies or preparing a salad, for which group members must work cooperatively and share kitchen tools, spices, plastic wrap, and so forth.

10. Topic:

Favorite recipes (their own or borrowed).

Activity/Method:

Members can look up recipes for various picnic foods or bring a familiar recipe to share with the group. Group members can discuss or teach their own method/recipe for the meal components, such as a favorite recipe for cookies or potato salad.

or

Members can use a worksheet to list one or more favorite homemade foods and answer discussion questions, such as if this food is healthy/unhealthy, a special treat, a childhood favorite, holiday related, how often it was available, emotions evoked, and so forth.

11. Topic:

Group members must decide how food will be packed (e.g., individual boxed lunches or shared platters of food).

Activity/Method:

List options on flip chart or white board and discuss. Consider factors such as food safety, decision making, cooperation.

12. Topic:

   After the outing, group members can discuss/critique the prepared food, picnic outing experience, and interaction with peers.

   Activity/Method:

   Have each client anonymously write a word or phrase on an index card describing their emotions regarding the picnic activity, such as fun, anxious, relaxing, stupid, and so forth, and place in a basket for discussion.

or

   Worksheet: Each client circles or checks off from a list describing how the client felt regarding the picnic and then discusses their choices.

or

   Worksheet: Rate each category (e.g., food, location, overall experience) on a scale from 0 to 10, then discuss.

13. Topic:

   Group members can discuss general feelings/attitudes toward food (e.g., emotional eating, comfort foods, healthy/unhealthy foods).

   Activity/Method:

   Worksheet: Have client write down specific foods that they usually eat in various designated situations, such as when feeling stressed, watching television, needing energy, as a reward/treat, and so forth.

Worksheet 8-3: Social Skills Group—Collage Craft

The OTA should encourage positive interaction among group members and provide feedback regarding appropriate/inappropriate language and behavior exhibited. Here are some suggestions to facilitate interaction among group members as they are making the collage.

1. Group participants must decide on a common theme such as "Happiness" or "Family." They may be provided with a list to choose from if more structure is needed.
2. Ask a group member who has made a collage before to teach others how to do the craft.
3. Limit materials so that clients will have to share (e.g., only one bottle of glue).
4. Ask group members to divide up the activity demands and decide who will do what aspects of the project (e.g., one person has to find magazines on the unit, another person has to clear and set up the work surface with newspapers).
5. Ask group members to explain why they chose the pictures they did.
6. Ask group members to comment on others' pictures.
7. Group members can be asked to collaboratively decide on picture placement.
8. Ask group members to decide on other possible art materials to decorate the collage (e.g., glitter, foam letters).
9. Ask group members to discuss or critique the finished product.
10. Create some situations to address frustration tolerance, facilitate problem-solving or decision-making skills, such as creating time constraints, running out of some materials, or establishing additional criteria (e.g., cannot use a picture of a person or all words must have red letters).
11. Ask group members to discuss their feelings regarding participation in this activity.
12. Ask group members to decide where to place the finished collage.

Worksheet 8-4: Therapeutic Responses

Resource: Rollnick et al., 2007

1. *"I hear you saying the Medicare rules and regulations are difficult to keep straight and it affects your ability to do your job."*
2. *"I can see how proud you are of your accomplishment. It is great that you were able to complete your very first attempt at a 5K."*
3. *"Please tell me more about the aspect of graduation that you are looking forward to the most."*
4. *"I think it is time for you to consider managing your alcoholism on your own. You do not seem ready to take help from anyone else."*
5. *"I know that things seem very difficult now, but I have worked with people who have also had significant strokes who have been able to return to many of their activities."*

Worksheet 8-5: Behavioral Observation Skills in Mental Health

Each client is different, but some of the following suggestions are presented as possible symptoms of depression that an occupational therapy practitioner might observe. Tufano (2003) urges caution when depressed clients show sudden peacefulness and behavioral changes along with sudden declaration that depression is resolved. This new vigor, for some clients, could be an indicator of suicidality (Tufano, 2003). Giving away of items can also be a warning sign. Laurie may exhibit other behaviors during her hospitalization or during group activities, but these are not noted in the case study.

1. Intrapersonal factors
- Expresses feelings of hopelessness, intense sadness, depression, or suicidal ideation (note specific statements); *Laurie states "Not good enough" to return to work and "Why bother?" Denies suicidal ideation.*
- Verbalizes negative attributes about self (note specific statements). *Laurie states "Not good enough" to return to work.*
- Expresses negative outlook regarding future or ability to cope (note specific statements). *Laurie states, "Why bother?" regarding contacting her boss and college.*
- Crying exhibited *Not noted in case scenario*
- Somatic complaints; *Laurie reports frequent headaches and muscle tension in her upper back*
- Inability to identify coping mechanisms for dealing with a depressed mood (e.g., does not identify people client can contact to discuss feelings, expresses unwillingness to exercise/go for a 15-minute walk). *Prior to admission Laurie stopped going to the gym and stopped answering emails, texts, or phone calls. However, the information presented does not indicate specifically if she can or cannot now identify the coping strategies that would be personally beneficial to her.*

2. Interpersonal behaviors
- Lack of eye contact (describe situation) *Not noted in case scenario*
- Flat affect/does not smile *Not noted in case scenario*
- Does not initiate conversation *Not noted specifically in case scenario*
- Uncommunicative or minimal level of engagement in conversation (note length and type of responses); *The scenario does not indicate if Laurie is presently not answering phone calls or responding to text messages or email. The scenario does indicate some level of responsiveness but does not specify the full extent.*

3. Task behaviors
- Refuses or minimally participates in group activities (note how often and for how long) *Not noted in case scenario*
- Poor task initiation *Not noted in case scenario*
- Poor decision making (describe what happens when presented with choosing an activity/craft project or components such as colors or materials) *Not noted in case scenario*
- Does not complete project/gives up *Not noted in case scenario*

- Poor attention to detail/does not recognize or correct errors (describe/give examples) *Not noted in case scenario*
- Low frustration tolerance (describe the situation and behavior) *Not noted in case scenario*

4. Areas of occupation
- ADLs
  - Change in appetite (note specific amount eaten and/or types of foods); *Laurie lost weight prior to admission due to decreased appetite. It is not noted if Laurie's eating patterns have changed since she was admitted.*
  - Specific weight loss or gain; *Laurie has lost weight recently due to decreased appetite although exact amount is not noted. This will need to be monitored on unit.*
  - Lacks initiation to get out of bed (note amount of cueing/assistance needed); *Prior to admission Laurie had stayed in bed all day. However, it is not noted if she is continuing this pattern of behavior on the unit.*
  - Lacks initiation to get dressed or shower (note amount of cueing/assistance needed); *Prior to admission, Laurie had stayed in bed all day in her pajamas. However, it is not noted if she is presently getting dressed on the unit.*
  - Inattention to grooming and hygiene (describe) *Not noted in scenario*
- Rest and sleep
  - Atypical amount of time sleeping or inability to sleep (note sleep patterns) *Current status not noted*
  - Reports poor sleep quality *Current status not noted*
- Leisure
  - Withdraws from regular leisure routine; *Laurie reports she had stopped her daily routine of going to the gym.*
  - Does not express interest in resuming leisure activities *Not specifically noted now*
  - Refuses or demonstrates limited participation in leisure activities on unit (specific tasks, length of time, level of participation *Not noted in scenario*
  - Expresses unwillingness to resume her exercise regimen or go for a 15-minute walk with staff *Not specifically noted*
- Work/education
  - Misses work or school; *Laurie reports prior to admission she had stopped attending her weekly college business class and for the past 2 weeks had also missed work.*
  - Expresses lack of desire to return to work and/or school; *Laurie states, "Why bother?"*
  - Difficulty with initiating contact with employer or teachers for a plan to return to work, complete studies, or arrange for a medical leave; *Laurie states, "Why bother?"*

References

Allen, C. K. (1985). *Occupational therapy for psychiatric diseases: Measurement and management of cognitive disabilities.* Little, Brown and Company.

American Occupational Therapy Association. (2020). Occupational therapy practice framework: Domain and process (4th ed.). *American Journal of Occupational Therapy, 74*(Suppl. 2), 7412410010. https://doi.org/10.5014/ajot.2020.74S2001

Cole, M. (2018). *Group dynamics in occupational therapy: The theoretical basis and practice application of group intervention* (5th ed.). SLACK Incorporated.

Early, M. B. (2009). *Mental health concepts and techniques for the occupational therapy assistant* (4th ed.). Lippincott Williams & Wilkins.

Morreale, M. J., & Amini, D. (2016). *The occupational therapist's workbook for ensuring clinical competence.* SLACK Incorporated.

Pfeiffer, J., & Jones, J. (1977). *Reference guide to handbooks and annuals* (2nd ed.). University Associates.

Rollnick, S., Miller, W., & Butler, C. (2007). *Motivational interviewing in health care: Helping patients change behavior.* The Guilford Press.

Ross, M. (1997). *Integrative group therapy: Mobilizing coping abilities with the five-stage group.* American Occupational Therapy Association.

Scaffa, M. E. (2019). Group process and group intervention. In B. A. Boyt Schell & G. Gillen (Eds.), *Willard and Spackman's occupational therapy* (13th ed., pp. 539-555). Wolters Kluwer.

Taylor, R. R. (2008). *The intentional relationship: Occupational therapy and use of self.* F. A. Davis Company.

Taylor, R. R. (2019). Therapeutic relationship and client collaboration. In B. A. Boyt Schell & G. Gillen (Eds.), *Willard and Spackman's occupational therapy* (13th ed., pp. 527-538). Wolters Kluwer.

Taylor, R. R. (2020). *The intentional relationship: Occupational therapy and use of self* (2nd ed.). F. A. Davis Company.

Tufano, R. (2003). Mental health occupational therapy (suicidality: section 6-31). In K. Sladyk (Ed.), *OT study cards in a box.* SLACK Incorporated.

Tufano, R. (2015). Group intervention. In K. Sladyk & S. E. Ryan (Eds.), *Ryan's occupational therapy assistant: Principles, practice issues, and techniques* (5th ed., pp. 445-462). SLACK Incorporated.

Demonstrating Knowledge and Skills for Different Practice Settings

Different types of occupational therapy settings require specialized knowledge and skills unique to those practice areas. Occupational therapists (OTs) and occupational therapy assistants (OTAs) working in hospitals, nursing homes, home care, and inpatient and outpatient rehabilitation facilities provide skilled interventions that address safety, improve or manage specific client factors/skills, and incorporate a variety of methods to support clients' health, wellness, and engagement in areas such as activities of daily living (ADLs), instrumental activities of daily living (IADLs), and work. In educational settings, occupational therapy focuses on the activities and occupations that the child needs to succeed in school. Interventions may include recommendations for the classroom (such as sensory strategies or assistive technology) or remediation of the student's underlying weaknesses or challenges that hinder educational performance. Early intervention addresses the needs of young children with (or at risk for) developmental delay, including the contexts that hinder or support development.

The worksheets and learning activities in this chapter focus on knowledge and skills necessary for understanding the needs of adults and children with physical conditions. OTs and OTAs should have an understanding of basic pharmacology, various health devices, and medical procedures impacting occupational performance. Practitioners must adhere to medical precautions/contraindications for various conditions and circumstances, and use professional reasoning to implement skilled interventions safely and effectively (Morreale & Amini, 2016). Note that space limitations in this chapter allow for only select initial evaluation data to be presented in these exercises. A "real" evaluation would include more complete information, such as the specific aspects of occupations needing assistance and the various factors, contexts, or performance skills hindering or supporting occupational performance. Answers to worksheet exercises are provided at the end of the chapter.

Contents

Morreale, M. J. Developing Clinical Competence:
A Workbook for the OTA, Second Edition (pp. 359-405).
© 2022 SLACK Incorporated.

Worksheet 9-1

Diseases and Conditions

List another applicable name for the following diseases and conditions listed.

1. Diplopia_____

2. Herpes zoster _____

3. Thrombus _____

4. Cerebrovascular accident _____

5. Ecchymosis _____

6. Lou Gehrig's disease _____

7. Dyspnea _____

8. Golfer's elbow _____

9. Degenerative joint disease _____

10. Adhesive capsulitis _____

11. Tennis elbow_____

12. Varicella _____

13. Conjunctivitis _____

14. Gamekeeper's thumb _____

15. Epstein-Barr virus_____

16. Ewing sarcoma _____

17. Barlow's syndrome _____

18. Decubitus ulcer_____

19. Hypoglycemia_____

20. Myocardial infarction_____

21. Hypertension _____

22. Hyperemesis _____

23. Colles fracture_____

Worksheet 9-1 (continued)

Diseases and Conditions

24. Hyperlipidemia _____

25. Hematuria _____

26. Osteogenesis imperfecta _____

27. Trisomy 21 _____

28. Strabismus _____

29. Rubella _____

30. Rubeola _____

Learning Activity 9-1: Defining Diseases and Conditions

Define the following diseases and conditions briefly.

1. Bell's palsy

2. Marfan syndrome

3. Pick's disease

4. *Clostridioides difficile*

5. Klinefelter's syndrome

6. Thoracic outlet syndrome

7. Williams syndrome

8. Charcot-Marie-Tooth disease

9. Orthostatic hypotension

10. Arthrogryposis

11. Kawasaki disease

12. Rett syndrome

13. Huntington's disease

14. Complex regional pain syndrome

15. Korsakoff's syndrome

16. Paget's disease

17. Tay-Sachs disease

18. Sjögren's syndrome

19. Myasthenia gravis

20. Guillain-Barré syndrome

21. Coronary artery disease

22. Ketoacidosis

23. Syncope

24. Atrial fibrillation

25. Congestive heart failure

Worksheet 9-2

Common Medications

Match each of the conditions in the following boxes to one of the brand name or generic medications listed. Although some of these medications may be used to treat multiple health problems, list each of the following conditions only once. Realize that other medications not listed here might be used to treat that same condition instead.

Multiple sclerosis	Infection	Pain	Angina
Osteoarthritis	Hypertension	Schizophrenia	Diabetes
Osteoporosis	Parkinson's disease	Gout	Thrombus
Atrial fibrillation	Cancer	Depression	Dementia
Fluid retention	Anxiety	Attention deficit disorder	Seizure
Shingles	Psoriatic arthritis	Crohn's disease	Asthma

1. Eliquis _____

2. Nitroglycerin _____

3. Naproxen sodium _____

4. Aricept _____

5. Risperdal _____

6. Atenolol _____

7. Cymbalta _____

8. Boniva _____

9. Levodopa _____

10. Topamax _____

11. Demerol _____

12. Methotrexate _____

13. Adderall _____

14. Lexapro _____

15. Proventil _____

16. Augmentin _____

17. Avonex _____

18. Acyclovir _____

Worksheet 9-2 (continued)
Common Medications

19. Humulin R _____

20. Lasix _____

21. Humira _____

22. Heparin_____

23. Enbrel _____

24. Allopurinol _____

Worksheet 9-3
Generic Medications

Match the brand name medications in the following box to the generic equivalent listed.

Neurontin	Aleve	Diovan	Valium
Advil	Lasix	Slow-FE	Tylenol
Tums	Coumadin	Cymbalta	Cardizem
Vasotec	Humulin R	Prozac	Klonopin
Prilosec	Ventolin	Vicodin	Paxil
Xanax	Norvasc	Lipitor	Tenormin

1. Warfarin _____

2. Omeprazole_____

3. Ibuprofen _____

4. Diazepam _____

5. Naproxen sodium _____

6. Hydrocodone bitartrate _____

7. Albuterol _____

8. Gabapentin _____

9. Atorvastatin calcium _____

10. Clonazepam _____

11. Enalapril maleate _____

12. Alprazolam _____

13. Insulin_____

14. Fluoxetine hydrochloride _____

15. Diltiazem _____

16. Acetaminophen_____

17. Paroxetine_____

18. Ferrous sulfate _____

19. Valstartin _____

Worksheet 9-3 (continued)
Generic Medications

20. Calcium carbonate _____

21. Atenolol_____

22. Furosemide _____

23. Amlodipine_____

24. Duloxetine _____

Learning Activity 9-2: Medical Devices

Clients with acute or chronic medical conditions may undergo special procedures or require temporary or long-term use of various medical devices. It is essential that occupational therapy practitioners working with those clients have knowledge of the particular devices and procedures used that can impact occupational therapy intervention and client recovery. Define the medical terms in the table below and list several conditions that would necessitate their use. For each device/condition listed, indicate any precautions impacting occupational therapy intervention and possible effect on a client's ADL performance (e.g., mobility, dressing, sexual activity).

Medical Devices and Procedures	Definition	Possible Conditions Requiring Use	Precautions	Effect on Occupational Performance
Left ventricular assist device (LVAD)				
Suprapubic catheter				
Foley catheter				
Central venous catheter/central line				
Peripherally inserted central catheter (PICC line)				
Implanted venous access port				
Tunneled central venous catheter				
Nasogastric tube (NG-tube)				
Percutaneous endoscopic gastrostomy (PEG)				
Gastric feeding tube (G-tube)				
Nasal cannula				
Percutaneous pinning				
External fixation device				
Tracheostomy				
Sequential compression device				
Neurostimulator/drug pump				
Halo				

Reproduced with permission from Morreale, M. J., & Amini, D. (2016). *The occupational therapist's workbook for ensuring clinical competence.* SLACK Incorporated.

Learning Activity 9-3: Medical Devices and Procedures Terminology

Define the following medical terms.

Incentive spirometer:

Nebulizer:

Hyperbaric oxygen therapy:

Bag-valve-mask:

Peak flow meter:

Pulse oximeter:

Endoscopy:

Gastrostomy:

Jejunostomy:

Enteral nutrition:

Gavage:

Lavage:

Stent:

Glucometer:

Insulin pen:

Morreale, M. J. (2022). *Developing clinical competence: A workbook for the OTA* (2nd ed.). SLACK Incorporated.

Insulin pump:

Sphygmomanometer:

Define stoma/stomata (surgical) and list five examples:

1.

2.

3.

4.

5.

Indicate several situations in which a client may be required to use a condom catheter instead of an indwelling catheter and the challenges associated with the use of that device.

1.

2.

3.

Worksheet 9-4

Wheeled Mobility

1. Michelle is a 62-year-old widowed female with a progressive neurological condition. She was referred to occupational therapy for a wheelchair assessment due to decline in functional status. She has been non-ambulatory for the past 3 months and requires moderate assistance to transfer. Michelle moved in with her sister who has a hard time pushing Michelle in a standard adult wheelchair because Michelle weighs 195 lb. The OT determined that Michelle's impairment in upper extremity function necessitates use of a joystick for wheeled mobility independence. Michelle has good functional cognition and states she would like to resume her part-time work as a greeter for a large discount store. She also desires to volunteer 1 day a week as a catechism teacher at her church. The city she lives in provides door-to-door transit service for wheelchair users. Which of the following mobility devices would be more suitable for Michelle to use?
   A. Power mobility scooter
   B. Reclining wheelchair with a Roho seat cushion
   C. Folding travel wheelchair with a foam seat cushion
   D. Tilt in space power wheelchair with a gel seat cushion

2. Derek, an 18-year-old-male weighing 185 lb, has a diagnosis of paraplegia due to a random drive-by shooting outside the local mall 4 months ago. Prior to the gun shot incident, Derek planned on attending college as a marketing major and was admitted on a full basketball scholarship. He is presently using a lightweight manual wheelchair independently. Which of the following types of wheelchairs is a possible choice for an occupational therapy practitioner to recommend to Derek?
   A. Power wheelchair
   B. Bariatric wheelchair
   C. Sports wheelchair
   D. Power mobility scooter

3. An OTA has collaborated with the OT and is ordering a wheelchair for a child with multiple needs. The child has unwanted movements due to poorly integrated primitive reflexes, kyphotic and left leaning posture due to poor trunk control, and excessive hip adduction. Which of the following is a possible choice for the OTA to specify in the wheelchair order?
   A. Pommel extending from in-between knees to groin
   B. Seat back at level of inferior angle of scapula
   C. Right lateral support insert
   D. Headrest and chest strap

4. Leticia, a 45-year-old female diagnosed with multiple sclerosis (MS), lives with her husband and 20-year-old daughter in a wheelchair-accessible apartment. Leticia can transfer independently but is unable to stand for more than several minutes or perform functional ambulation safely for long distances. Due to symptoms of MS and a chronic, painful left shoulder condition, Leticia fatigues easily when self-propelling her standard wheelchair. She desires to continue working as a school psychologist and maintain independence in IADLs such as driving and shopping. Which of the following mobility options would be more suitable for Leticia to use?
   A. Power mobility scooter
   B. One-arm-drive wheelchair
   C. Tilt in space power wheelchair
   D. Rollator

Worksheet 9-4 (continued)
Wheeled Mobility

5. Claudio, a 69-year-old male who is 5'6" and weighs 148 lb, has a diagnosis of left cerebrovascular accident (CVA) resulting in right hemiplegia. He was recently admitted to a rehabilitation hospital with expected discharge to home in approximately 2 weeks. The OT evaluation indicates Claudio does not have any functional cognitive deficits. One of Claudio's goals is wheeled mobility independence, as it is not likely he will be able to ambulate independently at time of discharge. Which of the following wheelchairs would be more suitable for an occupational therapy practitioner to recommend for him?
   A. Adult bariatric wheelchair
   B. One-arm-drive wheelchair
   C. Power wheelchair
   D. Ultralight wheelchair

6. For a client with bilateral lower extremity amputations, in which of the following ways is an "amputee" wheelchair different than a standard wheelchair?
   A. The rear wheel axles are in a more posterior position
   B. The rear wheel axles are in a more anterior position
   C. The caster wheels are larger than the rear wheels
   D. It has four anti-tippers attached

7. When an occupational therapy practitioner is measuring a client for a standard wheelchair, which of the following methods is correct?
   A. Seat depth should be 1.5 to 2 in. wider than client's hips
   B. Seat back height should be level with superior angle of scapula
   C. Armrest height should be measured with client's elbow placed in approximately 90 degrees of flexion
   D. The front edge of seat should reach to the back of client's knees

8. Andrew is a 42-year-old male carpenter who recently sustained an incomplete lumbar-level spinal cord injury (SCI) due to falling off a deck that he was working on. The OT and OTA determined that the safest way for Andrew to transfer is for him to use a sliding board. When ordering his wheelchair for home use, which of the following wheelchair options is probably less suitable to include?
   A. Removable front rigging
   B. Removable arm rests
   C. Scissors lock
   D. Toggle lock

9. Omar is an 80-year-old male admitted recently to a rehabilitation hospital with a diagnosis of Guillain-Barré syndrome. He is beginning to regain gross motor function in his upper extremities but has poor trunk control. The OTA observes that Omar tends to slide forward while seated in his wheelchair and is at risk for falling. A wheelchair lap belt with an attached buckle would be considered a restraint as Omar is not able to unfasten it independently. Which of the following is a possible choice for the OTA to try next to keep Omar seated safely in the wheelchair?
   A. Wheelchair seat alarm
   B. Adbuction wedge
   C. Lap belt with a loop Velcro closure
   D. Lap board

Worksheet 9-4 (continued)

Wheeled Mobility

10. When a client is about to perform a standing pivot transfer from wheelchair to bed, the OTA should instruct the client to do which of the following for safety?
    A. Disengage the toggle
    B. Lock the front rigging in place
    C. Close the footplates
    D. All of the above

Adapted from Morreale, M. J., & Amini, D. (2016). *The occupational therapist's workbook for ensuring clinical competence.* SLACK Incorporated.

Worksheet 9-5

Speech and Language

Indicate which of the following terms are typically used in documentation to describe speech and/or language.

1. _____ Dysarthria

2. _____ Dysphagia

3. _____ Dystonia

4. _____ Dysphonia

5. _____ Cadence

6. _____ Dysrhythmia

7. _____ Aspiration

8. _____ Intelligibility

9. _____ Shuttering

10. _____ Intonation

11. _____ Apraxia of speech

12. _____ Hemianopsia

13. _____ Aphasia

14. _____ Dysphasia

15. _____ Fluency

16. _____ Articulation

17. _____ Dysthymia

18. _____ Anomia

19. _____ Dysesthesia

20. _____ Pitch

Worksheet 9-6

Feeding and Eating

OTs and OTAs intervene with clients of all ages who have challenges in feeding and eating. According to estimates, approximately 590 million people or about 8% of the world's population are affected by dysphagia (Cichero et al., 2017). The American Occupational Therapy Association's (AOTA's) guidelines *The Practice of Occupational Therapy in Feeding, Eating, and Swallowing* (AOTA, 2017) outlines service delivery areas suitable for OT and OTA entry-level practice for these occupations and also delineates the specialized interventions requiring advanced-level knowledge and skills.

The International Dysphagia Diet Standardisation Initiative (IDDSI) is a non-profit organization that has established world-wide, standardized definitions and terminology for liquids and texture-modified foods for individuals of all ages with dysphagia (Cichero et al., 2017). The IDDSI's multi-professional group of international volunteers created a framework, released in 2015, that provides detailed guidelines for seven food levels and four drink levels using standardized, culturally sensitive nomenclature to improve dysphagia management and provide consistency in research and clinical practice (Cichero et al., 2017; IDDSI, 2019a). The IDDSI framework can be found at the IDDSI website at https://iddsi.org/ along with additional free resources for health care workers and patient education handouts. Answer the following multiple choice questions to test your basic knowledge in the area of feeding and eating.

1. When reviewing a client's chart today, an OTA sees the acronym NPO in the physician's orders. The OTA should understand this to mean which of the following?
   A. Nothing but puréed foods overnight
   B. No patient orders
   C. Keep nasopharynx open
   D. Nothing by mouth

2. Which of the following reflects the oral transit phase in a normal swallow?
   A. Lips close, food/liquid are manipulated within mouth with saliva mixing in
   B. The tongue moves the prepared bolus posteriorly
   C. Prepared bolus moves from base of tongue into the pharynx
   D. Bolus moves into the esophagus

3. Which of the following is a swallow study used by rehabilitation therapists with specialized training?
   A. Videofluoroscopy
   B. Peak flow test
   C. Colposcopy
   D. Spirometry

4. Rakesh is a 78-year-old male presently in a skilled nursing facility for short-term rehabilitation. He sustained a right CVA, which resulted in mild swallowing difficulties and hemiparesis of his left, non-dominant upper extremity and left lower limb. He has good functional cognition, fair dynamic sitting balance, and ability to transfer with minimum assistance. When working on self-feeding interventions with Rakesh, which of the following positions is more suitable for an OTA to place him in?
   A. Sitting in a reclined Geri chair with affected limb supported on tray rest and feet supported flat on footrest
   B. Sitting on side of bed with affected limb supported adjacent to food tray on the overbed table
   C. Sitting in bed with head of bed raised to 30 degrees and affected limb supported on a pillow
   D. Sitting in wheelchair at a table with affected limb supported on table and feet flat on floor

Worksheet 9-6 (continued)
Feeding and Eating

5. When working on self-feeding interventions with adults who have swallowing difficulties, which of the following is generally more suitable for an OTA to do?
    A. Instruct client to hyperextend neck when swallowing
    B. Have client take sips of water after each bite of food is swallowed
    C. Utilize tongue sweeps to promote oral pocketing of food
    D. Encourage multiple swallows after each bite

6. When an OTA is working on self-feeding interventions with an adult client, all except which of the following observations are possible warning signs that dysphagia is happening?
    A. Wet-sounding voice
    B. Use of dentures
    C. Pocketing of food
    D. Coughing while eating or drinking

7. Advanced techniques for swallowing require specialized training and include all except which of the following methods?
    A. Epley maneuver
    B. Valsalva maneuver
    C. Mendelsohn maneuver
    D. Supraglottic swallow

8. An adult client with dysphagia has physician orders for a diet using IDDSI guidelines for Level 6 soft and bite-sized foods. When working on self-feeding interventions, which of the following is a possible food choice for an OTA to use with the client?
    A. Plain white bread cut in no bigger than 2 cm by 2 cm pieces
    B. Soft, boiled vegetables no bigger than 1.5 cm by 1.5 cm cooked pieces
    C. Fresh pineapple
    D. Plain sticky rice that separates into individual grains when cooked and served

9. According to the IDDSI framework, which of the following statements is not correct about transitional foods?
    A. Tongue strength alone cannot break down these foods once softened
    B. They do not require biting
    C. They begin as one texture but change into another texture when moisture or temperature change occurs
    D. They require minimal chewing

10. A young child with dysphagia has physician orders for a diet using IDDSI guidelines for Level 3 liquedfied foods and moderately thick liquids. When working on self-feeding interventions, which of the following is a possible choice for an OTA to use with the child?
    A. Apple juice with a straw
    B. Infant formula with a bottle
    C. Grape juice with a sippy cup
    D. Runny rice cereal with a spoon

Worksheet 9-7

Home Care

1. An OTA arrives at a client's home for a scheduled occupational therapy visit. The OTA rings the doorbell several times, but no one answers. The OTA should perform which primary action?
   A. Use a cell phone to call 911
   B. Use a cell phone to call the OT
   C. Use a cell phone to call the client
   D. Leave and document that no one answered the door

2. An OTA arrives at an 80-year-old female client's home for a scheduled occupational therapy visit. A person answers the door and introduces herself as the client's niece who is visiting from out of town. She tells the OTA that the client is upstairs napping. The niece asks the OTA to explain why her aunt was hospitalized recently and wants to know what her aunt needs to work on in therapy. Which of the following should be the OTA's primary action?
   A. Help the client's niece to understand the client's condition and intervention plan
   B. Wake the client up and ask for permission to talk to her niece
   C. Call the OT and ask the OT to explain the intervention plan to the niece
   D. Cancel today's appointment, document the client is sleeping, and reschedule for tomorrow

3. For clients with Medicare who require that occupational therapy services be provided at their residence, the guidelines for home care must be followed except if the client is living in which of the following settings?
   A. A relative's home
   B. An assisted living facility
   C. A skilled nursing facility
   D. Subsidized apartment in senior housing complex

4. An OTA is providing home care services to a client diagnosed with Sjögren's syndrome, hypertension, and Type 2 diabetes. Today the client expresses that he is thirsty and nauseous, and the OTA observes that the client has labored breathing with a fruity breath odor. The OTA might conclude that the client is at possible risk for which of the following?
   A. Hypoglycemia
   B. Ketoacidosis
   C. Diaphoresis
   D. Orthostatic hypotension

5. A client diagnosed with congestive heart failure disease has Medicare and is receiving home care services following a recent hospitalization. He lives alone and exhibits deficits in endurance that limit his ability to perform IADLs, such as meal preparation, laundry, shopping, and yardwork. The client tells the OTA he has been driving himself to a local restaurant for dinner most nights and to a neighborhood dry cleaning establishment occasionally to get his laundry done. He also reported good results with using an electric scooter for the first time at a grocery store this week. Of the following choices, which is the OTA's best course of action (in collaboration with the OT)?
   A. Work on other community mobility activities
   B. Do not document that the client is driving because Medicare will deny home care services
   C. Document that the client no longer needs occupational therapy services
   D. Recommend outpatient occupational therapy services

Worksheet 9-7 (continued)
Home Care

6. For adult clients with Medicare or Medicaid receiving skilled rehabilitation home care services, which of the following outcome measures is required?
    A. OASIS
    B. COPM
    C. MDS
    D. FIM

7. According to Medicare guidelines, when a physician approves the plan of care, which of the following conditions must be met in order for an OTA to provide home care services?
    A. The OT is present during the OTA's session
    B. The physician must sign the OTA's progress notes at specified intervals
    C. The OT has established the plan and provides supervision
    D. The OTA cannot provide home care services for clients with Medicare

8. A client receiving home care services is recovering from bilateral lower extremity fractures. He requires assistance from his wife to use his wheelchair. When teaching wheelchair mobility in an area that lacks curb cuts, the OTA should instruct the client's wife to use which of the following methods with the wheelchair to descend a curb from the sidewalk?
    A. Approach curb with the wheelchair facing curb and tilted backward, castor wheels off the ground, and bring large wheels over the curb
    B. Approach curb with the wheelchair facing curb, lift large wheels off the ground, and bring castor wheels gently over the curb
    C. Approach curb with the wheelchair backward, ease large wheels over the curb, and tilt wheelchair backward to lift castor wheels over curb
    D. Approach curb with the wheelchair backward, tilt wheelchair forward to lift the large wheels, and ease castor wheels gently over the edge of curb

9. An OTA is working with a male client in home care who has a neurological condition. As the OTA begins today's session, the client begins to exhibit a seizure. Besides obtaining medical help, the OTA should perform which primary action?
    A. Try to restrain the client to minimize convulsions
    B. Adjust clothing around the client's neck to loosen it
    C. Place a washcloth or wallet in client's mouth to prevent him from biting his tongue
    D. Use smelling salts and place a cool washcloth on the client's forehead

10. Which of the following statements is accurate regarding hospice services?
    A. Palliative care is provided but not medications intended to help cure the primary illness
    B. Medicare will not reimburse for occupational and/or physical therapy because the client is not expected to have improved health or functional gains
    C. A physician must always certify that the client is within 1 month of expected death
    D. Most third-party payers will only provide reimbursement for hospice services if the diagnosis is cancer

Worksheet 9-8

Acute Care

1. A client in acute care has a Foley catheter in place. The collection bag is filled halfway with urine. When transporting the client in a wheelchair to the occupational therapy department, what should the OTA do with the catheter bag?
   A. Disconnect it
   B. Place it in the client's lap
   C. Attach it to the top of the wheelchair back support
   D. Attach it below the seat

2. A client in acute care contracted a nosocomial infection. This is normally classified as which of the following?
   A. An infection that causes a reversible coma
   B. A health care–associated infection
   C. An illness involving the nasal cavity
   D. Sarcoma causing a high fever

3. A client recovering from congestive heart failure has an intravenous line placed in left antecubital vein. When taking this client's vital signs, where should the OTA place the blood pressure cuff?
   A. On the client's right upper arm
   B. On the client's right forearm
   C. On the client's left upper arm
   D. On the client's left forearm

4. An OTA is working with a client who has hemiparesis and a nasogastric tube in place. Which of the following activities will more likely create a greater risk for dislodging the tube?
   A. Active range of motion of the affected upper extremity
   B. Donning and doffing a turtleneck sweater
   C. Using a transfer belt around the client's waist
   D. Retrograde massage to the affected arm

5. When preparing to transfer a client from a hospital bed to a wheelchair using the bed rail for support, which of the following is more suitable for the OTA to do?
   A. Move client's intravenous pole in order to maintain tension at infusion site
   B. Raise the hospital bed before locking it
   C. Swing away wheelchair front riggings
   D. Lower the bed rail

6. In acute care, when does discharge planning begin for most clients?
   A. After an occupational therapy evaluation is complete
   B. Upon admission
   C. After all nursing goals are met
   D. The day before discharge

Worksheet 9-8 (continued)

Acute Care

7. When working with a client who has orthostatic hypotension, an OTA might expect the client to have challenges with which of the following?
    A. Executive functions
    B. Bilateral dowel exercises to increase shoulder range of motion while seated
    C. Transferring sit to stand
    D. Using an upper body ergometer

8. A client with dementia confined to bed and weighing 130 lb requires assistance of two people for bed mobility. Which of the following methods is likely more suitable for the OTA and nurse to use together when attempting to position the client closer to the head of the bed?
    A. Utilize a trapeze
    B. Lift the patient up by holding under his arms and legs
    C. Hold onto a sturdy cloth beneath the client
    D. Mechanical lift

9. Which of the following isolation conditions require droplet precautions?
    A. *Clostridioides difficile*
    B. Tuberculosis
    C. Scabies
    D. Group A *streptococcus*

10. A 50-year-old client was admitted to the intensive care unit and is unable to communicate. The client's nephew has presented documentation to the hospital staff that indicates that he is the client's health care agent. The documentation the nephew presented is most likely which of the following?
    A. Life insurance beneficiary form
    B. Living will
    C. Do not resuscitate form
    D. Health care proxy

Worksheet 9-9

Skilled Nursing Facility

1. Which of the following ADL impairments is typically one of the earliest symptoms an individual may exhibit as an early sign of Alzheimer's disease?
   A. Incontinence
   B. Forgetting how to shave or brush teeth
   C. Forgetting how to operate a car
   D. Difficulty with remembering names or appointments

2. An OTA is working with a client, Josephine, diagnosed with Alzheimer's disease and functioning at Allen Cognitive Level 3. The client is recovering from a thoracic compression fracture due to a recent fall at the assisted living facility memory care unit where she resides. Josephine needs assistance for all ADLs and often asks when her mother, who is deceased, will be coming to visit. When implementing dressing interventions with Josephine, which of the following methods is probably less suitable for an OTA to do?
   A. Teaching use of a sock assist to don socks
   B. Using validation technique
   C. Using chaining technique to don a shirt
   D. Using task breakdown

3. Helene, a client with dementia, cannot remember to ask staff for assistance when she wants to get out of her wheelchair. She has poor fine-motor skills and is also at risk for falls due to poor balance and inability to remember to use her walker. Which of the following interventions is a possible choice for an OTA to suggest first as an alternative to a restraint while Helene sits in her wheelchair?
   A. Seat belt with buckle
   B. Vest restraint
   C. Seat alarm
   D. Lap board

4. An OTA in a skilled nursing facility is working with a client, Tariq, who exhibits left neglect following a CVA. Which of the following activities is less suitable for the OTA to do?
   A. Implement a symmetrical bilateral activity
   B. Implement an asymmetrical bilateral activity
   C. Have Tariq apply lotion to left arm
   D. When leaving the client's room, the OTA should tell Tariq the call bell is on the left side of the bed

5. An OTA is working with a client with dementia functioning at Allen Cognitive Level 2. The client is exhibiting agitation and keeps asking when her husband will arrive. The OTA knows that the client's spouse has been deceased for 10 years. Which of the following methods would likely be less effective for an OTA to use with this client?
   A. Reality orientation
   B. Therapeutic fib
   C. Redirect attention
   D. Validation

Worksheet 9-10

Rehabilitation Hospital—Total Hip Replacement Goals

Mary, a 79-year-old retired secretary, had left total hip replacement surgery (posterolateral approach) 5 days ago due to a hip fracture sustained in a fall. Left lower extremity has partial–weight-bearing status. Mary's medical history includes hypertension, coronary artery disease, and hyperlipidemia. She was transferred to a rehabilitation hospital yesterday, with expected discharge to home in 10 days. Here is some additional information taken from Mary's occupational therapy evaluation report:

- *Living situation*: Widowed and lives alone in a third-floor condominium with elevator access, in an adult retirement community. There is a shower stall in one bathroom and shower/tub in a second bathroom. Client's daughter lives in the next town, works full-time, and has two children in middle school. Mary also has a son who works full-time and lives approximately 100 miles away.
- *Prior level of function*: Independent in all ADLs and IADLs. Volunteers 1 day a week at a food pantry and is active in several church groups (choir and Bible study). Client uses the town's free senior transit service or has daughter/friend drive.
- *Cognition*: No functional deficits noted.
- *Upper extremity strength and range of motion*: Within functional limits.
- *ADLs*: Presently unable to perform lower body dressing and bathing due to total hip precautions. Client needs moderate assistance for transfers using a walker.
- *IADLs*: Dependent in household chores at this time.

Use a professional format to list four occupational therapy long-term goals for Mary.

1.

2.

3.

4.

Morreale, M. J. (2022). *Developing clinical competence: A workbook for the OTA* (2nd ed.). SLACK Incorporated.

Learning Activity 9-4: Spinal Cord Injury Interventions

Individuals diagnosed with SCIs do not necessarily have predictable and absolute outcomes as injuries sustained are often *incomplete*, rather than *complete*, lesions. Persons with incomplete lesions may vary greatly regarding specific viable client factors, present functional abilities, and ultimate outcomes for occupational participation. For this exercise, imagine three people who are diagnosed with complete spinal cord lesions, each at one of the three levels designated in the following chart. Choose 1 of the 10 activities/occupations listed and compare and contrast occupational therapy interventions for each of the three clients. Consider whether the client will likely achieve independence in this occupation or if the assistance of another person is needed to complete this task. Using activity analysis, consider how the client will perform each step. Determine the compensatory methods, equipment, or occupational adaptations that would be helpful, and any caregiver education required.

Activity/Occupation list:

1. Bowel and bladder management (including feminine hygiene)
2. Grooming (shaving face/legs, applying make-up, brushing teeth)
3. Lower body dressing (donning/doffing underwear, pants, socks, shoes)
4. Upper body dressing (donning/doffing button-down shirt, tie, bra, polo shirt, undershirt)
5. Upper and lower body bathing
6. Hair care (shampoo and style)
7. Feeding (managing finger foods, utensils, knife, cup)
8. Medication management (include oral medication and diabetic care)
9. Driving
10. Preparing lunch (frozen pizza and salad)

Occupation Requiring Intervention	Client With Complete C5 Lesion	Client With Complete C7-8 Lesion	Client With Complete T6 Lesion
Attainable assist level/desired outcome (e.g., modified independence, mod, max assist)			
Client position and where the intervention will take place (e.g., sitting upright in bed, sitting in wheelchair at sink, table)			
Mobility devices indicated			
Aspects of task requiring set-up/assistance			
Compensatory methods, orthotics, and/or adaptive equipment/durable medical equipment indicated			
Sequence of steps and instructional methods			
Caregiver education required for this task			

Worksheet 9-11

Amputations and Prosthetics

Determine if the following statements are true (T) or false (F).

1. T ____   F ____   Removal of all fingers on one hand except for thumb is termed a forequarter amputation.

2. T ____   F ____   Occupational therapy intervention for a person with a body-powered prosthesis includes training in prosthetic battery maintenance.

3. T ____   F ____   Benefits of a passive prosthesis include a lack of cables, low maintenance, and a lightweight consistency.

4. T ____   F ____   In documentation, an OTA might see the term transtibial amputation referred to as a below-knee amputation.

5. T ____   F ____   Increased sensory and proprioceptive input can be benefits of not wearing a prosthesis after amputation.

6. T ____   F ____   A hemipelvectomy involves removal of entire pelvis and distal structures.

7. T ____   F ____   The terms Chopart and Lisfranc refer to amputations at the wrist level.

8. T ____   F ____   When a primary purpose for using a prosthesis is cosmesis, a client may decide to use a passive prosthesis.

9. T ____   F ____   Due to the specialized knowledge required, the harness of a body-powered prosthesis is typically fabricated by an OT, not an OTA.

10. T ____   F ____   The part that connects the prosthesis to the residual limb is called the terminal device.

11. T ____   F ____   Following a Syme disarticulation, an otherwise healthy individual would likely have a harder time performing three-point and lateral pinch as a result.

12. T ____   F ____   A harness is not required for most kinds of myoelectric prostheses.

13. T ____   F ____   Using a body-powered prosthesis with a hook allows for better fine-motor prehension rather than a hand component as the terminal device.

Worksheet 9-11 (continued)

Amputations and Prosthetics

14. T ___ F ___   When the client with a transradial amputation tells an OT or OTA, "I feel like my hand is still there," this should be documented as phantom pain.

15. T ___ F ___   The pre-prosthetic phase follows the acute post-surgical phase.

16. T ___ F ___   Biofeedback is a primary method of training for the use of an externally powered prosthesis.

17. T ___ F ___   A main goal during the pre-prosthetic phase is shaping of the residual limb.

18. T ___ F ___   In documentation, an OTA might refer to a below-elbow amputation as a transhumeral amputation.

19. T ___ F ___   The hand component of a body-powered prosthesis typically has more grip strength than the hand component of an externally powered prosthesis due to torque force.

20. T ___ F ___   In general, children with congenital malformations should not receive an upper-limb prosthesis until age 5 years.

Worksheet 9-12

Clients With Chronic Conditions

1. A client is receiving occupational therapy at home following a healed transtibial amputation. The client also has end-stage renal disease and is on daily home peritoneal dialysis with an abdominal port. When performing showering interventions or when the client is self-connecting/disconnecting from the dialysis cycler machine, proper infection control procedures must be followed to primarily prevent which of the following from happening?
   A. Pericarditis
   B. Thrombocytopenia
   C. Peritonitis
   D. Osteomyelitis

2. An OTA is working on the cardiac care unit with a client who had a left ventricular assist device (VAD) implanted recently as destination therapy. Yesterday the client started sitting up in a wheelchair, but is deconditioned and needs assistance to transfer. Of the following statements, which is correct?
   A. When assessing vital signs, the OTA might find that the client does not have a palpable pulse
   B. The OTA should instruct the client to maintain a posterior pelvic tilt position when seated in wheelchair
   C. Inform the client that taking a bath can typically resume in approximately 5 to 6 weeks
   D. The OTA should have client perform wheelchair push-up exercises to increase independence in transfers

3. An OTA is working with a 10-year-old child who had a VAD implanted due to a congenital heart defect. In general, which of the following recommendations is more suitable for the OTA to give to the child's parents?
   A. To promote strength and endurance when therapy ends, child should participate in a non-contact sport such as swimming
   B. When dressing, button-down shirts may better accommodate the VAD driveline
   C. When the child is medically allowed to take a shower, a plastic grocery bag should be placed over the device to keep it dry
   D. Child should wear elastic waist pants directly over the driveline to better secure it in place

4. An OTA is reviewing the chart of a 40-year-old female client diagnosed with cubital tunnel syndrome. The OTA sees that the client's medical history includes osteopenia. The OTA might conclude that client is particularly at risk for developing which of the following conditions?
   A. Bone cancer
   B. Renal disease
   C. Type 2 diabetes
   D. Osteoporosis

5. When an OTA is assessing vital signs in an adult client, which of the following results could be indicative of hypoxemia and prehypertension?
   A. Blood oxygen saturation level 88% and blood pressure 135/88
   B. Blood oxygen saturation level 85% and blood pressure 125/75
   C. Blood oxygen saturation level 96% and blood pressure 140/90
   D. Blood oxygen saturation level 98% and blood pressure 130/90

Worksheet 9-12 (continued)

Clients With Chronic Conditions

6. An OTA is working in home care with a 74-year-old female client who has a femur fracture and Type 2 diabetes. The client reports she is starting to feel shaky and sweaty, and the OTA observes the client has become pale. The client tests her blood glucose level and obtains a result of 76. Which of the following choices is a more suitable action for the OTA to take?
   A. Have the client eat some nuts or cheese
   B. Call the referring physician
   C. Have the client drink some orange or apple juice
   D. Use smelling salts and have client sit with her head between her knees

7. An individual with chronic obstructive pulmonary disease, who requires supplemental oxygen, normally uses which of the following?
   A. Glucometer
   B. Nasal cannula
   C. Anti-embolism stockings
   D. Nasogastric tube

8. An OTA is reviewing the chart of a 66-year-old home care client, Ruby, who is diagnosed with head and neck cancer. The OTA reads that Ruby has a PEG tube following cancer surgery and radiation treatments. Which of the following items would the OTA expect to find in the client's home?
   A. Catheter bag
   B. Enterel nutrition products
   C. Oxygen tank
   D. Intravenous pole

9. An OTA is working with a client diagnosed with Ménière's disease. Which of the following items is suitable for the OTA to possibly recommend for symptoms associated with this condition?
   A. Tub seat/bench
   B. Large-print books
   C. Large-handle utensils
   D. An arm support

10. An OTA is reviewing the chart of a 4-year-old child who is diagnosed with a developmental delay and nystagmus. Upon meeting the child for the first time, the OTA might expect to observe signs of nystagmus in which anatomical structure?
    A. Spine
    B. Eyes
    C. Lips/mouth
    D. Hand

Questions 2 and 3 adapted from Morreale, M. J., & Amini, D. (2016). *The occupational therapist's workbook for ensuring clinical competence.* SLACK Incorporated.

Worksheet 9-13

Development of Hand Function

1. Which of the following choices reflect the typical developmental sequence of prehension from earlier to later?
   A. Radial palmar grasp, raking grasp, radial digital grasp
   B. Raking grasp, three-jaw chuck, developmental scissors grasp
   C. Radial digital grasp, three-jaw chuck, inferior pincer grasp
   D. Developmental scissors grasp, radial palmar grasp, inferior pincer grasp

2. An OTA was delegated the task of observing a first-grade student, Olivia, to ascertain the prehension pattern that Olivia uses for writing. The OTA observes Olivia holding the pencil in her right hand and using a static quadrupod grasp to complete a homework assignment. The OTA should inform the OT that Olivia is using what kind of grasp?
   A. Primitive
   B. Transitional
   C. Reflexive
   D. Mature

3. Which of the following activities normally entails using a lumbrical grasp?
   A. Using a cookie cutter
   B. Using a hand-held hair dryer
   C. Eating an apple
   D. Placing book vertically in bookcase

4. An OTA is working with a preschool child to promote development of an inferior pincer grasp. Which of the following activities is a possible choice to promote this specific type of grasp during a session at the child's home?
   A. Holding a spoon
   B. Pressing the pump of a liquid soap container to get the soap out for handwashing
   C. Using loop scissors
   D. Eating cheese puffs

5. Which of the following types of grasps would an OTA not expect to see in a 16-month-old child with typical development?
   A. Three-point pinch to hold a block
   B. Neat pincer grasp to hold a Cheerio
   C. Digital pronate grasp to hold a crayon
   D. Palmar supinate grasp to hold a marker

Worksheet 9-14

Pediatrics—Early Intervention

1. Under the Individuals with Disabilities Education Act (IDEA), the term *least restrictive environment* refers to which of the following conditions?
   A. Minimizing clutter in the home to enhance opportunities for motor development
   B. Avoiding the use of restraints when positioning the child
   C. A therapy room that has adequate space and supplies for necessary interventions, such as sensory integration equipment or orthotic device workstation
   D. Placing children with atypical development in settings with typically developing children

2. To better facilitate bilateral integration for a 7-month-old infant who is able to sit unsupported but does not demonstrate spontaneous use of the left upper extremity, which of the following positions is more suitable for an OTA to place the child in?
   A. Standing to push a toy shopping cart
   B. Supine to reach for a mobile
   C. Right side-lying to hold a stuffed animal
   D. Ring sitting to pick up 1-in. blocks

3. Which of the following children would not currently be eligible for early intervention services under Part C of IDEA?
   A. A 3-month-old infant born with low birth weight to a mother who drinks alcohol excessively
   B. A 6-year-old child diagnosed with Duchenne muscular dystrophy
   C. A 1.5-year-old child diagnosed with failure to thrive
   D. A 30-month-old child diagnosed with lead poisoning

4. An OTA at a preschool is working with a child diagnosed with a developmental delay. The OTA asks the child to name specific letters displayed on toy road signs and on an alphabet poster. The OTA also has the child pick out magnetic letters to spell the child's name. Which of the following is an underlying prewriting skill not being specifically addressed with these tasks?
   A. Visual closure
   B. Form constancy
   C. Visual memory
   D. Visual discrimination

5. A 4-year-old child with autism has difficulty adjusting to changes in his routine, such as going to the doctor or a family outing to an amusement park. Which of the following methods is a possible choice for an OTA to suggest to the child's parents to promote occupational participation?
   A. Have the child wear noise-blocking headphones
   B. Use negative reinforcement to change unwanted behaviors
   C. Have child wear a weighted vest
   D. Use a social story

Learning Activity 9-5: School Occupations

For each of the following student challenges in performance skills or client factors, list three educationally related activities that may be impacted by those challenges in a school setting. Examples are provided for each category.

Area Creating Challenge for Student	Educationally Related Activity That May Be Impacted in a School Setting
Tactile sensory processing	Art class project using glue 1. 2. 3.
Organizational skills	Writing down all homework assignments and developing a timeline for completion 1. 2. 3.
Proprioception	Applying appropriate amount of pressure to avoid breakage of pencil or crayon when writing or coloring 1. 2. 3.
Time management	Getting to next class in allotted time frame 1. 2. 3.
Fine-motor skills	Managing fastenings on clothing when changing for gym class 1. 2. 3.
Grip strength	Carrying lunch box 1. 2. 3.
Standing balance/tolerance	Standing in line to purchase lunch in cafeteria 1. 2. 3.
Shoulder ROM	Hanging clothing in locker 1. 2. 3.
Upper extremity strength	Carrying books 1. 2. 3.
Eye-hand coordination	Opening combination lock on locker 1. 2. 3.

Area Creating Challenge for Student	Educationally Related Activity That May Be Impacted in a School Setting
Crossing midline	*Turning pages in a large book* 1. 2. 3.
Spatial relations	*Buckling school bus seat belt* 1. 2. 3.
Bilateral integration	*Washing hands after toileting* 1. 2. 3.
Visual-motor	*Copying notes from the blackboard* 1. 2. 3.
Categorization	*Sorting school papers according to subject* 1. 2. 3.
Calculation skills	*Calculating cost of two items at school bake sale and the change back from $1.00* 1. 2. 3.
Emotional regulation	*When walking in a line going to the cafeteria or school bus, remaining calm when accidentally getting bumped by a classmate* 1. 2. 3.
Other	1. 2. 3.
Other	1. 2. 3.

Worksheet 9-15

Pediatrics—School Setting

1. An elementary school student with cerebral palsy is unable to turn pages in books due to spasticity in both upper limbs and poor hand function bilaterally. The student has good head control and can maintain upright symmetrical trunk position in wheelchair with minimal lateral supports and a seat belt. Which of the following is a possible choice as a low-tech assistive device in the classroom to aid student in page turning?
    A. Electronic book reader
    B. Mouth stick
    C. A classroom aide
    D. Electronic page turner

2. Steven is a second-grade student who has decreased pinch strength in his dominant right hand. As a result, he has challenges in handwriting such as sloppy letter formation, difficulty maintaining proper pencil grasp, and hand becoming tired. Steven's Individualized Education Program (IEP) delineates that an occupational therapy consultative model will be used to address these challenges. Which of the following actions is suitable for the OTA to take to implement the IEP?
    A. Work with Steven directly in the occupational therapy room to address fine-motor skills using media such as therapy putty and clothespins
    B. Work with Steven directly in the classroom to address fine-motor skills using media such as clay and a pegboard
    C. Suggest to the teacher that Steven use clay at play time and 1-in. pom-poms to erase a whiteboard
    D. Co-treat with the physical therapist to improve Steven's fine-motor skills more quickly

3. In a school setting, which of the following is less suitable as an IEP goal for a 14-year-old female student diagnosed with autism and dyspraxia, assuming the student has difficulty with all the following tasks?
    A. Ability to get from one class to another on time
    B. Ability to apply make-up independently
    C. Ability to manage feminine hygiene independently
    D. Ability to select and insert proper denomination of coins to use a cafeteria vending machine

4. An OTA is working in a school setting with Evan, a second-grade student who exhibits poor attention and fidgets frequently while seated at his desk. Which of the following is generally less suitable for the OTA to recommend to Evan's teacher?
    A. Have Evan sit directly under the bright overhead lighting to allow him to see better and improve concentration
    B. Have Evan use headphones to reduce ambient noise during independent tasks
    C. Have Evan help move a stack of books or classroom furniture
    D. Allow Evan to use a "fidget," such as a small squeeze ball, when seated at his desk

5. An OTA is working in a school setting with a 12-year-old student named Daisy who is diagnosed with a developmental disability. During today's occupational therapy session, Daisy begins to sob and states that her classmates are saying mean things about her on social media. Besides informing the OT, which primary action should the OTA take?
    A. Tell Daisy she is overreacting and should ignore the other student's comments
    B. Call the other children's parents
    C. Notify the police
    D. Ask Daisy for specific examples

Answers to Worksheets

Worksheet 9-1: Diseases and Conditions

1. Diplopia = Double vision
2. Herpes zoster = Shingles
3. Thrombus = Blood clot
4. Cerebrovascular accident = Stroke
5. Ecchymosis = Bruise
6. Lou Gehrig's disease = Amyotrophic lateral sclerosis
7. Dyspnea = Difficulty breathing, shortness of breath
8. Golfer's elbow = Medial epicondylitis
9. Degenerative joint disease = Osteoarthritis
10. Adhesive capsulitis = Frozen shoulder
11. Tennis elbow = Lateral epicondylitis
12. Varicella = Chicken pox
13. Conjunctivitis = Pink eye
14. Gamekeeper's thumb = Ulnar collateral ligament injury
15. Epstein-Barr virus = Mononucleosis
16. Ewing sarcoma = Bone cancer
17. Barlow's syndrome = Mitral valve prolapse
18. Decubitus ulcer = Pressure injury
19. Hypoglycemia = Low blood sugar
20. Myocardial infarction = Heart attack
21. Hypertension = High blood pressure
22. Hyperemesis = Vomiting excessively
23. Colles fracture = Distal radius fracture
24. Hyperlipidemia = Elevated lipid levels/high cholesterol
25. Hematuria = Blood present in urine
26. Osteogenesis imperfecta = Brittle bones
27. Trisomy 21 = Down syndrome
28. Strabismus = Cross-eyes
29. Rubella = German measles
30. Rubeola = Measles

Worksheet 9-2: Common Medications

Resources: Shields et al., 2020 and www.drugs.com

1. Eliquis = Atrial fibrillation
2. Nitroglycerin = Angina
3. Naproxen sodium = Osteoarthritis
4. Aricept = Dementia
5. Risperdal = Schizophrenia

6. Atenolol = Hypertension
7. Cymbalta = Depression
8. Boniva = Osteoporosis
9. Levodopa = Parkinson's disease
10. Topamax = Seizure
11. Demerol = Pain
12. Methotrexate = Cancer
13. Adderall = Attention deficit disorder
14. Lexapro = Anxiety
15. Proventil = Asthma
16. Augmentin = Infection
17. Avonex = MS
18. Acyclovir = Shingles
19. Humulin R = Diabetes
20. Lasix = Fluid retention
21. Humira = Crohn's disease
22. Heparin = Thrombus
23. Enbrel = Psoriatic arthritis
24. Allopurinol = Gout

Worksheet 9-3: Generic Medications

Resources: Shields et al., 2020 and www.drugs.com

1. Warfarin = Coumadin
2. Omeprazole = Prilosec
3. Ibuprofen = Advil
4. Diazepam = Valium
5. Naproxen sodium = Aleve
6. Hydrocodone bitartrate = Vicodin
7. Albuterol = Ventolin
8. Gabapentin = Neurontin
9. Atorvastatin calcium = Lipitor
10. Clonazepam = Klonopin
11. Enalapril maleate = Vasotec
12. Alprazolam = Xanax
13. Insulin = Humulin R
14. Fluoxetine hydrochloride = Prozac
15. Diltiazem = Cardizem
16. Acetaminophen = Tylenol
17. Paroxetine = Paxil
18. Ferrous sulfate = Slow FE
19. Valstartin = Diovan
20. Calcium carbonate = Tums

21. Atenolol = Tenormin
22. Furosemide = Lasix
23. Amlodipine = Norvasc
24. Duloxetine = Cymbalta

Worksheet 9-4: Wheeled Mobility

1. D. This option would allow for independent wheeled mobility for desired occupational roles, although other kinds of wheelchair cushions could also be appropriate. The client has ability to manage a joystick control and the tilt in space component would provide pressure relief throughout the day. A reclining wheelchair and travel wheelchair would not enable independent mobility. Also, although a travel chair is lighter than a standard wheelchair, it would be more difficult for her sibling to push due to smaller wheels.

2. C. This client's weight does not warrant a heavy duty (bariatric) wheelchair and he is able to use a manual wheelchair independently for general mobility. However, a sports wheelchair would allow this athletic client to play adapted sports such as basketball.

3. D. This client needs head and trunk support along with a *left* side support to maintain a more symmetrical upright position. The pommel should not extend all the way to the groin as that could be uncomfortable or possibly contribute to a pressure injury or urinary tract infection (Honaker & Campbell, 2017).

4. A. As this client has upper extremity function and ability to transfer and shift positions independently, she does not require a tilt-in-space component. A one-arm-drive wheelchair requires manual propulsion which would still cause fatigue. A power mobility scooter would be the most practical option to enable occupational participation.

5. B. This option would allow the client to propel and steer the wheelchair using only his uninvolved upper extremity. The client's weight and condition do not warrant a power wheelchair, heavy duty (bariatric) wheelchair, or special lightweight wheelchair.

6. A. The rear wheel axles are in a more posterior position to stabilize the wheelchair and compensate for the lost weight from lower limbs (Fairchild et al., 2018).

7. C. An occupational therapy practitioner performing a wheelchair assessment must ensure proper fit, support, optimal client positioning, and determine need for specialized seat cushion and/or any adaptations. Seat width (not depth) should provide slight clearance (1.5 to 2 in.) between the client's hips and the wheelchair side panels to avoid possible pressure injury. Proper seat depth will allow for approximately 2 in. of clearance between the edge of seat and popliteal space (back of knees). Armrest height is generally measured with elbow positioned at 90 degrees. Wheelchair back height should rest slightly below scapula inferior angles, although in some instances a higher back is needed for greater trunk support or a lower back height is sometimes indicated to allow for better propulsion (Bolding, et al, 2018; Fairchild et al., 2018).

8. D. Toggle brake locks can get in the way during sliding transfers. Scissors locks are a different kind of brake lock attached under the seat front and do not impede sliding transfers. When planning to transfer, the wheelchair front rigging with attached leg rest should be swung away/removed and wheelchair armrest also removed (Fairchild et al., 2018).

9. C. A lap belt secured with a loop Velcro closure will prevent client from sliding forward. It would also enable the client to place his hand/wrist through the loop and pull it open using gross movement. While an alarm can alert staff, it will not directly assist with the physical aspect of maintaining client's upright position in the wheelchair. Keeping the legs separated with an abduction wedge also does not really aid in upright positioning. A lap board may be considered a restraint as the client will probably not be able to remove that independently.

10. C. The footplates need to be in a closed/up position. Client needs to lock (engage) the toggle brake and unlock the front rigging to swing it away.

Adapted from Morreale, M. J., & Amini, D. (2016). *The occupational therapist's workbook for ensuring clinical competence*. SLACK Incorporated.

Worksheet 9-5: Speech and Language

Resource: American Speech-Language-Hearing Association (www.asha.org)

1. * Dysarthria
2. Dysphagia
3. Dystonia
4. * Dysphonia
5. * Cadence
6. Dysrhythmia
7. Aspiration
8. * Intelligibility
9. Shuttering
10. * Intonation

11. * Apraxia of speech
12. Hemianopsia
13. * Aphasia
14. * Dysphasia
15. * Fluency
16. * Articulation
17. Dysthymia
18. * Anomia
19. Dysesthesia
20. * Pitch

Reproduced with permission from Morreale, M. J., & Amini, D. (2016). *The occupational therapist's workbook for ensuring clinical competence.* SLACK Incorporated.

Worksheet 9-6: Feeding and Eating

Clients with dysphagia must have an individualized plan for dysphagia management and careful monitoring based on their physical and cognitive status. It is important to understand that clients with dysphagia are at risk for choking, aspiration pneumonia (and even possible death) if not observed and managed properly while eating/drinking or if given the wrong kinds of foods or liquids.

1. D.
2. B. The other choices reflect other phases of swallowing. The four phases of swallowing are: oral preparatory, oral transit, pharyngeal, and esophageal (American Speech-Language-Hearing Association, 2020; AOTA, 2017; Morawski et al., 2019).
3. A.
4. D. Client should be placed in a fully upright seated position. Due to deficits in sitting balance, his back should be supported so that he can better concentrate on safe swallowing.
5. D. Intervention should work toward minimizing, not promoting, pocketing of food. Clients with dysphagia may not be able to swallow thin liquids safely (Morawski et al., 2019).
6. B. Although the use of dentures could possibly contribute to difficulty with eating, such as pain or problems with chewing certain foods, they are not necessarily a sign of dysphagia.
7. A. (Morawski et al., 2019).
8. B. Pineapple is tough and fibrous, regular dry bread is a choking hazard and the rice needs moistening with an appropriate sauce (IDDSI, 2019a).
9. A. Some examples of transitional foods are cheese puffs, ice cream, and thin wafers (IDDSI, 2019b).
10. D. The other choices are thinner liquids which would not be safe for this child (IDDSI, 2019a).

Worksheet 9-7: Home Care

1. C. The client may be in the bathroom or might not have heard the doorbell, so the primary course of action would be to try and reach client by phone. If there is still no answer, the OTA should follow agency policy, such as contacting the OT and nurse case manager and document the situation.

2. B. An OTA must always adhere to the Health Insurance Portability and Accountability Act (HIPAA) guidelines for privacy and confidentiality. As the OTA must wake up the client for therapy, the OTA should ask the client for permission to discuss the client's medical information with her niece. The client may or may not want it disclosed.

3. C. According to Centers for Medicare & Medicaid Services (CMS, 2020b) guidelines, A, B, and D may be considered as the client's residence. If a client is in a skilled nursing facility, regulations for that setting would apply instead.

4. B. These may be symptoms of hyperglycemia, which can cause ketoacidosis (diabetic coma), which is a severe medical situation (George, 2018; Oakes, 2017).

5. D. If the client has ability to drive around the community independently, he may no longer ethically meet the Medicare criteria for being homebound and this should be discussed with the health team (CMS, 2020a). The client may still benefit from therapy to address his ADL deficits and can be referred to an outpatient clinic.

6. A. Medicare requires the Outcome Assessment Information Set (OASIS) be completed for home care (CMS, 2019b), although practitioners may utilize additional assessments, such as the Canadian Occupational Performance Measure (COPM), Functional Independence Measure (FIM), or others, depending on health discipline. The Minimum Data Set (MDS) is required by Medicare for clients in skilled nursing facilities.

7. C. Medicare guidelines for occupational therapy (CMS, 2019a, 2020c) require that an OT perform the assessment and establish, manage, and supervise the plan of care. The OT must also perform client reassessments at specified intervals. An OT does not have to be physically present when an OTA implements a delegated treatment session in between those intervals. While the physician must certify changes in the plan of care, there is no requirement that the physician sign treatment notes.

8. C. (Fairchild et al., 2018).

9. B. During a seizure, do not restrain the client or place objects in the client's mouth. Adjust clothing around the neck to help keep the client from having a restricted airway and call for medical assistance (George, 2018; Oakes, 2017).

10. A. Hospice provides comfort care and supportive, not curative, services. Typically, a client must be terminally ill with a prognosis of 6 months or less to receive hospice care, which a physician must certify. In addition to cancer diagnoses, hospice benefits are provided for other terminal conditions, such as congestive heart failure, failure to thrive, end-stage Alzheimer's or kidney disease, and so forth.

Worksheet 9-8: Acute Care

1. D. Do not place the bag on the client's lap. The urine collection bag should be below the bladder level to avoid backflow (Fairchild et al, 2018; George, 2018).

2. B. A more recent term for nosocomial is health care-associated infection, which includes conditions such as *Clostridioides difficile*, MRSA, and other infections from surgery or device placement (i.e., catheter).

3. A. Avoid placing the cuff above the intravenous insertion site (Fairchild et al., 2018).

4. B. The tube is inserted through the nose. Care must be taken so that donning and doffing an overhead sweater does not tug or pull at the tube.

5. C. The intravenous line should not be taut. The bed should be lowered so that the client's feet can reach the floor when seated on the edge of the bed for safety. Wheelchair footrests should be in the swing away position or removed. If a client is using bed rails to aid in transfers, the rails should be locked in the up position.

6. B. Lengths of stay in acute care are often very brief. As soon as the client is admitted, the team members consider if the client will be returning home, will need continued care or rehabilitation at another facility (e.g., skilled nursing facility, rehabilitation hospital), or will transfer to a different setting (e.g., relative's home, assisted living). This will give the discharge planner time to coordinate the transfer, order durable medical equipment if indicated, and help put into place other discharge recommendations. In acute care, not all clients will need or receive occupational therapy.

7. C. For some clients, sudden postural changes may cause the client's blood pressure to drop significantly and may cause lightheadedness or fainting.

8. C. A draw sheet under the client makes it easier for staff to move and position a client in bed who requires much assistance. Lifting a client up by the arms and legs poses greater risk for injury to both the client and health workers. While the client can attempt to assist by pulling up using a trapeze, that is not the best option in this situation.

9. D. In terms of isolation procedures, *Streptococcus A* requires droplet precautions, tuberculosis requires airborne precautions, and scabies and *C. difficile* require contact precautions (Siegel et al., 2019).

10. D. A health care proxy designates an individual who can make health care decisions on one's behalf in case of incapacitation.

Worksheet 9-9: Skilled Nursing Facility

1. D. Memory difficulty is an early sign for persons with Alzheimer's disease (Alzheimer's Association, 2020). While an individual in the early stages may still be able to physically operate a motor vehicle, a big concern is that the person may not be able to do this safely. The individual may have problems with following the rules of the road, spatial orientation, reaction time, or may easily get lost which all create significant safety concerns. Family education and other measures (e.g., take away keys, disable car) should be put in place to help keep an unsafe person from operating a motor vehicle.

2. A. A client functioning at Allen Cognitive Level 3 has poor problem-solving skills and diminished capacity for new learning, particularly when a device is unfamiliar (e.g., sock assist; Allen Cognitive Group, n.d.; Padilla, 2019a). For this client, the OTA's time would probably be better spent working on other aspects of dressing in which the client can better participate using task breakdown and chaining. Validation is an appropriate technique in this scenario to acknowledge that the client misses her mother (Padilla, 2019b).

3. C. A seat alarm would not restrain Helene but would alert staff if she begins to stand. As Helene has poor fine-motor skills, a seat belt with buckle and a lap board would be considered restraints if the client is unable to open or remove them independently.

4. D. For clients with unilateral neglect, it is useful for an OTA to incorporate activities that involve having the client use both upper extremities, such as using a rolling pin (symmetrical task) or holding toothpaste in one hand and applying it to a toothbrush held in the other hand (asymmetrical task). Applying lotion to the neglected side can also aid in bring awareness to it. The call bell should always be placed where the client can locate it easily when needed. In this situation, it should be placed to Tariq's right side, not the left.

5. A. A client functioning at Allen Cognitive Level 2 has severe cognitive impairment. Reality orientation would not be suitable in this instance as the client is unable to retain this information and could also become upset/agitated by the "news" her spouse is deceased. Answers B, C, and D present techniques that can be utilized with a caring approach to minimize the client's apparent emotional discomfort (Padilla, 2019b).

Worksheet 9-10: Rehabilitation Hospital—Total Hip Replacement Goals

Resources for goal writing: Gateley & Borcherding, 2017; Morreale & Borcherding, 2017; Sames, 2015

Goals need to specify a time frame, measurable criteria, and delineate a desired client behavior relating to function. Goals should reflect what the client needs to achieve, not what the occupational therapy practitioner will do as interventions. Here are some suggested goals for this client. Realize that different settings or practice areas may use slightly different formats or terminology, as shown in the various examples that follow. Of course, the actual goals and time frames may be different for a real client.

1. Client will complete lower body dressing with modified independence and adhere to all total hip precautions by expected discharge in 10 days.

    or

    By expected discharge in 10 days, client will don lower body garments independently using adaptive equipment and adhering to hip precautions.

2. Client will perform lower body bathing with modified independence and adhere to all total hip precautions by expected discharge in 10 days.

    or

    While seated on a tub bench and adhering to hip precautions, client will bathe lower body independently by expected discharge in 10 days.

3. While using walker in kitchen, client will demonstrate ability to heat items in microwave independently and adhere to all total hip precautions by expected discharge in 10 days.

4. In order to manage grooming tasks independently, client will demonstrate 8 minutes standing tolerance at sink using walker within 10 days.

5. Client will complete toilet transfers with modified independence (using walker, elevated seat, and grab bar) and adhere to all total hip precautions by expected discharge in 10 days.

6. Client will demonstrate ability to prepare a simple stove-top meal (e.g., eggs, soup) while standing with walker with contact guard assistance within 1 week.

Worksheet 9-11: Amputations and Prosthetics

1. F. Removal of all fingers on one hand except for thumb is termed a forequarter amputation.

    Forequarter amputation involves removal of entire upper extremity, clavicle, and scapula (Fairchild et al., 2018).

2. F. Occupational therapy intervention for a person with a body-powered prosthesis includes training in prosthetic battery maintenance.

    A battery is not involved with this type of prosthesis (Vacek, 2015).

3. T. Benefits of a passive prosthesis include a lack of cables, low maintenance, and a lightweight consistency. *(Vacek, 2015).*

4. T. In documentation, an OTA might see the term transtibial amputation referred to as a below-knee amputation. *(Fairchild et al., 2018).*

5. T. Increased sensory and proprioceptive input can be benefits of not wearing a prosthesis after amputation. *(Vacek, 2015).*

6. F. A hemipelvectomy involves removal of entire pelvis and distal structures.

    This describes a hemicorpectomy (Fairchild et al., 2018).

7. F. The terms Chopart and Lisfranc refer to amputations at the wrist leve.

    These terms refer to removal of part of foot (Fairchild et al., 2018).

8. T. When a primary purpose for using a prosthesis is cosmesis, a client may decide to use a passive prosthesis.

9. F. Due to the specialized knowledge required, the harness of a body-powered prosthesis is typically fabricated by an OT, not an OTA.

   The harness is normally fabricated by a prosthetist (Vacek, 2015).

10. F. The part that connects the prosthesis to the residual limb is called the terminal device.

    It is the socket (Vacek, 2015).

11. F. Following a Syme disarticulation, an otherwise-healthy individual would likely have a harder time performing three-point and lateral pinch as a result.

    Syme disarticulation is an amputation through ankle (Fairchild et al., 2018).

12. T. A harness is not required for most kinds of myoelectric prostheses.

    (Vacek, 2015).

13. T. Using a body-powered prosthesis with a hook allows for better fine-motor prehension rather than a hand component as the terminal device

    (Vacek, 2015).

14. F. When the client with a transradial amputation tells an OT or OTA, "I feel like my hand is still there," this should be documented as phantom pain.

    What the client is describing is phantom sensation (Vacek, 2015).

15. T. The pre-prosthetic phase follows the acute post-surgical phase.

    (Vacek, 2015).

16. T. Biofeedback is a primary method of training for the use of an externally-powered prosthesis.

    (Vacek, 2015).

17. T. A main goal during the pre-prosthetic phase is shaping of the residual limb.

    (Vacek, 2015).

18. F. In documentation, an OTA might refer to a below-elbow amputation as a transhumeral amputation.

    A transradial amputation is below-elbow, transhumeral is above elbow (Fairchild et al., 2018).

19. F. The hand component of a body-powered prosthesis typically has more grip strength than the hand component of an externally powered prosthesis due to torque force.

    The body-powered prosthesis hand component has less grip strength than that of an externally powered prosthesis (Vacek, 2015).

20. F. In general, children with congenital malformations should not receive an upper-limb prosthesis until age 5 years.

    Some children can receive a prosthesis as early as 2 months of age. Early and consistent prosthesis use will help promote typical development and spontaneous use in daily activities (Vacek, 2015).

Worksheet 9-12: Clients With Chronic Conditions

1. C. Because the dialysis port passes through the abdomen into the peritoneal cavity, it is essential to prevent germs from entering which can lead to peritonitis.

2. A. When working with clients who have a left ventricular assist device (LVAD; a mechanical pump connected to the heart implanted via a sternotomy), occupational therapy practitioners should have special training to understand proper care/use of this device and strictly adhere to relevant medical precautions/contraindications. A client with an implanted non-pulsatile VAD may not have a palpable pulse (University of California San Francisco Health, 2021b; Wells, 2013). A posterior pelvic tilt when seated may create kinks or pressure that could obstruct the driveline and impede blood flow (Abramson et al., 2012; McIntyre, 2007; Wells, 2013). The equipment cannot be submerged so client is unable to take baths, and sternal precautions should be followed (Abramson et al., 2012; Padmanabhan & Thankachan, 2011; University of California San Francisco Health, 2021a, 2021b; Wilson et al., 2009).

3. B. The abdomen upper quadrant is where the driveline exits the body so button-down shirts may be easier to accommodate it (Abramson et al., 2012). Direct pressure over the drive line (e.g., elastic waistbands) could possibly impede blood flow (Abramson et al., 2012; McIntyre, 2007). When the client is medically allowed to take a shower, a specialized manufactured waterproof bag/shower kit must be utilized (Abramson et al., 2012; Padmanabhan & Thankachan, 2011; University of California San Francisco Health, 2021a, 2021b). Because the equipment cannot get wet, the person using it cannot be immersed in water (i.e., swimming, baths) (Abramson et al., 2012; Padmanabhan & Thankachan, 2011; University of California San Francisco Health, 2021a, 2021b; Wilson et al., 2009). (Answers to questions 2 and 3 adapted from Morreale, M. J., & Amini, D. (2016). *The occupational therapist's workbook for ensuring clinical competence*. SLACK Incorporated.)

4. D.

5. A. Hypoxemia is a blood oxygen saturation level <90%. (Fairchild et al., 2018). Prehypertension range is 120 to 139 mm Hg for systolic blood pressure or 80 to 89 mm Hg for diastolic, with higher values possibly indicative of hypertension (Fairchild et al., 2018).

6. C. The client is approaching hypoglycemia which occurs when blood sugar levels are less than 70 mg/dL (American Diabetes Association, 2021). The client should ingest some quick-acting sugar and recheck glucose levels in 15 minutes to see if glucose levels have returned to a more normal range (American Diabetes Association, 2021). The OTA should inform the OT and nurse involved with the case. Of course, the OTA must always use professional reasoning to recognize if symptoms are worsening or blood glucose levels are dangerously low which could warrant a call to 911. Always follow your facility/agency policies and procedures regarding the handling of medical situations.

7. B. This is how supplemental oxygen enters the nose.

8. B. Percutaneous endoscopic gastrostomy is a type of feeding tube placed into stomach through abdomen.

9. A. This condition causes vertigo.

10. B. The OTA may observe rapid involuntary eye movements.

Worksheet 9-13: Development of Hand Function

Resource: Edwards et al., 2018

1. A.
2. B.
3. D.
4. D.
5. C.

Worksheet 9-14: Pediatrics—Early Intervention

1. D.

2. C. Positioning the child in right side-lying will partially limit motion of the uninvolved right arm. This can promote use of affected left arm to work together with right arm to play with the stuffed toy. Reaching for a mobile and picking up blocks does not necessarily involve simultaneous use of both hands, although these tasks could be used to encourage use of the involved arm. At 7 months, the child would not yet have ability to walk.

3. B. Under Part C of IDEA, early intervention services are provided from birth up to age 3 for children with, or at risk for, a disability. However, under IDEA Part B, related services and special education can be extended to age 21 (Center for Parent Information and Resources, 2017).

4. A. Visual closure is used in identifying an incomplete letter/figure or forming them (e.g., making clay letters, drawing shapes; Kaldenberg, 2017). In this situation the letters are already complete.

5. D. A Social Story can help prepare and explain to the child what to expect with specific upcoming events (Tanner, 2018). If the child has sensory challenges, a vest or headphones could possibly be beneficial also. Positive reinforcement could also be utilized.

Worksheet 9-15: Pediatrics—School Setting

1. B.
2. C. Occupational therapy practitioners using a consultative model provide direct recommendations to the teacher and other education staff regarding a specific student, such as strategies or activities the student would benefit from in the classroom. A direct service model provides designated therapy services to the child individually or in a group, for example, gross/fine-motor tasks, sensory integration activities, instruction in select ADLs, and so forth, to support participation in school occupations (Steva, 2017).
3. B. Goals in an IEP must pertain to necessary occupations/skills for the educational setting. Besides academics, these can include toileting and feminine hygiene skills, ability to get to class, managing a backpack, cafeteria functions (e.g., carrying a tray, purchasing school lunch, using a school vending machine), and so forth. While the student may desire to be able to apply make-up independently, it is not really an educationally related task unless associated with the school's drama club, for example.
4. A. A child with poor attention would benefit more from calming strategies, such as dim lighting and methods noted in answers B, C, and D (Gallagher, 2015).
5. D. Harassment, intimidation, and bullying (HIB) is a serious matter that should never be taken lightly. An OTA working in a school setting has a duty to report such behavior to help ensure the child's safety and emotional well-being. The OTA should ask the child about the general nature of the comments (i.e., teasing versus direct threat of bodily harm) and follow the protocol that the school district has in place for handling these situations.

References

Abramson, M., Harvey, J., Greenfield, M., Lauman, S., & Metzler, D. (2012). Partners in the journey: A case study of OT intervention for a recipient of a left ventricular assist device. *Advance for Occupational Therapy Practitioners, 28*(16), 16. http://occupational-therapy.advanceweb.com/Web-extras/Online-Extras/Partners-in-the-journey.aspx

Allen Cognitive Group (n.d.). *Allen scale/cognitive levels.* Retrieved June 22, 2021, from https://www.allencognitive.com/allen-scale/

Alzheimer's Association. (2020). *10 early signs and symptoms of alzheimer's.* www.alz.org/alzheimers_disease_10_signs_of_alzheimers.asp

American Diabetes Association. (2021). *Hypoglycemia (low blood sugar).* Retrieved June 22, 2021, from https://www.diabetes.org/diabetes/medication-management/blood-glucose-testing-and-control/hypoglycemia

American Occupational Therapy Association. (2017). The practice of occupational therapy in feeding, eating, and swallowing. *American Journal of Occupational Therapy, 71*(Suppl. 2), 7112410015. https://doi.org/10.5014/ajot.2017.716S04

American Occupational Therapy Association. (2020). Occupational therapy practice framework: Domain and process (4th ed.). *American Journal of Occupational Therapy, 74*(Suppl. 2), 7412410010. https://doi.org/10.5014/ajot.2020.74S2001

American Speech-Language-Hearing Association. (2020). *Feeding and swallowing.* https://www.asha.org/Practice-Portal/Clinical-Topics/Pediatric-Dysphagia/Overview/

Bolding, D., Hughes, C. A., Tipton-Burton, M., & Verran, A. (2018) Mobility. In H. M. Pendleton & W. Schultz-Krohn (Eds.), *Pedretti's occupational therapy practice skills for physical dysfunction* (8th ed., pp. 230-288). Elsevier Incorporated.

Center for Parent Information and Resources. (2017). *Building the legacy for our youngest children with disabilities: A training curriculum on part C of IDEA 2004.* Retrieved June 22, 2021, from https://www.parentcenterhub.org/legacy-partc/

Centers for Medicare & Medicaid Services. (2019a). *Medicare benefit policy manual (pub. 100-02: ch. 7, section 30.2.1).* www.cms.gov/Regulations-and-Guidance/Guidance/Manuals/Downloads/bp102c07.pdf

Centers for Medicare & Medicaid Services. (2019b). *Outcome and assessment information set: OASIS-C guidance manual (chapter 1).* https://www.cms.gov/Medicare/Quality-Initiatives-Patient-Assessment-Instruments/HomeHealthQualityInits/Downloads/OASIS-D-Guidance-Manual-final.pdf

Centers for Medicare & Medicaid Services. (2020a). *Medicare benefit policy manual (pub. 100-02: ch. 7, section 30.1.1).* https://www.cms.gov/Regulations-and-Guidance/Guidance/Manuals/Downloads/bp102c07.pdf

Centers for Medicare & Medicaid Services. (2020b). *Medicare benefit policy manual (pub. 100-02: ch. 7, section 30.1.2).* www.cms.gov/Regulations-and-Guidance/Guidance/Manuals/Downloads/bp102c07.pdf

Centers for Medicare & Medicaid Services. (2020c). *Medicare benefit policy manual (pub. 100-02: ch. 7, section 40.2.1).* www.cms.gov/Regulations-and-Guidance/Guidance/Manuals/Downloads/bp102c07.pdf

Cichero, J. A. Y., Lam, P., Steele, C. M., Hanson, B., Chen, J., Dantas, R. O. ... Stanschus, S. (2017). Development of international terminology and definitions for texture-modified foods and thickened fluids used in dysphagia management: The IDDSI framework. *Dysphagia 32,* 293-314. https://doi.org/10.1007/s00455-016-9758-y

Edwards, S. J., Gallen, D. B., McCoy-Powlen, J. D., & Suarez, M. A. (2018). *Hand grasps and manipulation skills: Clinical perspective of development and function* (2nd ed.). SLACK Incorporated.

Fairchild, S. L., O'Shea, R. K., & Washington, R. D. (2018). *Pierson and Fairchild's principles & techniques of patient care* (6th ed.). Elsevier Incorporated.

Gallagher, S. (2015). A third-grader with attention deficit hyperactivity disorder. In K. Sladyk & S. E. Ryan (Eds.), *Ryan's occupational therapy assistant: Principles, practice issues, and techniques* (5th ed., pp. 204-221). SLACK Incorporated.

Gately, C. A., & Borcherding, S. (2017). *Documentation manual for occupational therapy: Writing SOAP notes* (4th ed.). SLACK Incorporated.

George, A. H. (2018). Infection control and safety issues in the clinic. In H. M. Pendleton & W. Schultz-Krohn (Eds.), *Pedretti's occupational therapy practice skills for physical dysfunction* (8th ed., pp. 141-154). Elsevier Incorporated.

Honaker, D., & Campbell, M. (2017). Positioning in pediatrics: Making the right choices. In A. Wagenfeld, J. Kaldenberg, & D. Honaker (Eds.), *Foundations of pediatric practice for the occupational therapy assistant.* (2nd ed., pp. 117-1410. Slack Incorporated.

International Dysphagia Diet Standardisation Initiative. (2019a). *Complete IDDSI framework detailed definitions 2.0/2019.* https://ftp.iddsi.org/Documents/Complete_IDDSI_Framework_Final_31July2019.pdf

International Dysphagia Diet Standardisation Initiative. (2019b). *IDDSI consumer handouts: Transitional foods.* https://ftp.iddsi.org/Documents/Consumer_Handouts_for_Adults_All_Levels.pdf

Kaldenberg, J. (2017). Visual-perceptual dysfunction and low-vision rehabilitation. In A. Wagenfeld, J. Kaldenberg, & D. Honaker (Eds.), *Foundations of pediatric practice for the occupational therapy assistant* (2nd ed., pp. 249-262). SLACK Incorporated.

McIntyre, M. (2007). Keeping VAD patients functional. *ADVANCE for Occupational Therapy Practitioners, 23*(5), 43. http://occupational-therapy.advanceweb.com/Article/Keeping-VAD-Patients-Functional-1.aspx

Morawski, D. L., Davis, T., & Padilla, R. (2019). Dysphagia and other eating and nutritional concerns with elders. In H. L. Lohman, S. Byers-Connon, & R. L. Padilla (Eds.), *Occupational therapy with elders: Strategies for the COTA* (4th ed., pp. 255-267). Elsevier Incorporated.

Morreale, M. J. & Amini, D. (2016). *The occupational therapist's workbook for ensuring clinical competence.* SLACK Incorporated.

Morreale, M. J., & Borcherding, S. (2017). *The OTA's guide to documentation: Writing SOAP notes* (4th ed.). SLACK Incorporated.

Oakes, C. (2017). Safety and support. In K. Jacobs & N. MacRae (Eds.), *Occupational therapy essentials for clinical competence* (3rd ed., pp. 161-174). SLACK Incorporated.

Padilla, R. (2019a). Occupational therapy practice models. In H. L. Lohman, S. Byers-Connon, & R. L. Padilla (Eds.), *Occupational therapy with elders: Strategies for the COTA* (4th ed., pp. 84-102). Elsevier Incorporated.

Padilla, R. (2019b) Working with elders who have dementia and Alzheimer's disease. In H. L. Lohman, S. Byers-Connon, & R. L. Padilla (Eds.), *Occupational therapy with elders: Strategies for the COTA* (4th ed., pp. 282-297). Elsevier Incorporated.

Padmanabhan, K., & Thankachan, S. (2011). Occupational therapy in cardiac care: Left ventricular assistive devices. *OT Practice, 16*(22), 15-20.

Sames, K. (2015). *Documenting occupational therapy practice* (3rd ed.). Pearson Education.

Shields, K. M., Fox, K. L., & Liebrecht, C. M. (2020). *Pearson nurse's drug guide*. Pearson Education.

Siegel J. D., Rhinehart, E., Jackson, M., Chiarello, L., & the Healthcare Infection Control Practices Advisory Committee. (2019). *2007 guideline for isolation precautions: Preventing transmission of infectious agents in healthcare settings*. https://www.cdc.gov/infectioncontrol/guidelines/isolation/index.html

Smith, J. (2018). Eating and swallowing. In H. M. Pendleton & W. Schultz-Krohn (Eds.), *Pedretti's occupational therapy practice skills for physical dysfunction* (8th ed., pp. 669-700). Elsevier Incorporated.

Steva, B. J. (2017). Interventions to enhance occupational performance in school and work. In K. Jacobs & N. MacRae (Eds.), *Occupational therapy essentials for clinical competence* (3rd ed., pp. 399-419). SLACK Incorporated.

Tanner, K. (2018). Interventions for improving social skills and social participation for individuals with ASD. In R. Watling & S. L. Spitzer (Eds.), *Autism across the lifespan: A comprehensive occupational therapy approach* (4th ed., pp. 405-414). American Occupational Therapy Association.

University of California San Francisco Health. (2021a). *FAQ: Living with a ventricular assist device (VAD)*. Retrieved May 23, 2021, from https://www.ucsfhealth.org/education/faq-living-with-a-ventricular-assist-device

University of California San Francisco Health. (2021b). *Ventricular assist device (VAD)*. Retrieved May 23, 2021, from https://www.ucsfhealth.org/treatments/ventricular-assist-device

Vacek, K. M. (2015). Upper extremity prosthetics. In B. M. Coppard & H. Lohman (Eds.), *Introduction to orthotics: A clinical-reasoning & problem-solving approach* (4th ed., pp. 424-439). Elsevier Incorporated.

Wells, C. L. (2013). Physical therapist management of patients with ventricular assist devices: Key considerations of the acute care physical therapist. *Physical Therapy, 93*(2), 266-278. https://pubmed.ncbi.nlm.nih.gov/23043149/

Wilson, S. R., Givertz, M. M., Stewart, G. C., & Mudge, G. H. (2009). Ventricular assist devices: The challenges of outpatient management. *Journal of the American College of Cardiology, 54*(18), 1647-1659. https://pubmed.ncbi.nlm.nih.gov/19850205/

Understanding Department Management

The worksheets and learning activities presented in this final chapter address a variety of areas applicable to occupational therapy department management. Topics include billing and reimbursement, developing a business plan, budget basics, quality management, and the marketing/promotion of occupational therapy services. Answers to worksheet exercises are provided at the end of the chapter.

Contents

Morreale, M. J. Developing Clinical Competence:
A Workbook for the OTA, Second Edition (pp. 407-426).
© 2022 SLACK Incorporated.

Worksheet 10-1

Billing and Reimbursement

1. An 85-year-old client receiving outpatient rehabilitation services has Medicare B as his primary health insurance. Today the occupational therapy assistant (OTA) and physical therapist assistant (PTA) are working together with the client for 30 minutes to instruct the client in safe transfers. The physical therapist (PT) plans to bill Medicare for two units of therapy. How many units should the supervising occupational therapist (OT) bill Medicare for this co-treatment?
   A. 0
   B. 1
   C. 2
   D. 3

2. A client in a skilled nursing facility has Medicare B as his primary health insurance. An OTA works with the client in occupational therapy, providing 20 minutes of activities of daily living (ADL) training. How many units can Medicare be billed for the therapy provided?
   A. 1
   B. 2
   C. 4
   D. 20

3. An OTA is working in an acute care hospital with a 65-year-old inpatient who is a retired executive. Of the following choices, which is likely the third-party payer for this client's hospital care?
   A. Medicare Part A
   B. Medicare Part B
   C. Medicare Part D
   D. Social Security

4. An OTA is working on an acute behavioral health unit with a 72-year-old client who is a retired factory worker. The client's primary health insurance is Medicare. The facility will most likely be reimbursed through which of the following?
   A. Medicare Part A Prospective Payment System
   B. Medicare Part B Physician Fee Schedule
   C. Medicare Part D Rehabilitation Fee Schedule
   D. Medicare Part B Therapy Cap

5. An outpatient client in occupational therapy is 45 years old and has private insurance that pays 80% of health care costs after a $150 deductible is met. The client's occupational therapy evaluation last week cost $100 and today is the client's first intervention session, which costs $70. The client has not had any other health services this calendar year. How much money out-of-pocket will the client have to pay for today's session?
   A. $20
   B. $54
   C. $56
   D. $70

Worksheet 10-1 (continued)

Billing and Reimbursement

6. Which of the following is a mandatory insurance that businesses pay to cover the health costs of workers who are injured on the job?
   A. TRICARE
   B. Unemployment insurance
   C. Medicare Part C
   D. Workers' compensation

7. Which of the following does not meet the Medicare criteria to be classified as durable medical equipment?
   A. Wheelchair
   B. Commode
   C. Tub seat
   D. Quad cane

8. A 14-month-old child with a developmental delay could be entitled to receive occupational therapy services resulting from which legislation?
   A. OBRA
   B. IDEA Part B
   C. IDEA Part C
   D. FERPA

9. Jana is an unmarried 28-year-old U.S. citizen who has been unemployed for 12 months. She is pregnant and has no assets. Which of the following choices is a fit as a third-party payer source for Jana's prenatal care?
   A. Unemployment insurance
   B. Supplemental security insurance
   C. Workers' compensation
   D. Medicaid

10. An OTA is providing 30 minutes of therapy to a 50-year-old outpatient client who is recovering from a shoulder fracture. The OTA is unsure as to what the proper billing codes are for therapeutic exercises and ADL retraining. Which of the following would be a better resource to obtain this information?
    A. International Classification of Diseases manual
    B. Medicare Benefit Policy manual
    C. Current Procedural Terminology manual
    D. Minimum Data Set

Learning Activity 10-1: Billing Codes

Current Procedural Terminology (CPT) are standard billing codes that are part of the Healthcare Common Procedure Coding System and used to bill insurance companies for individual skilled health services, such as outpatient occupational therapy (Centers for Medicare & Medicaid Services [CMS], 2016). Billing for some therapy procedures is based on units of time (in 15-minute increments). Other procedures are considered untimed and billed only one unit regardless of the time provided for that service (CMS, 2016). Use a CPT manual (found at a library, fieldwork site, or online) to find the correct billing codes for the following occupational therapy interventions listed. Determine what general intervention category correlates with each specific task, if it is considered a timed service, and if constant attendance or one-on-one care by the occupational therapy practitioner is required or not. An example is provided.

Occupational Therapy Intervention Implemented	Billing Category	Is This Intervention Considered Timed or Untimed?	Is This Intervention Considered as Only a Supervised Modality or Is It Classified as Requiring Constant Attendance or One-on-One With an Occupational Therapy Practitioner?	Current Procedural Terminology Billing Code
Example: Upper extremity coordination exercises	Neuromuscular reeducation	Timed	One-on-one intervention	97112
Teaching use of a button-hook				
Measuring a client for a wheelchair				
Instruction and practice using worksheets to improve sequencing and problem solving				
Using a hot pack				
Checking and modifying an orthotic device				
Assessing upper extremity strength				
Teaching compensatory techniques for cooking				
Educating a client in sliding board transfers				
Hand strengthening using a hand gripper and therapy putty				
Assessing a client's home for safety				
Teaching coping strategies to a client who uses alcohol excessively				
Teaching a client how to propel and use a wheelchair				
Paraffin treatment				

Learning Activity 10-2: Diagnosis Codes

The World Health Organization (WHO) maintains a standard, universal listing of codes for diseases and conditions, called the International Classification of Diseases (ICD). ICD is a coding system used around the world by more than 100 countries, including the United States, and is periodically revised (WHO, 2020). The current version being used in U. S. health care settings is ICD-10-CM, which stands for International Classification of Diseases, Tenth Revision, Clinical Modification (American Academy of Professional Coders [AAPC], 2021). A new version, ICD-11, was released by WHO in 2018 and is expected to be implemented in 2022 (WHO, 2021).

Instructions: For the following conditions listed, use a current ICD manual to look up each of the diagnosis codes. Realize that the condition may be listed as a synonym in the ICD manual.

1. _____ Parkinson's disease

2. _____ A cut to the index finger

3. _____ Marfan syndrome

4. _____ Middle cerebral artery subarachnoid hemorrhage

5. _____ Cubital tunnel syndrome

6. _____ Down syndrome

7. _____ Failure to thrive (child)

8. _____ Schizophrenia

9. _____ Glaucoma

10. _____ Ulnar shaft open fracture

Worksheet 10-2

Department Management

Occupational therapy practitioners planning to establish a private practice therapy program or clinic must first create a sound business plan. Multiple factors must be thoroughly considered in this process such as the potential client base, likely funding sources (e.g., Medicare, workers' compensation, early intervention, private insurance, client self-pay), available working capital, and budget. Reimbursement from third-party payers is normally contingent on meeting strict criteria in order to bill that insurer for therapy services, for example, becoming a Medicare-certified agency or being part of an insurer network. In addition, there are many legal and logistical considerations that are involved with owning or managing a program or clinic.

Instructions: As a creative exercise, imagine that you and an OT have decided to open a private outpatient therapy clinic together. Consider the following factors regarding this endeavor.

1. **Vision**: Determine what your vision is for this new program and decide on a name for the program or facility. Consider the geographic area (e.g., town, county, entire state, multiple states) and client population that the clinic will likely serve (e.g., infants, school-age children, adults, older adults). Decide on the specific types of services that will be offered (e.g., health and wellness, adult rehabilitation, sensory integration, driver rehabilitation, low vision, hand therapy). Looking toward the future, consider if your plans would include eventually expanding the clinic or establishing other sites.

Vision for private practice: _____

_____

A. Name of facility: _____

B. Geographic area: _____

C. Type of practice area: _____

D. Population served:_____

E. Services offered: _____

_____

F. Likely funding sources (third party payers): _____

_____

G. Future plans: _____

_____

Worksheet 10-2 (continued)

Department Management

2. **Space:** Besides the cost, determine at least 10 criteria to consider when looking for a suitable space to rent or buy.

A.

B.

C.

D.

E.

F.

G.

H.

I.

J.

3. **Equipment and supplies:** Assume you have rented empty space and now need to purchase all the equipment and supplies for this clinic. Brainstorm a list of items that will be needed. Prioritize the items into three categories: Items that are essential for day 1, items that are needed but do not have to be purchased immediately, and a "wish list" of items that will be purchased as revenue increases. Do not include professional expenses such as insurance, building permits, and licensing fees in this list.

Category	Essential Items	Needed but Can Be Deferred	Wish List
Safety			
Office furniture			
Office equipment			
Office supplies			
Evaluation tools			
General supplies			
Exercise equipment			
ADL equipment			
Adaptive equipment			
Physical agent modalities			
Orthotic devices/supplies			
Other:			
Other:			

Worksheet 10-2 (contiued)

Department Management

4. **Possible staff and professional services needed:** Besides possibly hiring other occupational therapy practitioners, list at least eight other disciplines or services you may need to hire/pay for when starting or owning a private practice. Do not include other rehabilitation disciplines, such as physical or speech therapy.

   A.

   B.

   C.

   D.

   E.

   F.

   G.

   H.

5. **Methods of marketing:** Identify at least five ways to market/promote your business that do not involve television, radio, or newspaper ads.

   A.

   B.

   C.

   D.

   E.

Worksheet 10-3

Budget

Determine if the following statements are true (T) or false (F).

1. T ___ F ___ A fiscal year goes from January 1 to December 31.

2. T ___ F ___ An example of an occupational therapy capital budget expenditure is a transfer tub bench.

3. T ___ F ___ Revenue equals total income minus expenses.

4. T ___ F ___ Rent and a copying machine lease are examples of fixed costs.

5. T ___ F ___ Accounts receivable includes the money due from an insurance company.

6. T ___ F ___ Example of variable expenses include personal protective equipment, hook and loop fastener, and client-issued therapy putty.

7. T ___ F ___ Non-profit means that the organization does not make enough money to meet its total expenses.

8. T ___ F ___ Total costs subtracted from revenue equals profits.

9. T ___ F ___ Occupational therapy department budgets always allocate money for staff to attend continuing education seminars to maintain National Board for Certification in Occupational Therapy (NBCOT) certification.

10. T ___ F ___ Costs for items ordered but not paid for, such as evaluation forms and adaptive equipment, are considered accounts payable.

11. T ___ F ___ Thermoplastic materials, gauze, and paraffin are considered direct-use supplies.

12. T ___ F ___ Cash flow consists of pending money due from third-party payers.

13. T ___ F ___ Expenses not associated directly with productivity levels, such as monthly utilities and yearly service contracts, are called overhead.

14. T ___ F ___ Productivity refers to the amount of billable services that an individual provides.

15. T ___ F ___ Accounts payable include money that clients owe the business, such as copayments and coinsurance.

Learning Activity 10-3: Mission Statements

Choose two health-related facilities in your community, such as a hospital, doctors' group, or outpatient rehabilitation clinic. One facility should be classified as a nonprofit organization and the other a for-profit organization. Using the company websites, locate the mission statements for both facilities and compare and contrast them.

	Nonprofit Health Facility	*For-Profit Health Facility*
Name of facility/organization		
Is this facility part of a larger network or organization? If so, describe.		
Overall philosophy (i.e., religious, philanthropic, social justice)		
Population served (geographic area and/or types of diagnoses)		
List three primary services provided to the community it serves		
List five words from the mission statement that best convey the values of the organization		
Stated vision for the future		
Other:		
Other:		

Quality Improvement

Health facilities and agencies often have a quality improvement (QI) committee to ensure that client care is appropriate and meets clinical, ethical, and professional standards. A QI committee might consist of members from various disciplines in that setting and may include an occupational therapy practitioner or the rehabilitation supervisor. Accrediting agencies such as The Joint Commission and certifying bodies such as CMS are interested in certain performance metrics that reflect a setting's level of care, including but not limited to hospital readmission rate, incidence of falls, and prevalence of hospital-acquired infections. QI committees strive to attain quality benchmarks in addition to looking for and solving problems in client care. All staff employed in the health setting should be empowered to suggest or help make positive changes to enhance safety, reduce medical errors, improve efficiency, and ensure high care standards (Morreale & Borcherding, 2017).

As part of the on-going QI process, facilities might require that, at specified intervals, each discipline identify particular problem areas in their own department for which a plan can be created to improve safety, provide value-based care, attain better health outcomes, and/or enhance client satisfaction. While not an all-inclusive list, the following are examples of possible concerns that an occupational therapy department might choose to address from a quality standpoint:

- Adaptive equipment or orthotic devices go missing in the facility
- After therapy, clients in wheelchairs are lined up like a train with excessive wait times to be brought back to their rooms
- Clients are noncompliant with orthotic device or adaptive equipment use
- Clients are missing their appointments
- Specific pieces of equipment are faulty or unsafe (e.g., temperature gauge not working, pinch meter broken, presence of sharp/jagged edges)
- Required productivity levels limit time necessary for clinical documentation

When a specific problem is identified, the QI team collaborates with the relevant department(s) to determine possible solutions, develop an action plan, implement new procedures to tackle the problem, and establish measures for acceptable outcomes. Once systems and procedures are in place, designated staff will then track whether these new methods are effective in meeting desired benchmarks over certain time periods (e.g., quarterly, yearly). To attain a better understanding of the quality improvement process, complete Learning Activity 10-4.

Learning Activity 10-4: Quality Improvement

Describe an issue that has a negative impact on client satisfaction, safety, or care that you have either (a) personally experienced while receiving health services or (b) that you have observed on fieldwork or on the job at a health facility/agency. For example, perhaps you find that you have to wait at your doctor's office for at least an hour before you are seen for a scheduled appointment, your department is out of certain essential supplies when you need them, or that your outpatient clients forget to bring their orthotic devices to their follow-up therapy sessions. Once you have identified an issue needing QI, use the following worksheet to develop an action plan to address the issue.

1. Identified problem: _____

_____

2. Describe why this is a problem (i.e., safety concern, client satisfaction): _____

_____

3. Brainstorm possible solutions:

   a.

   b.

   c.

   d.

   e.

4. Choose one idea from your list that you think will be the best solution: _____

_____

5. Develop an action plan. List the steps needed to implement your plan, the staff member(s) who will be responsible (e.g., rehab aide, secretary, OT, nursing), and possible factors limiting implementation (e.g., cost, staff time):

Action Plan Steps	Staff Member(s) Responsible	Factors Limiting Implementation

6. Identify a method to evaluate, measure, or track the effectiveness of your intended plan: _____

_____

_____

Learning Activity 10-5: Client Satisfaction Survey

A method used by health providers to help assess quality of care often entails having consumers of health services complete questionnaires (client satisfaction surveys). These feedback forms are completed upon discontinuation of care and/or during the intervention phase and help health providers gauge overall client satisfaction and perception regarding care received. They also allow for specific problems and recurring areas of concern to be identified. Additionally, surveys are a way to attain suggestions for positive changes and recognize specific staff members for exceptional service. Depending on the setting, surveys can be specific to one department or might reflect totality of care received from the entire facility or agency. Some questionnaires can be quite detailed and lengthy, addressing a wide variety of areas. Other feedback forms are short and basic, consisting of only a few generic questions. An example of an occupational therapy client satisfaction questionnaire is presented in Figure 10-1. You can use an internet search engine to find and compare various feedback forms.

Instructions: Recall your last visit to a health provider (e.g., doctor, dentist, physical therapist, nurse practitioner, chiropractor). Complete the client satisfaction survey in Figure 10-1 based on your experience, adapting the form to reflect the discipline you chose. After completing the questionnaire, create a list of five additional questions that you feel would be beneficial to include on this survey.

Additional questions to add to this survey:

1.

2.

3.

4.

5.

We Really Care Rehabilitation Facility
Occupational Therapy Department

Thank you for choosing to receive rehabilitation services at our facility. Please answer the following questions based on your experience here and return this survey in the postage-paid envelope provided. We appreciate your feedback.

	Strongly Agree	Agree	Neither Agree nor Disagree	Disagree	Strongly Disagree
I was able to schedule my initial appointment in a timely manner.	◯	◯	◯	◯	◯
Parking was convenient.	◯	◯	◯	◯	◯
I was seen on time for scheduled appointments.	◯	◯	◯	◯	◯
The facility was clean/sanitary.	◯	◯	◯	◯	◯
I was treated with courtesy/respect.	◯	◯	◯	◯	◯
My privacy and confidentiality were well protected.	◯	◯	◯	◯	◯
My concerns were listened to and addressed satisfactorily.	◯	◯	◯	◯	◯
My OT/OTA spent sufficient time with me.	◯	◯	◯	◯	◯
Treatment was clearly explained.	◯	◯	◯	◯	◯
Therapy helped the problem(s) I was being treated for.	◯	◯	◯	◯	◯
I would not have gotten better without therapy.	◯	◯	◯	◯	◯
I would recommend this facility.	◯	◯	◯	◯	◯

How did you hear about us? Physician ☐ Family member/friend ☐ Internet ☐

Newspaper ☐ Other ☐ _____

Comments/suggestions: _____

_____

Name and contact information (optional): _____

_____

Figure 10-1. Client satisfaction survey.

Worksheet 10-4

Marketing

An occupational therapy manager scheduled a staff meeting to elicit ideas for marketing the hospital's outpatient occupational therapy program. During the brainstorming session, the OTs and OTAs suggested the following ideas. Critique each idea and explain the rationale for why it may or may not be feasible to execute. Discuss factors that would affect implementation, such as specific costs, personnel requirements, and ethical or legal considerations. Create two additional marketing ideas to critique also. Develop a marketing plan for the idea you think would work out the best.

1. Host a breakfast or lunch for a group of physicians to explain the unique value of occupational therapy.
2. Contact potential referring physicians and offer a referral bonus for each client that the physician refers to the occupational therapy department.
3. Develop an informational brochure about the occupational therapy department and send it to physicians in the surrounding area.
4. Create a commercial for the local television station.
5. In the lobby or next to the hospital cafeteria, host an occupational therapy event, such as an exhibition of adaptive equipment or wellness activities.
6. Write an article for the local newspaper about occupational therapy and the specific occupational therapy services provided at the hospital.
7. Provide educational sessions to local organizations such as support groups for individuals with arthritis, Alzheimer's disease, or Parkinson's disease.
8. Provide free occupational therapy screenings to members of the community.
9. Other:
10. Other:

Answers to Worksheets

Worksheet 10-1: Billing and Reimbursement

Resource: Morreale & Borcherding, 2017

The American Occupational Therapy Association website (www.aota.org) contains useful information about public policy and reimbursement of occupational therapy services. Further information about Medicare can be found at www.medicare.gov, and information about Medicaid can be found at www.medicaid.gov. The CMS manuals can also be found online at www.cms.gov. CMS Publication 100-02: Medicare Benefit Policy Manual (Chapter 15, Section 220) delineates criteria for reimbursement of outpatient occupational therapy services.

1. A. According to CMS guidelines for co-treating, the total units billed by both disciplines cannot exceed the allowable units based on time: 30 minutes equals 2 units. Occupational and physical therapy can each bill Medicare for 1 unit, or the entire 2 units can be billed by *either* occupational or physical therapy.

2. A. According to CMS, 1 unit of a timed service equals 8 to 22 minutes (CMS, 2016).

3. A. Medicare Part A covers inpatient acute stays, although there are some out-of-pocket expenses.

4. A. Inpatient hospital stays using Medicare Part A is reimbursed through the Prospective Payment System, which pays a predetermined per-diem rate.

5. B. The client must pay the full cost of the deductible before the insurance provides any reimbursement. To meet the deductible, the client must pay in full for the evaluation ($100), plus $50 for the second visit. For the remaining $20 owed for the second visit, the insurance pays 80% ($16) and the patient must pay the remaining $4. Thus, the total out-of-pocket cost for the second visit is $54 ($50 + $4).

6. D.

7. C. Answers A, B, and D are classified as durable medical equipment (DME). Items such as tub seats, grab bars, reachers, sock aids, and the like are not DME, as they are considered self-help or hygienic devices and not considered medical in nature (CMS, 2014). Strict criteria must be met for Medicare reimbursement of DME.

8. C. IDEA Part C pertains to eligible children under 3 years of age while IDEA Part B pertains to eligible preschool and school-aged children (Center for Parent Information & Resources, 2014)

9. D. Medicaid covers health care costs for eligible individuals who meet low-income guidelines. Unemployment insurance, supplemental security insurance, and workers' compensation are separate programs that do not cover health care costs directly.

10. C. CPT are billing codes for health care services provided. ICD-10 contains diagnosis codes. The Minimum Data Set is an assessment tool used in skilled nursing facilities. The client is not likely eligible for Medicare.

Worksheet 10-2: Department Management

Resources: Ellexson, 2011; Giles, 2011

1. *Vision*

2. *Space*: Here are suggestions when choosing a space but you may come up with others:

- Meets requirements for local zoning and building codes
- Available client base in area
- Proximity to competitors in area
- Wheelchair accessibility
- Parking

- Space adequate for types of services to be provided/number of rooms are sufficient
- Outdoor facilities/space if required (e.g., playground equipment for sensory integration or gross-motor tasks)
- Bathroom facilities present in therapy clinic or building
- Adequate electrical outlets and supply
- Adequate water supply for hand hygiene, orthotic device fabrication, and so forth.
- Overhead lighting

3. *Equipment and supplies:* The specific equipment and supplies required will depend on the type of practice setting, space, and available budget. Some considerations are noted below but should not be considered an all-inclusive list.

- Safety—Personal protective equipment (e.g., gloves, gowns, masks), fire extinguisher, smoke and carbon monoxide detectors, soap and paper towels, hand sanitizer, first-aid kit, wheelchair, and so forth.
- Furniture for staff office and client waiting area—Chairs, desk, table, mat, plinth, and so forth.
- Office equipment—Computer, phone, fax, copier, file cabinets, staff refrigerator, washer/dryer (for linens), and so forth.
- Office supplies—Pens, paper, toner, envelopes, stapler, paper clips, folders, postage, and so forth.
- Evaluation tools—Specific formal/informal assessments, goniometer, tape measure, dynamometer, pinch meter, volumeter, specific sensory tests, and so forth.
- General supplies—Bandages, treatment table paper, pillows, pillowcases, towels, crayons, toys, lotion, and so forth.
- Exercise equipment—Putty, weights, exercise bands, pegboard, cones, hand grippers, and so forth.
- Physical agent modalities—Paraffin unit, paraffin, hydrocollator, hot packs, cold packs, terrycloth covers, tongs, timer, thermometer, and so forth.
- ADL equipment—Refrigerator, stove, microwave, coffee maker, laundry basket, pots/pans, utensils, and so forth.
- Adaptive equipment—Reachers, buttonhooks, long-handle shoehorns, built-up utensils, and so forth.
- Orthotic supplies—Heat pan, heat gun, thermoplastics, hook and loop fastener, scissors, spatula, pre-fabricated orthotic devices, and so forth.

4. *Possible staff or professional services needed* (non-inclusive list):

- Accountant
- Attorney
- Janitor/handyperson
- Cleaning person
- Electrician/plumber/carpenter (will depend on renovations required)
- Engineering service/technician to calibrate or repair medical devices/equipment
- Billing service
- Secretary
- Marketing professional/web designer
- Information technology specialist
- Landscaper/snow removal
- Rehabilitation aide
- Laundry service

5. *Methods of marketing* (non-inclusive list):

- Social media
- Brochure
- Local magazine article/advertisement
- Join a speakers bureau
- Chamber of Commerce membership
- Letters to physicians
- Promotional emails
- Health fair participant

Worksheet 10-3: Budget

Resources: Braveman, 2019; Ellexson, 2011

1. F. A fiscal year goes from January 1 to December 31.
    An organization determines its own fiscal time frame consisting of a 1-year period, such as October 1 to September 30.
2. F. An example of an occupational therapy capital budget expenditure is a transfer tub bench.
    A capital expense is larger cost item meant for long-term use (e.g., a Fluidotherapy machine, mat table, computer, hydrocollator) that can be considered an asset and usually depreciated for tax purposes. A tub bench comes under a lower cost category of general equipment and supplies and does not meet those criteria.
3. F. Revenue equals total income minus expenses.
    Revenue equals total income before expenses.
4. T. Rent and a copying machine lease are examples of fixed costs.
    Fixed costs do not vary during a specified time-period (e.g., fiscal year) and are not impacted by volume of services.
5. T. Accounts receivable include the money due from an insurance company.
6. T. Examples of variable expenses include personal protective equipment, postage, and client-issued therapy putty.
7. F. Nonprofit means that the organization does not make enough money to meet its expenses.
8. T. Total costs subtracted from revenue equals profits.
9. F. Occupational therapy department budgets always allocate money for staff to attend continuing education seminars to maintain NBCOT certification.
    Companies choose whether they will or will not provide a continuing education benefit to employees.
10. T. Costs for items ordered but not yet paid, such as evaluation forms and adaptive equipment, are considered accounts payable.
11. T. Thermoplastic materials, gauze, and paraffin are considered direct-use supplies.
12. F. Cash flow consists of pending money due from third-party payers.
    Cash flow is the real money that comes in and out of the business available presently for use.
13. T. Expenses not associated directly with productivity levels, such as monthly utilities and yearly service contracts, are called overhead.
14. T. Productivity refers to the amount of billable services that an individual provides.
15. F. Accounts payable include money that clients owe the business, such as copayments and coinsurance.
    Copayments and coinsurance owed are accounts receivable.

Worksheet 10-4: Marketing

Here are some suggestions although you may come up with others. As you can see by the answers that follow, some ideas should not be implemented because they may be impractical or unethical.

Marketing Idea	*Costs Incurred*	*Tasks/Personnel Needed*	*Other Considerations*
Host a breakfast or lunch for a group of physicians to explain the unique value of occupational therapy.	Food and beverages Paper goods Invitations/Postage Staff time	Create list of potential referral sources Create and send out invitations Keep track of responses Order and set-up food and beverages Host event	Costs may not be reflected in department budget Participating staff will not be able to implement client interventions during this time Determining a mutually agreeable time and suitable space
Contact potential referring physicians and offer a referral bonus for each client that the physician refers to the occupational therapy department	-----------------------------	-----------------------------	***This is unethical*** because anti-kickback laws are in place regarding Federal funds such as Medicare and Medicaid (U.S. Department of Health and Human Services, n.d.)
Develop an informational brochure about the OT department and send it to physicians in the surrounding area.	Cost of preparing brochure/postage Services of a marketing professional or IT professional Staff time	Create brochure Create list of potential referral sources Mail or email brochure	Costs may not be reflected in department budget
Create a commercial for the local television station.	Cost of ad time Services of a marketing professional, videographer, actors	Coordinate with the facility's public relations/marketing department Create ad Purchase air time	Costs probably not reflected in department budget Suitable space and time for filming Obtain releases from persons in ad
In the lobby or next to the hospital cafeteria, host an OT event such as an exhibition of adaptive equipment, wellness activities, etc.	Decorations Giveaways or prizes Poster boards Brochures/copies of marketing materials Staff time	Determine agenda Reserve space Set-up and host event Create poster boards or marketing materials	Costs may not be reflected in department budget Participating staff will not be able to implement client interventions during this time Determine suitable time frame and space

Marketing Idea	Costs Incurred	Tasks/Personnel Needed	Other Considerations
Write an article for the local newspaper about occupational therapy and the specific occupational therapy services provided at the hospital.	Staff time Photographer	Write article Collaborate with facility public relations/marketing department Contact newspaper Take pictures	Obtain releases from persons in pictures
Provide educational sessions to local organizations such as support groups for individuals with arthritis, Alzheimer's disease, or Parkinson's disease.	Staff time Transportation costs if offsite Handouts, brochures/copies of marketing materials	Collaborate with facility public relations/marketing department Contact appropriate agencies Create handouts or PowerPoint presentations	Participating staff will not be able to implement client interventions during this time Determine if these sessions will be pro bono or not
Provide free occupational therapy screenings to members of the community.	Cost of particular assessments or materials used Transportation costs if offsite Handouts, brochures/copies of marketing materials Staff time	Collaborate with facility public relations/marketing department Schedule appointments if needed Set-up event/screening area Administer screenings	Participating staff will not be able to implement client interventions during this time Obtain suitable space Privacy concerns That state's OT practice act regarding OT screenings

Reproduced with permission from Morreale, M. J., & Amini, D. (2016). *The occupational therapist's workbook for ensuring clinical competence.* SLACK Incorporated.

References

American Academy of Professional Coders. (2021). *What is ICD-10?* Retrieved May 22, 2021, from https://www.aapc.com/icd-10/

Braveman, B. (2019). Management of occupational therapy services. In B. A. B. Schell & G. Gillen (Eds.), *Willard and Spackman's occupational therapy* (13th ed., pp. 1118-1133). Wolters Kluwer.

Center for Parent Information & Resources. (2014). *Part C of IDEA: Early intervention for babies and toddlers.* Retrieved May 22, 2021, from https://www.parentcenterhub.org/partc-

Centers for Medicare & Medicaid Services. (2014). *Medicare national coverage determinations (NCD) manual (pub. 100-03: ch. 1, section 280.1).* https://www.cms.gov/Regulations-and-Guidance/Guidance/Manuals/Downloads/ncd103c1_Part4.pdf

Centers for Medicare & Medicaid Services. (2016). *Medicare claims processing manual (pub. 100-04: ch. 5, section 20.2).* https://www.cms.gov/Regulations-and-Guidance/Guidance/Manuals/Downloads/clm104c05.pdf

Centers for Medicare & Medicaid Services. (2019). *11 Part B billing scenarios for PTs and OTs (individual vs. group treatment).* Retrieved May 22, 2021, from www.cms.gov/Medicare/Billing/TherapyServices/billing_scenarios

Ellexson, M. T. (2011). Financial planning and budgeting. In K. Jacobs & G. L. McCormack (Eds.), *The occupational therapy manager* (5th ed., pp. 113-125). American Occupational Therapy Association.

Giles, G. M. (2011). Starting a new program, business, or practice. In K. Jacobs & G. L. McCormack (Eds.), *The occupational therapy manager* (5th ed., pp. 145-166). American Occupational Therapy Association.

U.S. Department of Health and Human Services (Office of Inspector General). (n.d.). *A roadmap for new physicians: Fraud & abuse laws.* Retrieved June 22, 2021, from https://oig.hhs.gov/compliance/physician-education/01laws.asp

World Health Organization. (2021). *International classification of diseases and related health problems (ICD).* Retrieved May 22, 2021, from https://www.who.int/classifications/classification-of-diseases

Index